The Adolescent and Pregnancy

The Adolescent and Pregnancy

Margaret-Ann Corbett, M.S., C.N.M.

Associate Professor of Nursing
Yale University School of Nursing
New Haven, Connecticut

Jerrilyn H. Meyer, R.N., M.S., C.N.M.

Former Assistant Professor of Nursing
Yale University School of Nursing
New Haven, Connecticut

Blackwell Scientific Publications

BOSTON ■ OXFORD ■ LONDON ■ EDINBURGH ■ PALO ALTO ■ MELBOURNE

Blackwell Scientific Publications

Editorial Offices
52 Beacon Street, Boston, Massachusetts
  02108, USA
Osney Mead, Oxford OX2 0EL, England
8 John Street, London, WC1N2ES, England
23 Ainslie Place, Edinburgh, EH3 6AJ,
  Scotland
107 Barry Street, Carlton, Victoria 3053,
  Australia
667 Lytton Avenue, Palo Alto, California
  94301, USA

Distributors
USA
  Year Book Medical Publishers, Inc.
  35 East Wacker Drive
  Chicago, Illinois 60601
Canada
  Blackwell Mosby Book
    Distributors
  120 Melford Drive
  Scarborough, Ontario M1B 2X4
Australia
  Blackwell Scientific Publications,
  Pty., Ltd.
  107 Barry Street
  Carlton, Victoria, 3053
Outside North America and Australia
  Blackwell Scientific Publications, Ltd.
  Osney Mead
  Oxford OX2 0EL
  England

Typeset by Ampersand, Inc.
Printed and bound by the Maple-
Vail Book Manufacturing Group.

Blackwell Scientific Publications,
Inc.
© 1987 by Blackwell Scientific Publications,
  Inc.
Printed in the United States of America
87 88 89 5 4 3 2 1

Library of Congress Cataloging in
Publication Data

**Library of Congress Cataloging-in-
Publication Data**

Corbett, Margaret-Ann, 1933–
  The adolescent and pregnancy.

  Includes index.
  1. Pregnancy, Adolescent. 2. Pregnancy,
Adolescent—Social aspects. 3. Obstetrical
nursing. I. Meyer, Jerrilyn H., 1952–   .
II. Title. [DNLM: 1. Obstetrical Nursing. 2.
Pregnancy in Adolescence—nurses'
instruction. WY 157.3 C789a]
RG556.5.C67   1987   618.2'0088055
87-862
ISBN 0-86542-013-0

To all adolescents, especially Sharon and Pam.

Contents

Contributors

Lane Michelle Holland, M.S.N., C.N.M.

Assistant Professor
Maternal-Newborn Nursing/Nurse Midwifery Program
Yale University School of Nursing
New Haven, Connecticut

Mary Alice Johnson, M.S.N., C.N.M.

Assistant Professor
Yale University School of Nursing
New Haven, Connecticut

Lois Siebert Sadler, R.N., M.S.N., C.P.N.P.

Pediatric Nurse Practitioner
Assistant Professor of Nursing
Yale University School of Nursing
New Haven, Connecticut

Preface

This book is written for clinicians who manage the health care of both the pregnant and nonpregnant adolescent. It is also written for those who wish to learn such practice. As with all clinical books, this book is intended to be comprehensive. Clinical management is constantly evolving, however, and when this fact is combined with publishing deadlines, it is difficult to be as current as we might wish to be. Such was the case with Acquired Immune Deficiency Syndrome—too late for this book but of such importance in adolescent health care. Indeed AIDS may become the Damocles sword and reduce adolescent pregnancy rates, although the immortality view of adolescents tends to dissipate deadly threats.

Psychosocial aspects of adolescent care are included as part of comprehensive health care. They are not, however, emphasized or addressed in depth in this book because many other books have been written exclusively on this topic. Our concern is to emphasize the other components of care not previously detailed.

Some readers will find this book more beneficial than others, but all, who as professional colleagues identify with the following passage, will understand what this book is all about:

> The staff works hard on Fridays ... to help these young women help themselves ... and to prepare for childbirth. This entails new tasks for the adolescents, learning to communicate with others, identifying feelings, and taking on responsibility. Such demands also challenge the health care provider to listen attentively, reach out lovingly, and to touch others in a different way.*

Nothing more needs to be said.

*Meyer, J. The Women's Center: Education and Concern. *Nursing Update.* New Haven: Yale-New Haven Hospital. 1980; 1(3):7.

Acknowledgments

We wish to acknowledge first and foremost the adolescents who have contributed so much to the authors' thinking.

We also wish to thank those special loved ones and friends whose tremendous patience and input have helped to see the book through its various stages. The list is long, but Tad and Helen were particularly important figures in helping us reach the zenith called "the end." We are grateful.

We wish to express a special word of acknowledgment to our professional colleagues who contributed to this book: Helen Varney Burst, C.N.M., M.S.N., D.H.L. (Hon.); Anne Malley-Corrinet, C.N.M., M.S.; Lane M. Holland, C.N.M., M.S.N.; Mary Alice Johnson, C.N.M., M.S.; and Lois S. Sadler, P.N.P., M.S.N.

This acknowledgment could never be considered complete without an expression of our sincere appreciation to our Editor-in-Chief, Richard Zorab. Without Richard's prodding and guidance the book would never have reached fruition. In addition, we wish to thank Patricia Sheehan who inspired us to try.

Margaret-Ann Corbett
Jerrilyn H. Meyer

1 Introduction

Adolescent pregnancy is a multidimensional topic. It reduces human and financial resources and is setting a social precedent whose long-range effects are still largely unknown. Concern is worldwide. It is estimated that close to half of the world's population is under 20 years of age (1). This age factor combined with the incidence of out-of-wedlock pregnancy concerns society in general and the adolescent and her child in particular. In a 1982 report (2) commissioned by the World Health Organization (WHO) Maternal and Child Health Division, it was calculated that there were about 450 million females between the ages of 15 and 19 in the world. Collectively, this group accounts for 20 percent of the world population and 6 percent to 18 percent of all births annually.

Definition

Adolescence is a unique period of life commonly described as transitional. The WHO defined adolescence at its 1976 conference on adolescent pregnancy as a period when: 1) the individual progresses from the point of the initial appearance of the secondary sex characteristics to that of sexual maturity; 2) the individual's psychological processes and patterns of identification develop from those of a child to those of an adult; and 3) a transition is made from the state of total socioeconomic dependence to one of relative independence (3). Consequently, adolescence is a period when one moves from childhood to adulthood and develops the realization that adulthood includes the acceptance of responsibilities as defined by one's individual society or culture.

Defining adolescence is often controversial. Cultures and societies differ in their concepts as individuals do. Hence, a wide spectrum of interpretation of this period exists. Erikson (4) referred to it as a period when one establishes an identity and eliminates conflicting and confusing issues associated with it. His concept includes the ability to envision oneself as an individual separate from others while still capable of developing successful relationships with peer groups. To be successful, Erikson's identity processing also includes the development of a purpose in life and the ability to identify with a specific philosophy (4). Some believe that a pregnancy during this period may significantly alter the success of this transition.

Hence, pregnancy may disrupt the normal formation of adolescent identity. Moreover, a successful transition from adolescence to young adulthood includes the development and search for independence, whereas pregnancy is a time when women feel a need to be dependent. The conflict is obvious.

Parenting requires the capability to nurture psychologically another human being. Erikson (4) believes that this is an intimacy beyond the reach of most adolescents unless they have proceeded through their identity formation. However, if they have developed a personal identity, the fact that are already adolescent and pregnant may not be so pertinent.

Another factor is the social isolation pregnancy imposes on the adolescent. Since many teenagers elect to attend special school programs developed to meet their pregnancy needs, they are often sequestered from their peers. Even those who elect to remain in a regular school program may feel "different" and hence isolated. As Erikson suggests, identity formation includes acceptance and association with one's peers, which adolescent pregnancy often precludes.

Incidence

The problem of adolescent pregnancy is particularly apparent in the United States. America's adolescent pregnancy rates in 1978 ranked it eighth out of 31 industrialized countries (5). This extraordinary fact was reflected in 1.1 million teenage pregnancies in the United States—554,000 of which resulted in live births (5). The actual number of births has declined since then, reflecting a decline in the population of U.S. teenagers ages 15–19 since 1976. Although the pregnancy rate has risen from 94 pregnancies per 1000 women in 1972 to 109 pregnancies per 1000 women in 1984, when adjusted for sexual activity the rate actually declined during the same period, from 272 pregnancies per 1000 women to 233 pregnancies per 1000 women. So as the pregnancy rate increased in the total population of adolescent girls, the actual pregnancy rate among sexually active girls decreased. These figures reflect the decrease in the total adolescent population, the increase in the number of sexually active girls, the greater use of contraception, and the increased number of abortions (6).

These statistics make it obvious that the American adolescent is sexually active. In 1948, Kinsey (7) reported that 14 percent of all males under age 15 were sexually active and 20 percent of those age 16 to 20 had had intercourse. He found in 1953 (8) that for females 15 years and under, 7 percent reported sexual intercourse and 31 percent of those 16 to 20 had had intercourse. In the late 1970s, 46 percent of all teenage females in urban areas acknowledged having intercourse (9). On the other hand, Zelnik and Kanter (10) found that sexual initiation does not necessarily imply sexual frequency or promiscuity. Of those interviewed in their study, 51 percent of the "non-virgin" girls age 15 to 17 had not had sex for four weeks and most reported only one partner (10). The sporadic activity may blind the adolescent to the need for effective contraception. Sadly, most do not elect to use contraception in the first year of sexual activity, and this results in one-fifth becoming pregnant one month after commencing coitus and one half within six months (11). Further, even though the number of adolescents using contraceptives increased by 1982, these adolescents continued to be inconsistent users, with nearly 40 percent only using contraceptives "sometimes" (6).

Many factors contribute to the increased teenage sexual activity: peer pressure, sex-oriented media, minimal or no parental supervision, mobility, and a transient society that does not allow time for neighbors to know each other. The result is a young, inexperienced population enticed to the sexual threshold without adequate preparation. Unfortunately, once they have crossed that threshold, there is for many no turning back.

Additional factors may include the younger age of menarche and an older marital age. It is tempting to assume that the younger age of menarche is a crucial factor in adolescent pregnancy rates, but as Zelnik (12) suggests, individual studies must be done first to determine if there is a relationship between the ages of menarche and initiation of coitus. He believes we cannot assume such a relationship until this is analyzed (12). If such a relationship does exist and assuming the trend to delay marriage continues, it is easy to see that the risk of premarital intercourse will increase and more teenage pregnancies will occur.

With the availability of contraception and abortion, many find it difficult to understand the phenomenon of adolescent pregnancy, which prompts the question, "Does the pregnant adolescent deliberately select motherhood?" The answer is unclear. Because contraception and abortion are available, rational thinking suggests that the pregnant teenager has. However, most health clinicians disagree. Instead, they believe these pregnancies have resulted from ignorance about conception and contraception, or from the fear of discovery if contraception is sought and used. Although statistics support that belief, it is imperative to note that teenagers are using contraception more effectively today than in the past. Further, nearly 40 percent of all adolescent pregnancies end in abortion (6). Subsequently, both pregnancy rates and the number of births among the sexually active declined from 1972 to 1984 by approximately 14.5 percent (6). Acknowledgment of this fact forces one to recognize that some teenagers have made a deliberate choice to become pregnant and give birth. If this is true, Baldwin and Cain (13) theorize that these adolescents are motivated to become parents and therefore the current statistics reflecting poor outcomes for teenage pregnancies are not as applicable to this group. In other words, the statistics associated with negative outcomes for adolescent pregnancy are not an appropriate standard to apply to teenagers motivated to become parents (13).

Outcomes and Consequences

Statistics are ironic because their accuracy is limited to the past; to apply them to current or future generations may be futile. On the other hand, when statistics show a consistent year-to-year pattern they help us understand the present and give us some direction for the future. Certainly statistics have helped us identify risks associated with adolescent pregnancy. For example, they consistently have revealed a low-birthweight outcome for infants born to teenagers. This results in a staggering cost to society in intensive care to support the premature or intrauterine-growth-retarded infant. Moreover, because mental retardation is frequently associated with low birthweight (as are cerebral palsy, epilepsy, and increased perinatal mortality and morbidity), the cost to society increases. When this low-birthweight risk is combined with the fact than many adolescents do not obtain adequate prenatal care, the low-birthweight risk increases even more. This is verified by Stickle (14) who reported a 26.4 percent incidence of low birthweight among mothers under age 18 who did not obtain proper prenatal care. Mothers under 15 are twice as likely to have premature or low-birthweight infants (5).

Both maternal and infant mortality rates are higher for the adolescent mother than they are for women in their 20s. For example, pregnant adolescents under 15 have a maternal death rate that is 2.5 times that for mothers ages 20–24 (5). Teenagers who have an induced abortion, however, have a lower incidence of complications and overall death rates than do adult women (15). Statistics documented by Trussel and Menken (16) indicate that those who begin childbearing in their teens have more children in rapid succession and have more unwanted children than do their counterparts who begin reproducing at a later age.

At one time statistics inferred that pregnancy generally curtailed the adolescent's opportunity to continue school. Certainly this is still true, but not to the extent previously thought. Statistics now suggest that if the adolescent comes from a stable family environment and has emotional and financial support from that source, the return-to-school rate is high. If, however, she moves away from her family, the school drop-out rate increases. In these situations there is an obvious need for day care, which, if unmet, means that the teenager remains at home. If this results in a year's absence from school, little incentive may remain to return, especially if the adolescent's former classmates are in an advanced grade.

Certainly the reduced educational opportunities will impose a lifetime of lost advantages. A longitudinal study done by Card and Wise (17) showed that adolescent parents (male and female) are more apt to terminate their education than their peers. This study also found that the impact was greater on the female (16). Consequently, this teenage mother may lack the educational criteria to enter the labor force. In a technology-emphasized era where the need for manual labor is low, this teenager has little hope of anything but an economically deprived life. Poor nutrition, unsanitary living conditions, and poor health habits may result, which will inevitably affect the physical and spiritual well-being of both her and her children.

Furthermore, because the pregnant teenager begins childbearing at such an early age, she will bear more children than her counterparts who reproduce at a later age. This fact will increase the economic burden on an already poor income and may affect the quality of maternal input the pregnant teenager has to offer her offspring.

It is generally acknowledged that the survival rates of teenage marriages are not good. Approximately half of all pregnant adolescents are married at the time they give birth (18). On the whole, older adolescents (18- and 19-year-olds) are far more likely to legitimize birth than are younger adolescents, especially if they are white (6). Subsequent separation and divorce rates, however, are high. The black population, on the other hand, does not marry as frequently to legitimize a birth. Whether married and divorced or unmarried, the cumulative result is a single-parent family usually of low income that resides in urban dwellings where the neighbors are generally strangers. Isolation and loneliness often result. It is little wonder that some teenage parents develop drug problems and their children exhibit learning deficiencies in cognitive development as well as social and emotional malaise. Baldwin and Cain (13) reported that learning deficiencies occur most frequently when a child is raised solely by the teenage mother without help from adults or from the child's father. There is also some limited evidence that a child's score on intelligence, achievement, and other cognitive functioning tests and performance in school is affected by the age at which the mother gave birth and consequently her level of completed education (6).

Inevitably, a teenage mother will feel the need to express this emotional trauma and hence may seek nurturance through sexual activity, and another unplanned pregnancy often results. Her anger and frustration with yet another pregnancy may lead to child abuse and neglect if her new baby fails to meet her expectations and need for love.

Cultural Influences

The many ethnic groups in the United States often prompt us to question the cultural role background plays in adolescent pregnancy. It is tempting to speculate that culture is a factor; however, evidence does not support this thought. Certainly, all cultures desire children, but no American culture promotes premarital pregnancy and childbirth, especially among its teenagers. On the contrary, most cultures in America are concerned when adolescent pregnancy occurs.

Mead (18) described culture as "a systematic body of learned behavior which is transmitted from parents to children" but predicted a worldwide culture would result if the impact of the media continues to influence society. Such an outcome could threaten individual cultures and conceivably remove the culture's ability to discipline and mold future values of its young generations.

Certainly cultures incorporate social change over the years as each generation contributes new concepts and subsequently revokes former traditions. As Benedict (20) pointed out, if one is to interpret an individual's behavior one cannot ignore the historical process by which the society has accepted or rejected different concepts. Therefore, if we are to look at adolescent pregnancy on an individual basis, we must look at the history of the particular culture of that adolescent.

Social mores concerning out-of-wedlock pregnancy are changing in America. This is especially true for older single women (21). As the number of single parents increases, older single female parents may begin to be socially accepted into the culture. Single teenage parents, however, are a different story in spite of the fact that they generally keep their children. Wisconsin adopted legislation in late 1985 that illustrated this difference and addressed the issue of single teenage parents. The legislation required that the grandparents of a teenager's baby to accept legal responsibility for the child's financial needs. In the words of Wisconsin's governor, "Young people and parents of young people have a responsibility for their [the former's] actions" (22). Obviously, this legislation does not promote unwanted teenage pregnancy or suggest that the local culture in Wisconsin is ready to condone the concept of single parenting among teenagers.

American culture is as diverse as the nation and differs not only geographically, but also between its urban and rural areas. Thus the cultural heritage of an American youth born and bred in New York City—regardless of his or her ethnic background—will differ considerably from the cultural heritage of one raised in a rural area of America. The cultural experience, although labeled "American," differs in its ideas and standards depending on one's locale in the nation. Consequently, American adolescents are not only bound by their national culture, but also by their local American culture, their ethnic culture, and their peer culture. As a result many adolescents may experience conflict and confusion when they attempt to identify a pertinent value system.

Who does one listen to? If Mead is right, one listens to one's parents. If, however, a child is raised in a home by an older sibling or neighbor, because his/her parent(s) work or are not in the home, the television set often becomes a substitute parent and reduces the degree of learned behavior normally transmitted from parent to child. Hence, a scriptwriter's values have the potential to become a child's major source of information about the cultural values in the United States, and the role models with whom he or she identifies become those viewed on a television screen. In most cases these characters are flamboyant, glamorous, and successful; they enjoy sex on a frequent and often casual basis, are never heard to discuss the need for contraception, and seldom experience an unwanted pregnancy. This is true even when intercourse has occurred in a spontaneous and unprotected manner. When such media exposure is combined with peer pressure to "make it," and when parents are reluctant to discuss sex seriously and sensitively with their teenagers, a confused outcome such as pregnancy is an inevitable result.

No American culture actively encourages adolescent pregnancy. However, American culture as portrayed and interpreted by television, movies, magazines, and popular music can undermine this value. In addition, adolescent peer pressure, which develops much of its values from the media's interpretation and presentation, may force sexual intercourse on girls at an early age. Thus, poorly prepared by improper role models and grossly ignorant about contraception, they lack the ability and foresight to say "no." This outcome has little to do with cultural values of ethnic groups. Other than the value all cultures place on children (including adolescents), little can be found to suggest that a teenager's cultural background is a factor in increased pregnancy rates for American adolescents.

Conclusion

Our literature is replete with the phrases "lost generation," "lost potential," and "lost horizons." All generate vague and negative images. When nothing but an ambiguous awareness of loss can be identified, one is tempted to rely on such mental images. We do not know what potential is lost to society and to an individual when an adolescent pregnancy occurs. The risk varies in each situation, which makes generalized statements difficult to measure. Many pregnant teenagers are on welfare, and some of their infants will require expensive and intensive care after birth. Because the death risk in the first year of life for these children is so high, the need for medical supervision and emergency care is critical. Additionally, the children of teenage parents who suffer from learning disabilities will require more expensive teaching in school. All of this costs money. And, most profoundly, without sufficient role models, these children are prone to imitate the lifestyles of their parents and thus will begin to have children at an early age.

Society's demands may seem endless and at many times impossible, but the needs of the pregnant teenager and her offspring can be met. Society must first recognize that adolescent pregnancy is an existing problem. Once this is done, the full spectrum of its negative potential can be understood, and it can be acknowledged that an adolescent population informed of the risks of pregnancy is superior to the current flotilla of unwanted teenage pregnancies.

It is also necessary that society address its own double standards and recognize the impact of the media and altered family lifestyles on the current incidence of sexual activity among teenagers. Moreover, attention must be given to developing training programs for postpartal teenagers who elect not to return to a formal school setting. Such readily available programs will facilitate the adolescent's entry into the job market and prepare her for a more productive life. Furthermore, nonpregant adolescents, male and female, should be informed about the risks of pregnancy. Much has been written in the medical literature about the ramifications of teenage pregnancy and implications for offspring, but little has been shared comprehensively with teenagers in a language they can understand.

Today's teenagers are more at risk than ever of becoming pregnant. The concept of "forced fruit" comes to mind because it is unfair to place teenagers in a position in which they are forced to ask for direction when it is too late. Statements such as "When you try to be a mother and go to school, it is like waking up to misery. I wish I knew someone who could solve my problem" (23), "Not knowing what to do is like a panic. It's like asking yourself 'When? Where? Why? How? Try to find the correct answer. Can you pick the right one?" (23), and "I try my best to look the other way, but there is no one to tell me what to do" (23) should never occur. It does not have to be this way. If adult consultation on the subject of sex is sincere, nonjudgmental, and available to teenagers, pregnancy will become less of a risk for the American teenager.

References

1. Burst HV. Adolescent pregnancies and problems. *J Nurse-Midwif* 1979;24(2): 19–24.
2. Hofman AD. Biological and Psychological Correlates of Contraception in Adolescence: A Review. Report submitted to the Maternal and Child Health Division of the World Health Organization, Geneva, Switzerland, March 18, 1982; testimony before the U.S. Senate Subcommittee on Aging, Family and Human Services, Washington, DC, April 19, 1982.
3. Pregnancy and abortion in adolescence. *World Health Organization Technical Report Series No. 583.* Geneva: WHO, 1975.
4. Erikson E. H. *Identity, Youth and Crisis.* New York: WW Norton, 1968.
5. *Teenage Pregnancy: The Problem That Hasn't Gone Away.* New York: The Alan Guttmacher Institute, 1981.
6. National Research Council (Hayes CD, ed). *Risking the Future: Adolescent Sexuality, Pregnancy, and Childbearing.* Washington, DC: National Academy Press, 1987.
7. Kinsey AC, Pomeroy WB, Martin CE. *Sexual Behavior in Human Males.* Philadelphia: WB Saunders, 1948.
8. Kinsey AC, Pomeroy WB, Martin CE. *Sexual Behavior in Human Females.* Philadelphia: WB Saunders, 1953.
9. Zelnik M, Kanter JF. Sexual activity, contraceptive use and pregnancy among metropolitan teenagers: 1971–1979. *Family Planning Perspectives* 1980; 12:230.

10. Zelnik M, Kanter JF. Sexual and contraceptive experience of young married women. *Family Planning Perspectives* 1977; 9:55–71.
11. Zabin LS, Kanter JF, Zelnik M. The risk of adolescent pregnancy in the first months of intercourse. *Family Planning Perspectives* 1979; 11:215–222.
12. Zelnik M. Sexual activity among male adolescents. *Birth Defects* 1981; 17(3):19–34.
13. Baldwin W, Cain VS. The children of teenage parents. *Family Planning Perspectives* 1980; 12:34–43.
14. Stickle G. Overview of incidence, risks and consequences of adolescent pregnancy and childbearing. *Birth Defects* 1981; 17(3):5–18.
15. Cates W Jr et al. The risks associated with teenage abortion. *New England Journal of Medicine* 1983; 309:621–624.
16. Trussel J, Menken J. Early childbearing and subsequent fertility. *Family Planning Perspectives* 1978; 10:209–218.
17. Card JJ, Wise LL. Teenage mothers and teenage fathers: The impact of early childbearing on the parents' personal and professional lives. *Family Planning Perspectives* 1978; 10:199–205
18. O'Connell M, Rogers CC. Out-of-wedlock births, premarital pregnancies, and their effects on family formation and dissolution. *Family Planning Perspectives* 1984; 16:157–162.
19. Mead M. A new preface by Margaret Mead. In: Benedict R. *Patterns of Culture.* New York: New American Library, 1934.
20. Benedict R. *Patterns of Culture.* New York: New American Library, 1934.
21. *Quarterly Vital Statistics Review.* New York: New York State Department of Health, 1984.
22. Wallis, C. Children Having Children. *Time* 1985; Dec. 9:79.
23. Statements made by pregnant adolescents and adolescent mothers in the Yale-New Haven Young Mothers' Program. Yale-New Haven Hospital, New Haven, Connecticut.

Bibliography

Brown SV. Early childbearing and poverty: implications for social services. *Adolescence* 1982;397–408.

Cobliner WG. Prevention of adolescent pregnancy: a developmental perspective. *Birth Defects* 1981;17(3):35–47.

Finkel ML, Finkel DJ. Male adolescent contraceptive utilization. *Adolescence* 1978; 13(51):445–452.

Forrest JD, Sullivan E, Tietze C. Abortion in the United States, 1977–1978. *Family Planning Perspectives* 1979;11:329–341.

McCarthy J. Social consequences of childbearing during adolescence. *Birth Defects* 1981;17(3):107–122.

Patten M. Self concept and self esteem: factors in adolescent pregnancy. *Adolescence* 1981;16:64.

Protinski H, Sporakorski M, Atkins P. Identity formation: pregnant and nonpregnant adolescent. *Adolescence* 1982;17:65.

Roberts J, Engel A. Family background, early development, and intelligence of children aged 6–11 years. Rockville, MD: National Center for Health Statistics, 1974;11:142.

Schneider S. Helping adolescents deal with pregnancy: a psychiatric approach. *Adolescence* 1982;17(66):285–289.

Whiting B. *Six Cultures.* New York: John Wiley & Sons, 1963.

2 Physiological Aspects of Adolescence

Practical Concepts of Growth and Development

Why look at the physiological events of puberty in a book about adolescent pregnancy? Although pregnant, the adolescent is still very much an adolescent who must continue her own growth and development while experiencing the additional changes occurring with pregnancy and later lactation. The stage of her own maturation is an integral part of her physiology for the nine months she is pregnant. To separate the pregnant adolescent from her normal growth and development by considering her solely as a pregnant being is not only an injustice, but this view often results in negligence of the adolescent's total health care needs. An understanding of the relationship between the normal physiological changes of puberty and the changes of pregnancy may lead to appropriate health care management during and after adolescent pregnancy. Although a review of puberty can be found in textbooks in varying degrees of depth and detail, here, the physiological processes and the sequence of pubertal events are described.

Puberty is the ongoing process of sexual maturation. It involves psychological, physical, and sexual development and growth. It is much easier to state what happens during puberty than why or how it happens; there are still many unknowns. Simply stated, puberty results from the secretions of the hypothalmus, the gonadotropins and the sex steroids, probably at the time of the maturation of the hypothalmus and central nervous system. During childhood, the immature ovaries secrete low levels of estrogen which prohibit the hypothalmus from producing gonadotropin releasing factor (GRF). This negative feedback mechanism functions at maximal sensitivity at about 4 years of age. Prior to the onset of puberty and secondary sexual characteristics, the sensitivity of the negative feedback mechanism changes. With increasing age, and the influence of the growth hormone, there are increased amounts of catecholamines in the hypothalmus and increased sensitivity of the pituitary to the GRF.

During puberty, the hypothalmus produces the GRF which stimulates the pituitary to release follicle stimulating hormone (FSH) and luteinizing hormone (LH) initially in night-time surges. Sex steroids are now produced at an accelerated rate, which begins a new positive feedback system. With this

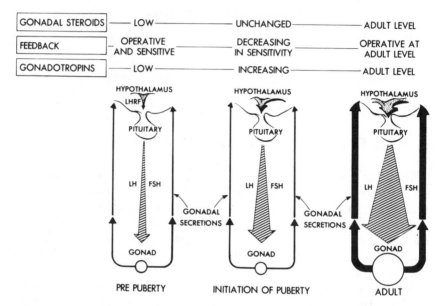

Figure 2.1. The changes in sensitivity of the hypothalamic gonadostat. In prepuberty, the concentration of gonadal steroids and gonadotropins is low; the hypothalamic gonadostat is functional but highly sensitive to low levels of gonadal steroids. With the initiation of puberty, there is decreased sensitivity to the hypothalamus to negative feedback by gonadal steroids, increased release of LRF, and enhanced secretion of gonadotropins. In the negative feedback mechanism, the hypothalamus is less sensitive to feedback by gonadal steroids (adult set point), and adult gonadotropin and gonadal steroid levels are present. (Reproduced with permission from John Wiley & Sons, Inc. Grumbach MM, Roth JC, Kaplan SL, Kelch RP. Hypothalamic pituitary regulation of puberty in man: evidence and concepts from clinical research. In: *Control of the Onset of Puberty.* Grumbach MM, Grave GD, Mayer FE (eds). New York: John Wiley & Sons, Inc., 1974:128.

increase in the gonadotropins there is stimulation of the ovaries, resulting in follicular development, which in turn increases the estrogen level resulting in the development of secondary sexual characteristics. Estrogen stimulates breast development and the maturation of the uterus, vagina, and external genitalia. An increase in adrenal androgens is associated with the appearance of pubic and axillary hair. With the increased production of sex steroids and this corresponding response, a new positive feedback mechanism is formed. During mid- to late puberty, this positive feedback mechanism matures, resulting in the LH surge and menarche (Fig. 2.1).

Finkelstein (1) divides and defines the stages of puberty as follows:

1. *Late prepuberty.* Neither physical nor hormonal changes have occurred, but a change in the sensitivity of the gonadostat has taken place. The growth hormone is low.

2. *Very early puberty.* No physical signs of sexual maturation are present. There is an increase in the release of gonadotropins and sex steroids during sleep, and an increase in the secretion of adrenal sex steroids.

3. *Early Puberty.* Sleep augmentation of gonadotropin continues. The concentrations of sex steroids increases and some increase in the growth hormone secretion may occur, as well as some change in the thyroid function. Early physical changes appear.

4. *Midpuberty.* Development of sexual characteristics increases. There is concentration of gonadotropins and sex steroids during wakefulness and a continuation of sleep augmentation. Achievement of peak height velocity in females occurs with the increased release of growth hormone.

5. *Late puberty.* Menarche occurs, and reproductive capacity and maturation is almost complete. Sleep augmentation of gonadotropins and growth hormone secretion is maximal.

6. *Adulthood.* Physical and sexual maturation is complete. Sleep augmentation of gonadotropins disappears. Gonadotropin secretory episodes are dissociated, and growth is complete in females.

Thelarche

Thelarche, the beginning of breast development, is usually the first event of puberty which signifies the production of estrogen in the ovary. The onset of breast development corresponds with the beginning of the initial spurt of growth, and it is followed by the appearance of pubic hair. Breast and pubic hair development usually occur within the same year, although a two year separation may occur.

Stages for breast development during adolescence have been defined by Tanner (2) as follows:

Stage 1. Preadolescent: elevation of papilla only.

Stage 2. Breast bud stage: elevation of breast and papilla as small mound and enlargement of areolar diameter.

Stage 3. Further enlargement and elevation of breast and areolar, with no separation of their contours.

Stage 4. Projection of areolar and papilla to form a secondary mound above the level of the breast.

Stage 5. Mature stage: projection of papilla only, due to recession of the areolar to the general contour of the breast.

Breast budding, or breast stage 2, occurs at an average age of 11 years and within a range of 9.0–13.0 years for 95 percent of the population. The breast bud stage may last from 6 months to 2 years. The average interval between the appearance of the breast bud and menarche is 2.5 years, with a range of 6 months to 5.75 years. The average interval between breast budding and peak height velocity is one year. It takes approximately one year from the first appearance of the breast bud to stage 3, and another four years to adult stage 4. The stage 4 development of the areolar mound may not occur in one fourth of all females, and may occur only slightly in another fourth. Most breast development is caused by the deposition of fat in the connective tissue of the lobules, as well as some increase in the number and size of the epithelial ducts. The development of the aveoli does not occur until pregnancy.

By using Tanner's classification system, the stages of breast development can be assessed for normalcy. Breast development prior to age 8–9 would suggest precocious puberty, while the abscence of breast development by the age of 13–14 years would suggest delayed puberty.

Adrenarche

Adrenarche is the growth of pubic and axillary hair, whereas pubarche is the isolated appearance of pubic hair. The growth of pubic hair is the result of the gradual increase of adrenal androgens beginning at age 6–9, which culminates in the appearance of pubic hair at an average age of 11–12. Pubic hair usually occurs after breast budding, but because of the early presence of the adrenal androgens, pubic hair may be the first sign of puberty in 20 percent of the population. Stages of pubic hair growth in females have been described by Tanner (3) as follows:

Stage 1. Preadolescent: the vellus over the pubes is no further developed than over the abdominal wall (i.e., no pubic hair).

Stage 2. Sparse growth of long, slightly pigmented downy hair, straight or only slightly curled, appearing chiefly along the labia.

Stage 3. Considerably darker, coarser and more curled, the hair spreads sparsely over the junction of the pubes.

Stage 4. Hair now resembles adult in type, but the area covered by it is still considerably smaller than in the adult. No spread to the medial surface of the thighs.

Stage 5. Adult in quantity and type with distribution of the horizontal pattern and spread to the medial surface of thighs but not up the linea alba or elsewhere above the base of the inverse triangle.

It takes an average of 3–4 years, with a range of 2–6 years, from the beginning of pubic hair growth to its completion. Stage 5 of pubic hair development is reached between the ages of 12–17 years. In 10 percent of females, the pubic hair growth extends beyond stage 5 into other patterns described as either sagittal, acuminate or disperse. This development is usually not completed until after puberty and is rated as stage 6.

Axillary hair usually appears within two years after the onset of pubic hair growth, during breast stage 3-4 and stage 4 of pubic hair development. Occasionally, however, axillary hair appears shortly before pubic hair. Circumoral hair, on the perineum, appears shortly before axillary hair and is independent of pubic hair growth. The apocrine glands of the axilla and vulva begin to function at approximately the same time hair appears.

Growth Rate

The first event of puberty is often a general increase in the growth rate of the skeleton, muscles and viscera, an increase commonly known as the adolescent growth spurt. The beginning of this growth spurt is seldom noticed. During puberty, this gradual acceleration in the growth rate can be divided into three general stages: minimum growth velocity, peak height velocity (PHV), and a stage of decreased velocity where the epiphyseal fusion occurs, resulting in growth cessation.

Prior to reaching PHV and shortly afterward, the growth rate is 4-6 cm (1.6-2.4 inches) per year. PHV usually occurs around the age of 12 with a range of 10-14 years. In relation to other pubertal events, PHV occurs a year after the onset of breast development, 1.5 years prior to menarche and, in 25 percent of the population, prior to the development of pubic hair. The linear growth spurt reaches PHV soon after breast stage 2 and occasionally before it. It is often reflected in breast development in that 40 percent of the population reach PHV before breast development is beyond stage 2, 50 percent in breast stage 3, and 10 percent in breast stage 4. During PHV, there is 7-11 cm (2.8-4.3 inches) of growth per year with an average of 9 cm (3.5 inches) per year, stimulated by the ovarian steroids. Therefore, females may grow 25 cm (9.8 inches) during this growth spurt. Peak weight velocity, occurring at a mean age of 12.9 years is 8.8 kg (4 lbs) per year.

Another index of growth and maturation is bone age. After the age of 12, with the continual influence of the ovarian steroids, there is fusion of the epiphyses in the hand. Bone age correlates with menarche, in that ossification of the iliac crest and epiphysis begins at the time of menarche (approximately 13 years) and continues until complete fusion takes place (at approximately 23 years).

Since PHV occurs prior to menarche, there is only a limited growth potential postmenarcheal of approximately 6 cm (2.4 inches) per year. The postmenarcheal gain is relatively independent of menarche occurring early or late. Because of the correlation between the growth spurt and age at menarche, Frisch and Nagel (4) were able to develop a chart that predicts the adult height of females from their age and height at menarche. In the final step of puberty, growth ceases 1-2 years postmenarcheal.

A normal growth rate is a sign of normal development. The absence of a growth spurt, even with signs of thelarche and adrenarche, may be ominous. If the growth spurt occurs early, the physiological events will generally occur early as well. If the growth spurt occurs late, the physiological events will also occur late. After menarche, at the end of the growth spurt, there is a flattening of the systolic blood pressure curve to the adult level, a sharp fall in the basal metabolic rate to adult values, and a gradual decline in the heart rate (5).

With the onset of puberty, there is a noticeable change in the body composition relating to weight and fat distribution. In females, the areas of most change are within the hips, calves, thighs, and chest. From the initiation of the growth spurt until menarche, whether early or late, females will gain approximately 17 kg (or 7.7 lbs). Weight more than doubles between the ages of 10 and 20 due to this pubertal growth. The accumulation of body fat during puberty continues after menarche and by age 16, females may have twice as much body fat as males do. The growth resulting from fat distribution is sex specific. Females have a greater increase in hip width without a corresponding increase in shoulder width, and less growth of the body as a whole.

Sexual differentiation can be observed from conception through puberty in the rate of maturation variations between the sexes. Half-way through the fetal period, the female skeleton is approximately three weeks more advanced than is the male. At the time of birth, there is a 4–6 week advancement in the female, and by the beginning of puberty the difference in maturation is two years. Also, permanent teeth appear earlier in females. Fifty percent of adult height is reached at an earlier age in females. Females begin their height spurt considerably earlier than males, and reach their PHV approximately two years earlier. The first appearance of pubic hair occurs nine months earlier in females, and pubic hair stage 3 is reached 1.5 years earlier in females. The first appearance of breast changes precedes the first changes in the testes by six months. Females usually reach PHV while in breast stage 2, while it is unusual for males to reach PHV until the genitalia have reached stage 4. The primary reason for the difference in the overall body size between the sexes is the delay in growth in males, allowing an 8–10 cm (3.1–3.9 inches) extra prepubertal growth. The actual height gained during puberty is exceeded in males by only 3–5 cm (1.2–2.0 inches), bringing the total growth potential of males to 11–15 cm (4.3–5.9 inches) during this period. Therefore, the maturational processes for females and males contain the same sequence of events but occur at varying intervals. One exception to the "females earlier" rule is at 7–8 weeks gestation during which the male gonad becomes recognizable as testes two weeks before the female gonad becomes identifiable as an ovary (6).

Menarche

Menarche, or the first menstrual period, also contains the Greek root "arche," translated as "beginning." Menarche begins when the hormonal stimulation during puberty produces endometrial hyperplasia which breaks down when estrogen support is withdrawn. The average age of menarche is 12.8–13.2 years with a range in chronological age of 9.1–17.7 years (some use 10–15), and a range in bone age of 14.5 years. It occurs relatively late in puberty at the time of maximal deceleration of height velocity and during Tanner's stages 3–4 of breast and pubic hair development.

Menarche is evidence of a mature stage of uterine development and a patent genital tract. It does not signify the attainment of full reproductive functions. The early menstrual cycles which are often irregular, may be anovulatory for 12–18 months postmenarche. Because of this fact, many adolescents erroneously think they cannot become pregnant and therefore do not use contraception. This period of adolescent sterility or partial sterility, however, does not occur in all females.

There are many influences which affect the age of menarche, some known and some unknown. Menarcheal age has become progressively earlier at the rate of 3–4 months each decade over the past 100 years as seen in studies of Norway, Germany, Finland, Sweden, Denmark, Great Britain and the United States (7). During the mid-1800s, the mean menarcheal age was 17 years, while in the 1950s, the mean menarcheal age was 11–12 years (in the United States, 13 years). This secular trend is believed to be related to improved nutrition, especially during infancy. This trend, however, is diminishing in the more prosperous areas of Great Britain and in Norway. Some suggest that the decreasing age of menarche is associated with the correlative increase in height and weight. Frisch (8) further speculated that an earlier menarche was associated with the attainment of a critical weight. She found that the mean weight of females at the initiation of the adolescent growth spurt was 30 kg (66 lbs). At the peak velocity of weight gain, the mean weight was 39 kg (86 lbs). Menarche occurred at a mean body weight of 17 kg (103.5 lbs). Earlier menses was associated with the earlier attainment of a critical weight usually found in cases of obesity. Later menarche was associated with slower pre- or postnatal growth where the critical weight was reached later, as in the menarche of twins, which occurs later than that of singletons. Zacharias et al. (9), however, considered the age of menarche more closely associated with body shape rather than size and weight. Early menarche, they believed, was associated with a short, stout body shape. Later menarche was, on the other hand, associated with a tall, thin body shape. Further study has presented exceptions to both these theories. In the case of obesity in excess of 30 percent normal weight, menarche was earlier, but severe obesity resulted in delayed menarche (10). Other studies have discredited the relationship between the initiation of menses and the attainment of a particular body weight or size, including the ratio of body fat contributing to body size and weight.

The age of menarche is determined by a variety of hereditary and environmental factors. The differences in the menarcheal age of identical twins varies only within 2.2 months, whereas that of dizygotic twins varies by 8.2 months. In families, there is a correlation between the menarcheal age of mothers and daughters and among siblings. Menarche occurs later in females in accordance with the number of siblings. In large families, however, females born later reach menarche earlier by 0.1 year per older sibling. The differences in the menarcheal age and birth order may be, however, more closely associated with social and nutritional factors. Environmental influences relating to class often affect the age of menarche. Those of the lower to middle class often have a later menarche, while those of the upper class generally experience an earlier menarche. In Europe and America, however, many of these distinctions have disappeared. In general, improved economic conditions and smaller family size result in an earlier menarche, whereas malnutrition frequently delays menarche. It has also been demonstrated that menarche occurs later in higher altitudes than those nearer sea level and that it occurs later in rural areas than in urban communities (11).

Heredity and Environmental Factors

Many factors influence puberty, the most prominent of which are changes in living conditions and nutrition. Improved diet and environment result in taller, heavier, and earlier maturing offspring. As previously stated, the secular trend toward lower menarcheal age and earlier puberty appears to be halting in some areas. Prenatal factors, both genetic and environmental, are now being carefully screened. The effects of harmful agents, drugs, injury, radiation, industrial accidents, nuclear exposure, atmospheric conditions, and temperature, as well as the health and parity of the mother, multiple pregnancies, intervals between pregnancies, and birth weights are all being monitored for any pubertal effects. Postnatal factors including climate, seasonal variations, nutrition, health, disease, stress and socioeconomic factors are also being closely studied.

The variations in growth and development during puberty are summarized below with reference to Tanner's nine factors of hereditary and environmental influences on growth (12).

THE GENETICS OF SIZE, SHAPE, AND THE TEMPO OF GROWTH

Body shape appears to be more resistant to environmental pressure than is body size. A body is shaped by the way cells are distributed; its size results from the sum of the sizes of the various cells—their number being fixed at an early stage. Increases in body size are related to a faster tempo of growth and puberty. Early puberty growth usually indicates that growth will also cease earlier.

THE EFFECTS OF NUTRITION ON GROWTH AND THE TEMPO OF GROWTH

Malnutrition delays growth and the onset of puberty. The associated factors of infection and the restriction of physical activity and social interaction lead to delayed physical, intellectual, and social development.

THE DIFFERENCE AMONG RACES

Populations differ in their body shape, average adult size, and tempo of growth. The differences may be a reflection of the environmental factors present.

CLIMATIC AND SEASONAL EFFECTS ON GROWTH

Ecological and climatic conditions have produced adaptive characteristics within populations. There is a linear correlation between peoples and the average annual temperature of their environment. Higher altitudes result in a larger chest circumference and larger lungs as well as a later menarche. Climate and length of daylight appear to play only a minor role in the rate of growth and the onset of menarche. Later menarche in tropical climates may be a result of a low nutritional level related to the rainy/dry periods that affect food supply and the frequency of infections. Some seasonal variations in growth have been noted. Height growth is faster during the spring and summer months and more weight is gained in the autumn and winter months. Blind children do not seem to be affected by the seasonal variations, as the length of daylight plays a minor role in synchronizing the seasonal and climatic variations in growth.

EFFECTS OF DISEASES

The effect of minor diseases on the growth of well-nourished children is minimal. For inadequately nourished children, however, even minor diseases may slow or delay growth. A catch-up period of growth usually occurs when the disease is resolved. Continual minor diseases coupled with malnutrition result in smaller size. In these cases, factors of economic depression and social disorganization are usually associated. Major or chronic diseases such as diabetes, renal disease, tuberculosis, and other debilitating illnesses can slow growth and delay sexual maturation, although the effects are seldom permanent.

PSYCHOSOCIAL STRESS

Stress may inhibit the secretion of growth hormone, and generally retards sexual maturation, most probably by increasing the adrenal androgen production. With the removal of the stress, the secretion of growth hormone is increased and there is a period of catch-up growth.

EFFECTS OF URBANIZATION

In urban areas, offspring are larger and have a more rapid tempo of growth. This is thought to result from a regular food supply, effective health and sanitation services, and adequate educational, recreational and welfare facilities. This is not true for areas of high population density or slums, however. The age of menarche is earlier in urban environments. In rural environments, more energy is spent in physical activity and the total caloric intake is frequently less than that in urban areas.

EFFECTS OF SOCIOECONOMIC STATUS AND SIZE OF FAMILY

There is a difference in size and the tempo of growth among socioeconomic levels in every society except the urban areas of Sweden. Upper socioeconomic levels, categorized by the father's occupation, result in larger children with a faster tempo of growth. In European countries, differences in growth are seen between manual and nonmanual occupations, while in developing countries, differences have been seen between the educational status of the parents. In all countries, the student population is the tallest group by 2–3 cm (0.8–1.2 inches). The first-born is usually taller and demonstrates a faster tempo of growth.

SECULAR TREND

There has been a noteworthy increase in size, including height and weight, and an earlier rate of maturation in succeeding generations. The decrease in the age of menarche has been related to improved nutrition, less disease, increase in adult size, and possibly an increase in psychosexual stimulation.

Conclusion

The maturational process of puberty lasts from 1.5 to 5 years. The height acquired during adolescence contributes to 15–20 percent of the adult height, and during the ages of 10–20, the weight more than doubles. The adolescent growth spurt, the development of breasts, and the growth of pubic hair are relatively concurrent. Menarche occurs in the later half of this period of growth and development. The relationship between thelarche and adrenarche is variable, not simultaneous. The first sign of puberty, whether it is breast development or pubic hair growth, occurs between 8.5 and 13 years in 95 percent of females. The breasts mature between 11.8 and 18.9 years,

Table 2.1. *Mean Onset of Female Pubertal Changes in the United States*

Age	Characteristic
9–10	Beginning of height spurt Growth of bony pelvis Female contour fat deposition Budding of nipples
10–11	Budding of breasts Appearance of pubic hair (may precede breast budding in 10%)
11–12	Appearance of vaginal secretions Growth of internal and external genitalia Increase in vaginal glycogen content, lowering of pH
12–13	Pigmentation of areolae Growth of breasts
13–14	Appearance of axillary hair Increase in amount of pubic hair Acne (in 75–90%) Menarche
15–16	Arrest of skeletal growth

Reproduced with permission from JB Lippincott/Harper & Row. Goldfarb AF. Puberty and menarche. *Clin Obstet Gynecol* 1977;20:629.

the mean PHV is 12.14 years, and the mean age at menarche is 13.47 years (Table 2.1).

The changes during puberty in the anatomy and physiology of the reproductive tract can be seen in Table 2.2.

Table 2.2. *Changes to the Reproductive Tract During Puberty*

	Early Puberty	Mid-Puberty	Late Puberty
Breast	Budding occurs.	Separation of breast and areolar tissue. More glandular tissue appears and ductal structure develops.	Continues to enlarge. Distinction between areola and breast is still present.
Uterus/cervix	Enlarges, corpus and cervix are the same length. Endometrium not	Substantially larger; corpus longer than cervix.	Continues to enlarge and corpus is now distinctly larger than cervix. Cervix now

(continued)

Table 2.2 (*continued*)

	Early Puberty	*Mid-Puberty*	*Late Puberty*
	developed. No glandular secretory activity.		adult shape and size. Copious secretions are produced by the cervical epithelium and ferning can be detected.
Ovaries	Enlarge.	Continue to enlarge; will increase from 3–4 g to 6 g at menarche.	Continue to enlarge.
Tubes		Increase in diameter, more complex folds appear in mucosa. Developing a ciliated epithelial lining.	
Vagina	Estrogenization of mucosa, reddish in color.	pH becomes acid. Increase in size from 4 cm to 7–8.5 cm. Mucosa thickens and is pink in color. Secretions appear. Bartholin glands become active.	Continues to elongate and mucosa thickens. Average length is 15 cm.
Labia	Wrinkling, increased vascularity, developing hair follicles on labia majora.	Labia minora enlarge. Pubic hair appears on labia majora and occasionally on the mons. Toward the end of this period, coarse, curly pubic hair present in moderate amounts on mons and labia majora. Apocrine activity present.	Labia minora elongated. Pubic hair course, curly, and abundant spreading over the mons and labia majora.
Body fat	Changes in distribution begin.	Changes striking.	Changes in distribution now obvious.
Axillary hair		Begins to appear toward the end of	Present.

Table 2.2 *(continued)*

	Early Puberty	*Mid-Puberty*	*Late Puberty*
		this period. Apocrine activity present in axillae.	
Skin		Sebaceous glands, especially in the face and back are active. Acne present.	
PHV		Attained.	
Miscellaneous		Pelvic cavity enlarges to allow ovaries, uterus and tubes to be lower in the pelvis. Goiters may be noticed.	Slight hair growth on outer edges of upper lip. Menarche occurs.

Adapted from Finkelstein JS. The endocrinology of adolescence. *Pediatr Clin North Am,* 1980; 27:53–69.

References

1. Finkelstein JW. The endocrinology of adolescence. *Pediatr Clin North Am* 1980; 27:53–69.
2. Tanner JM. *Growth at Adolescence.* Oxford: Blackwell Scientific Publications, 1962;37.
3. Tanner JM. *Growth at Adolescence.* Oxford: Blackwell Scientific Publications, 1962;32–33.
4. Frisch RE, Nagel JS. Predictions of adult height of girls from age of menarche and height at menarche. *J Pediatr* 1974;85:838–841.
5. Tanner JM. *Growth at Adolescence.* Oxford: Blackwell Scientific Publications, 1962;156.
6. Tanner JM. *Growth at Adolescence.* Oxford: Blackwell Scientific Publications, 1962;36.
7. Tanner JM. *Growth at Adolescence.* Oxford: Blackwell Scientific Publications, 1962;153.
8. Frisch RE. Critical weight at menarche, initiation of the adolescent growth spurt, and control of puberty. In: *Control of the Onset of Puberty.* Grumbach MM, Grave GD, Mayer FE (eds). New York: John Wiley & Sons, 1974:403–423.
9. Zacharias L, Wurtman RJ, Schatzoff M, et al. Sexual maturation in contemporary American girls. *Am J Obstet Gynecol* 1970;108:833–846.
10. Styne DM, Kaplan SL. Normal and abnormal puberty in the female. *Pediatr Clin North Am* 1979;26:123–148.

11. Eveleth PB, Tanner JM. *Worldwide Variations in Human Growth*. Cambridge: Cambridge University Press, 1976: 259, 419.
12. Tanner JM. *Foetus into Man: Physical Growth from Conception to Maturity*. London: Open Books, 1978: 119–153.

Bibliography

Brook CGD (ed). *Clinical Pediatric Endocrinology*. Oxford: Blackwell Scientific Publications, 1981.

Ducharme JR, Collu R. Pubertal development: normal, precocious and delayed. *Clin Endocrinol Metabol* 1982;11:57–87.

Falkner F, Tanner JM (eds). *Human Growth: Vol. 2: Postnatal Growth*. London: A Baillière Tindall, 1978.

Frisch RE, Revelle R. Height and weight at menarche and a hypothesis of menarch. *Arch Dis Child* 1971;46;695–701.

Gardner LI. *Endocrine and Genetic Diseases of Childhood and Adolescence* (2nd ed). Philadelphia: W.B. Saunders Co., 1975.

Goldfarb AF. Puberty and menarche. *Clin Obstet Gynecol* 1977;20:625–631.

Gysler M, Cowell CA. Gynaecological endocrinology of the paediatric and adolescent age group. *Clin Endocrinol Metabol* 1982;11(1):253–265.

Marshall WA. *Human Growth and Its Disorders*. London: Academic Press, 1977.

Marshall WA, Tanner JM. Variations in the patterns of pubertal changes in boys. *Arch Dis Child* 1970;45:13–23.

Marshall WA, Tanner JM. Variations in the patterns of pubertal changes in girls. *Arch Dis Child* 1969;44:291–303.

Reiter EO, Kulin HE. Sexual maturation in the female. *Pediatr Clin North Am* 1972;19:581–603.

Speroff L, Glass RH, Kase NG. *Clinical Gynecologic Endocrinology and Infertility*. Baltimore: Williams & Wilkins, 1981.

Tanner JM. *Education and Physical Growth*. London: Hodder & Stoughton, 1978.

Tanner JM. Population differences in body size, shape and growth rate: 1976 review. *Arch Dis Child* 1976;51:1–2.

Tanner JM, Whitehouse RH, Takaishi M. Standards from birth to maturity for height, weight, height velocity, and weight volume: British children 1965. *Arch Dis Child* 1966;41:454–471, 613–635.

Weideger P. *Menstruation and Menopause*. New York: Alfred A. Knopf, 1976.

Zacharias L, Wurtman RJ, Schatzoff M, et al. Sexual maturation in contemporary American girls. *Am J Obstet Gynecol* 1970;108:833–846.

Zacharias L, Wurtman RJ. Age at menarche: genetic and environmental influences. *New Engl J Med* 1969;280:868–875.

3 Primary Care and Preventive Health Services for the Normal Adolescent

The Pubertal Examination

It has been estimated that a practitioner might expect 1 of 10 gynecological patients to be adolescents—a statistic that appears to be equally applicable to obstetric care. Other than pregnancy, reasons given by adolescents for seeking health care include 1) menstrual disorders; 2) genital tract infections, and postpartum, postabortion, or postoperative referrals; 3) lower abdominal pain; 4) routine examination; 5) contraception; and 6) referrals for asymptomatic adnexal mass (1). Periodic health visits establish a trust relationship with the adolescent that set the tone for health care encounters throughout life. Such a relationship may well encourage a compliance with health advice and preventive care through anticipatory guidance and health education.

Before approaching the adolescent in the health care setting a clear picture of her social, psychological, and medical history is obtained. The World Health Organization (2) has identified certain health and social problems occurring during adolescence (Table 3.1). In addition, the summarized Report of the Task Force on Pediatric Education in the U.S. (1978) formulated the following adolescent needs (3):

1. Knowledge about their own physical, mental, and emotional processes.
2. Sexual education, including information on pregnancy, birth control, gender preference, and venereal disease.
3. Screening for precursors of adult disease.
4. Living, career, and parenting skills.
5. Education in how to use health services appropriately and effectively.
6. Prevention and treatment of substance abuse (alcohol, drugs, tobacco).
7. Management and counseling for long-term illnesses and handicapping conditions.
8. Prevention and treatment of obesity and undernourishment.

Table 3.1 *Examples of Health and Social Problems Occurring During Adolescence*

Type of Problem	Determinant Factors	Prevention and Management of Problems
Malnutrition	Poverty	A. Strengthening maternal and child health educational services:
Repeated infections	Unemployment of parents	
Total abandonment of the child	Deficient diet	Supplementary feeding Maternal and child
Partial abandonment of the child (psychosocial deprivation) leading to nutritional dwarfism decrease in intellectual performance	Insufficient health and other social services	health care, immunizations
	Insanitary environment	Organization of creches and other preschool institutions
	Parents' lack of information	Environmental sanitation
behavioral disturbances	Cultural blocks	Health, nutrition, and family life education, including family planning
social maladaptation	Employment of mothers away from home	
Frequent accidents (risk-taking behavior)	Irresponsible parenthood	B. Additional activities and services:
Truancy	Abandonment of home by parents	Extending maternity benefits
Drug addiction	Disrupted families	Local services for employment arrangements
Abuse of alcohol and tobacco	Shortage of personnel for community services	Comprehensive care services for abandoned children
Juvenile delinquency		Services for adoption
Early pregnancy in young adolescents	Hormonal and other biological changes	Legislation to protect women, children, and family
Abortion	Frequent need for readaptation	Voluntary organization work for assisting mothers and young children
Venereal diseases	Lack of understanding by family environment	
Prostitution		Specialized adolescent health care:
High incidence of tuberculosis	Ignorance about sexuality and family life	Appropriate units in schools of medicine
	Inadequate school syllabus	Inclusion of subjects relating to adolescence in other professional training
Unemployment of young people		
Emotional distress	Lack of recreational and creative opportunities	Education of parents

Table 3.1   (*continued*)

Type of Problem	Determinant Factors	Prevention and Management of Problems
Presence of a handicap or chronic illness	Social frustration Lack of working opportunities Lack of rehabilitation facilities and of sheltered workshops for the handicapped	about adolescents' health and social needs and problems Education of adolescents about sexuality, family life, responsible parenthood, drug addiction, etc. Sports and recreational projects (youth camps, hobbies) Rationalization of school syllabus Promotion of voluntary activities *for* and *by* adolescents Protection of totally and partially abandoned young adolescents, training and employment opportunities for them Special open institutions for rehabilitation of juvenile delinquents (academic and vocational training Introduction of subjects relating to adolescence into the regular school curriculum Application of existing and creation of new legislation for the protection of children, young people, and families rehabilitation and employment opportunities for handicapped and chronically ill

Table 3.1   *(continued)*

Type of Problem	Determinant Factors	Prevention and Management of Problems
		adolescents supportive social measures and relevant legislation

Reproduced by permission from the World Health Organization. Health Needs of Adolescents. *World Health Organizations Technical Report Series No. 609.* Geneva: WHO, 1977; 26–27.

9. Learning to cope with death and dying.
10. Services for runaways, including alternative living arrangements.
11. Mental health services in schools as well as in community health centers and physicians' offices.
12. Improved management of conversion symptoms, depression, delinquency, truancy, and vandalism.
13. Prevention of suicide.

These reports give a clear view of the health needs of the adolescent as seen by the practitioner and health care agencies. Adolescents themselves have also identified major areas of concern they may directly or indirectly communicate to the health care provider. In one study, adolescents identified certain areas of anxiety such as social, sexual, and psychological feelings toward self, parental problems, school problems, problems with alcohol and drugs, and other issues relating to racial prejudice and physical handicaps (4).

When all of this information is considered it becomes evident that the periodic health visit becomes an important and integral part of the growth and development of the adolescent. To provide comprehensive care for the adolescent the following services may be considered.

1. Health care services: prenatal, postnatal, family planning, gynecological services, including pap smears, venereal disease testing and treatment, pregnancy testing, abortion/adoption information and referral, rape counseling and referral.
2. Health education: nutrition, dental care, weight control, normal growth and development, reproductive information.
3. Counseling: psychosocial factors of parental and peer relationships, future plans, environmental safety, substance abuse, sexuality, and parenting.

4. Provision for services: physical examination for athletics, work and school, and immunizations.

The biosocial screening examination for health maintenance in the adolescent cannot be routine or "just the essentials." The adolescent requires a direct and personal level of primary care to meet her many needs. The biosocial screening examination presented in this text will cover those areas which are specifically pertinent to the adolescent. For information about complete physical assessment and examination there are several excellent, detailed texts (5, 6, 7). Besides the general overview of adolescent health needs, a few areas in the following examination may need clarification.

A positive history of in utero exposure to diethylstilbestrol (DES) may still occur as this drug was prescribed to prevent miscarriages up until 1971. When exposed to DES, adenocarcinoma and squamous cell dysplasia most frequently occur shortly after puberty. Screening procedures begin at any of the following points: within three cycles after the onset of menarche, unusual vaginal bleeding at any age, or by 14 years of age (8).

The immunization status of adolescents also requires investigation. There is a significant number of adolescents who lack sufficient immunization and who are vulnerable to diphtheria-tetanus, polio, measles, mumps, and rubella. Adolescents who have never had mumps or measles or who have never been immunized require immunizations. All female adolescents should be screened for rubella immune status, immunized if susceptible, and provided with appropriate contraception during this time. The diphtheria-tetanus booster is also recommended every 10 years. Although the incidence of tuberculosis has decreased, the initial infection has become relatively frequent in adolescents and young adults. The chance of developing chronic pulmonary tuberculosis is greater in females, especially within two years of menarche. Adolescents who have symptoms of tuberculosis or are in contact with carriers should be screened. Routine screening usually takes place in any area where the local incidence of tuberculosis is 1 percent or greater (9).

Cardio-respiratory screening in adolescence may seem excessive, but the health risks associated with smoking, obesity, and hypertension occur during adolescence as well as in adulthood. Adolescents who are heavy smokers may show symptoms of chronic productive cough, shortness of breath, and abnormal respiratory flow rates indicative of small airway disease. Pulmonary function tests may be used in assessing the symptomatic adolescent. Also, a family history of coronary heart disease or stroke may indicate a need for screening of triglyceride, cholesterol and lipoprotein levels. Sustained hypertension in adolescence occurs in approximately 1 percent to 2 percent of the population, usually a mild form of essential hypertension (9).

The complaint of severe pleuritic pain in the young sexually active female, in association with tenderness under the rib cage on the right side, may be a sign of Fitz-Hugh-Curtis syndrome or gonococcal perihepatitis. The pleuritic upper quadrant pain arises from adhesions between the front surface of the liver and the abdominal wall or diaphram. Gonococcal perihepatitis may occur in up to 5 percent of females with gonococcal pelvic inflammatory disease (PID) and may also occur with nongonococcal PID, especially where an intrauterine device is present (10).

During the biannual pelvic examination, the cervix fundus ratio of puberty is 1:1, becoming 1:3 in late adolescence. Anteversion and anteflexion of the uterus do not occur until menarche. The adnexal structures may or may not be palpable during early adolescence (8). Prior to the pelvic examination, the hymen is inspected for common variations. A thin strand bifurcating the hymenal opening may occur in 6 percent to 8 percent of female adolescents, causing pain, bleeding and possible fear of penetration, especially if tampon use has been attempted (11).

Cervical cytology is proving to be an integral part of the health assessment of the sexually active adolescent. Kaufman and others (12, 13) screened over 10,000 adolescents and found 23 per 1000 demonstrated significant atypia in cervicovaginal smears, with carcinoma in situ in 1 per 2000. In 1 of every 1000 there were signs of severe dysplasia, in 5.6 per 100 there were changes suggestive of either severe dysplasia or carcinoma in situ (12, 13). Also, Hein (14) and others reported early neoplastic changes in 35 per 1000 sexually active adolescent females screened, and Feldman and others reported dysplasia in 70 per 1000 adolescents (14, 15). Pap smears are a normal component of the initial examination and may be taken annually. Pap smears are recommended annually for the first two years and, if negative, once every three years until age 35.

A common orthopedic condition in female adolescents is scoliosis. Inspection and palpation of the spine for abnormalities as well as observation for body asymmetry are also essential assessments (9).

Periodic screening for vision problems or referral to an ophthalmologist is advisable during adolescence (9). By late adolescence, one fifth of the population have defective acuity of 20/40 or less without correction. The incidence of myopia is three times greater between the ages of 12 and 17 than during the ages of 6 and 11.

Depression is common among adolescents and suicide is the third leading cause of death during adolescence. It is estimated that for each adolescent suicide, 200 attempts were made. Nonparticipation, numerous bodily concerns, and depression may be indicators of suicidal behavior in the adolescent (9).

The biosocial screening (Table 3.2) begins with an identification of primary language spoken, grade completed in school, and the ability to read and write English.

Table 3.2.   *The Biosocial Screening*

Medical History
Childhood illness
  Measles, mumps, chicken pox
  Communicable diseases
  Febrile illness
  Rheumatic heart disease or other heart disorder
  Kidney disease
Immunizations
  Primary and boosters (tetanus-diphtheria, typhoid; polio; measles-mumps-rubella)
  Influenza
Major illness, surgery, hospitalizations
Injury/accidents
  Broken bones
  Motor vehicle accidents
  Unconsciousness
Sensory impairment
  Use of glasses/contacts (last vision examination)
  Hearing impairment (last hearing examination)
  Speech impairment
  Use of orthodontics (last dental examination)
Emotional disorders
  Depression
  Suicide
  Emotional disturbances
  Therapy
Weight gain/loss
Sleep pattern
Infectious diseases

Sexually transmitted diseases/venereal diseases
Vaginitis/cervicitis/cystitis
Exposure to tuberculosis
Medications
  Prescription
  Over-the-counter
Substance use/abuse
  Nicotine
  Alcohol
  Marijuana
  Caffeine
  Other drugs
Date and results of last physical examination
Date and results of last Pap smear
Previous abnormal Pap smear
Previous abnormal breast examination
Previous abnormal pelvic examination
DES exposure and follow-up

Family History
Parents and siblings
  Age
  Health status
  Education
  Occupation
Significant illness of members
  Cardiovascular disease, arteriosclerosis
  Cancer of breasts and/or reproductive tract
  Problems of the

breasts and/or reproductive tract, (miscarriages, sexually transmitted diseases, structural abnormalities, menstrual abnormalities, infertility)
  Obesity
  Hypertension
  Diabetes
  Renal disease
  Migraine headaches
  Epilepsy
  Mental/emotional disturbances/illness
  Sickle cell anemia

Social History
Progress with development tasks
  Independence
  Gender role and sexuality
  Identity and role in society
Relationships
  Parents/siblings
  Peers
  Intimate partner(s)
  General adjustments
Emotional temperment
Acheivement
  Education
  Job/career
  Assets/skills
Place of residence/conditions

Habits
Diet
Exercise/physical activity
Nail-biting, thumb-sucking
Stutter/lisp

(continued)

Table 3.2 (*continued*)

Tics
Enuresis
Sleep/dreams/insomnia
Current drug usage
  Pattern and length
  Reasons
  Role drugs play in life
Self breast exam
Menstrual calendar

Menstrual History
Age of menarche
Interval and duration
Amount and character-
  istics of flow
Discomforts
  PMS
  Dysmenorrhea
  Dysmenorrhagia
  Intermenstrual
    bleeding/spotting
Last menstrual period/
  previous menstrual
  period
Sanitary pads/tampons:
  TSS

Hygiene
Leukorrhea
  Duration and time
    present in menstrual
    cycle
  Character, color, odor
Use of commercial
  products (toiletries)
Vaginal sprays
Douches
Perfumed soaps and
  powders
Cleaning front to back
  (vagina to anus)
Clothing
  Cotton/synthetic
    underwear
Panty hose/pants
Shaving of axillary and/
  or pubic hair
Foreign bodies in

vagina or rectum
Urinary tract infections
  cystitis and/or
  vaginal infections

Sexual History
Sexual activity
  Initial/onset
  Frequency and type(s)
  Number of partner(s)
Satisfaction with
  sexual activity and/
  or relationship
Pain or bleeding with
  coitus or postcoitus
Availability of privacy
Orgasm
Presence of sexual
  dysfunction/
  problem
Masturbation
Sexual preference
  (heterosexual, ho-
  mosexual, asexual/
  bisexual/transexual)
Use of stimulants
  (pornography, vibra-
  tors, other devices)
Knowledge of
  reproduction
Duration of sexual
  exposure with and
  without contra-
  ception
Previous/recent/
  current sexual
  trauma
Sexually transmitted
  diseases
  Syphillis or gonorrhea
  Herpes
  Venereal warts
  Other
Abstinence

Contraceptive History
Present method
  Satisfaction

Duration of use
  Side effects/problems
  Understanding of
    method and com-
    pliance
Previous methods
  Type and duration of
    use
  Satisfaction
  Side effects/problems
  Understanding of
    method and com-
    pliance
  Reason(s) for
    discontinuing
Contraceptive failures

Obstetric History
Gravity/parity (live
  births, miscarriages,
  abortions, still
  births)
Description of ante-
  partum, intrapar-
  tum, and postpar-
  tum course(s)

Review of Systems
General
  Appearance and
    nutritional status
  Recent emotional/
    mental status
  Recent weight gain
    or loss
  Bodily concerns
  Physical activity (par-
    ticipation in sports,
    exercise, fatigue/
    malaise)
Chief complaint
  Onset and recurrence
  Description of each
    symptom
  Relation to time,
    activity, menses,
    bodily functions
  Relation to recent

Table 3.2   *(continued)*

events, social activity, school/home crises
Skin
  Acne
  Hair distribution
  Scars
Head
  Headaches/migraines
  Syncope (fainting)
  Ear aches
  Epistaxis (nosebleeds)
  Colds, sore throats
  Hay fever, asthma
  Mouth (toothaches, bleeding gums, orthodontics, difficulty swallowing)
Cardiorespiratory
  Dyspnea (shortness of breath) or cough
  Chest pain, palpitation or trachycardia
  Right-sided tenderness under rib cage
Breasts
  Development
  Pain, lumps, discharge, changes
  Use of a bra
  Lactation experience
Gastrointestinal system
  Diet
  Appetite
  Signs of obesity/anorexia nervosa
  Food allergies
  Use of cathartics, laxatives, antacids or antiemetic drugs
  Constipation/diahrrea
  Rectal pain/bleeding
Urinary system
  Dysuria, frequency discharge
  Pain, nocturia

Incontinence (normally, with athletic activities)
Muscular-skeletal-vascular systems
  Joint pain
  Backache
  Athletic injuries
  Scoliosis
  Limitation of motion or activities
  Edema
Nervous system (coordination, reflexes)

Physical Examination
Physical measurements
  Height
  Weight
  Blood pressure
  Pulse
  Skinfolds (optional)
Maturational rating
  Recent changes in height and weight/growth spurt
  Tanner breast and pubic hair stages
  Hair distribution patterns
  Distribution of adipose tissue
  Acne
  Leukorrhea
Skin
  Scars
  Lesions
  Rashes
Mouth and throat
  Oral hygiene
  Gums, caries, fillings, occulsions
  Tonsils
  Thyroid
Thorax
  Deformity

Breath sounds
Spine
  Posture (curvature, scoliosis, pilonidal depression)
Heart
  Rhythm
  Murmur
Breasts
  Developmental rating
  Asymmetry
Abdomen
  Liver/spleen
  Masses/tenderness
  Surgical scars
Genital examination
  Speculum, rectal examination, biannual palpation
  Developmental rating
  Discharge
  Structures (hymen, vagina, uterus, ovaries, pelvic or adnexal masses)
Extremities
  Edema
  Bruising
  Hands/feet for infection
Neurological
  Gait
  Coordination
  Balance
  Reflexes

Laboratory Examination
Blood work
  Complete blood count or hemoglobin/hematocrit
  As indicated (sickle cell trait, G_6 PD, VDRL, GTT, thyroid functions, triglycerides, choles-

(continued)

Table 3.2   (*continued*)

terol, lipoprotein, Rh titer)	Pap	PPD or tine test for tuberculosis
Urine	Herpes culture	Chest x-ray
Urinalysis, culture, and sensitivity	Wet mount preparations for vaginitis	Vision screening
Pregnancy test as indicated	Vaginal maturation index (estrogen effect)	Audiogram
Cultures/smears GC	Other screening tests (as indicated)	Step test Pulmonary functions

The Adolescent and Nutrition

Before considering the nutritional needs of the pregnant adolescent, an initial review of the nutritional requirements of the normal adolescent is necessary. Once a clear understanding of these nutritional needs has been established, the additional dietary demands required by the pregnant or lactating adolescent can be examined.

Adolescents, particularly between the ages of 10 and 16, have the poorest and most unsatisfactory nutritional status. They need good nutrition in order to satisfy the body's growth demands for energy, protein, fat, vitamins, and minerals—demands that markedly increase at this time of rapid weight gain and linear growth. Normal adolescent development requires adequate nutrition, sleep, exercise, and psychological stimulation. Nutritional reserves must not be depleted by an inadequate diet. Healthy living habits must be established and reinforced to provide the necessary amounts of exercise, sleep, and mental stimulation. Nutritional needs are at their highest during adolescence, as the body seeks to meet the growth needs of puberty, which are accompanied by an increase in both muscle and adipose tissue. Failure to meet dietary needs during this growth period can potentially retard growth and delay sexual maturation.

As noted earlier, the nutritional status of adolescence is the poorest of any age group. The typical American diet is high in saturated fats, sugar, and salt—a diet that not only fails to promote and support growth and development, but also may lead to diseases such as cancer, hypertension, coronary artery disease, diabetes, obesity, or dental caries. The consumption of fast foods, so popular with adolescents, provides a diet high in fat and salt, but low in vitamins C and A, folic acid, and fiber. This nutritional imbalance has been implicated in the etiology of degenerative diseases in later life. Vegetarian diets, also popular with adolescents, are a source of concern as well because the absence of animal foods reduces the amounts of B_{12}, B_6, riboflavin, and the minerals calcium, iron, and zinc. Such diets often create nutritional problems for the adolescent, with overnutrition, undernutrition, and iron-deficiency anemia the most common. Overnutrition results in early maturation and menarche and greater skeletal growth. Undernutrition, on the other hand, can contribute to delayed menarche and a prolonged growth period, with the most pronounced retardation occurring just prior to menarche.

Many factors influence the nutrition of the normal adolescent. Some are related to the social and economic status of the adolescent and her family, such as the adequacy of food supplies and the cultural importance of food. In homes where the mother prepares breakfast daily, the adolescent tends to eat a regular breakfast and lunch when away from home. In low-income families, these influences become crucial. The lack of money to purchase food, inadequate facilities for food storage and preparation, limited knowledge of nutrition and food management, dependence upon others for food preparation, unusual eating patterns, and ethnic language barriers all contribute to inadequate nutrition for the adolescent. Other factors revolve about the individual adolescent's response to her environment and her ability to deal with diverse influences. Such influential factors include family food patterns, ethnic and cultural food preferences, desire for independence, and personal food preferences. Several factors also affect the adolescent's appetite. Not only do psychological, social, and cultural pressures alter the adolescent's response to food, but physiologically the demand for nutrients increases during the adolescent growth spurt.

The complexities of the adolescent appetite are a response to competing influences. The typical adolescent diet is irregular: meal skipping (particularly breakfast), between-meal snacking, increased eating away from home, and eating sparingly throughout the day and trying to catch up in the late evening. Often in conflict with the adolescent's increased needs for food are food fads; fast foods; diets; erratic work, school, and social schedules; and athletic training. The adolescent is also concerned about appearance and especially desires slimness and to prevent acne. There may also be dietary restrictions involved in the wearing of braces. Adolescents are also great imitators of people they admire and like to use these people as role models. This is often reflected by the adolescent in adopting such food preferences as seasonings (particularly sugar and salt), artificial sweeteners, high-fat and high-cholesterol foods, food supplements, chronic dieting, and the use of drugs (especially alcohol and nicotine). Both smoking and alcohol consumption alter the appetite, which displaces food in the diet and can affect the gastrointestinal tract by changing the transport, metabolism, and storage of nutrients, thereby leading to nutritional deficiency. For social, cultural, religious, and moral reasons, the adolescent may also be attracted to speciality diets such as vegetarian, organic, kosher, and health foods that may or may not provide the necessary nutrients for this period of growth and change. If adolescents diet, they do so for appearance, athletics or because of economic problems, but not usually for health reasons. Not all adolescents are aware of the inherent dangers in some food products: food processing, dyes, chemical additives, food-borne toxins, and radioactivity. There are also other factors that affect nutritional requirements: the presence of disease, degrees of physical activity, adolescent body size and composition, age, and climate.

Nutritional Deficiencies

Most authorities agree that adolescents are deficient in vitamin A, vitamin C, riboflavin, thiamine, calcium, iron, zinc, and folic acid. In many areas, the impact of these deficiencies upon the adolescent is still not clear. These deficiencies may be related to the adolescent's eating habits or preferences for meats, grains, pastries, dairy products, and fast foods. When necessary nutrients are missing from the adolescent diet, resistance to infection is lost and puberty delayed, which can reduce the lean body mass, the cell numbers, and the protein:DNA ratio in the muscle. Caloric demands peak at menarche then slowly decline. Protein intake peaks about age 12 with a secondary rise at age 17. While there is a steady increase in fat intake between the ages of 8 and 12, there is then a decline that parallels the total caloric intake. The Recommended Daily Allowances (RDAs) for adolescents have been estimated by adjusting the adult requirements to meet the increased nutrient needs of adolescence. Many of these estimates are based on body weight and height, which are influenced by biological maturity, genetic factors, and nutrition. Nutritional requirements, therefore, are dependent upon the developmental stage rather than the chronologial age of the adolescent. Physical activity versus a sedentary lifestyle, body size and composition, sexual maturity, and consumptive patterns all influence the balance of the RDAs necessary for the individual adolescent's nutritional requirements.

Energy requirements are greatly influenced by the velocity of growth during adolescence, as well as physical activity levels, body size, climate, and ecological factors. The adolescent seems more sensitive to caloric restrictions than the child or adult probably because body mass almost doubles during puberty. The highest energy intake of 2550 Kcal occurs during 12–13 years. By 17–18 years energy intake decreases by 300 Kcal.

In females, energy intake decreases at the sexual maturity rating of 4 and 5, when the period of most rapid growth has passed. Protein supplies a constant 12 percent to 14 percent of the energy intake throughout childhood and adolescence. If energy intake is limited, protein is used and therefore not available for synthesis of new tissue. This can lead to a reduction of the growth rate, even with an adequate dietary protein intake. Peak protein intake (80 mg per day) coincides with the peak energy intake in females at age

12–13 years. The requirements for proteins vary according to the amounts needed for body maintenance, as well as growth of new tissue during this period.

Many adolescents are deficient in the minerals calcium, zinc and iron. This deficiency occurs simultaneous with an increased demand for these minerals during the adolescent growth spurt. Calcium is necessary for development of skeletal mass; iron, for the expansion of muscle mass and blood volume; and zinc, for the generation of both skeletal and muscle tissue, and sexual maturation. A typical American diet contains 300 mg of calcium daily, but the adolescent RDA ranges from 500–1200 mg per day. To meet these requirements, up to six cups of milk may be needed daily. As many as 50 percent of adolescent females consume less than two thirds of the recommended dietary intake of calcium. Both calcium and phosphates are needed during maximum growth periods for rapid bone development. There is some controversy, however, about the evidence of calcium deficiency and the need for dietary calcium supplementation in the normal or pregnant adolescent (16).

A zinc deficiency is now considered a health risk, because the resulting retardation of growth and delayed sexual maturation have been clearly seen. Not only is zinc essential for the growth process, but it also plays a role in insulin metabolism, nucleic acid and protein synthesis, gonadal development, wound healing, and enzyme reactivity. Adolescents on vegetarian diets are particularly susceptible to zinc deficiency. Over one third of adolescent females consume less than two thirds of the 11–15 mg daily requirement for dietary intake of zinc.

Requirements for dietary intake of iron increase during adolescence with the acceleration of blood volume and muscle mass and with the onset of menses. Iron is needed to cover losses in iron supplies as well as to meet the increased need in the growth of red cell mass and tissues during puberty. Few adolescents consume the recommended 18 mg–20 mg of iron per day. Five percent to 15 percent of adolescents, of both low and high income families, have iron-deficiency anemia with an increased incidence in the black population. Ingesting sources of vitamin C with iron-rich foods can increase the absorption of iron. Anemia during adolescence is a worldwide nutritional problem relating to chronic iron loss often from parasitic infection or by malabsorption.

Adolescence increases the demand for dietary vitamins. With the greater energy demand there is an increased need for thiamine, riboflavin, and niacin for energy metabolism. As tissue synthesis increases with the adolescent growth spurt, there is an increased demand for folacin and vitamin B_{12}, which are required for normal DNA and RNA metabolism. Folacin plays a role in DNA synthesis and in cell replication and growth. B_{12} is required for the rapid growth of cells during adolescence, and it also plays a role in fat, carbohydrate, and protein metabolism. Increased amounts of vitamins A, C, D, and E, which are essential for skeletal growth, are also needed. Vitamins are needed to maintain the homeostasis of calcium and phosphate in the mineralization of bone. The amounts of vitamins needed may depend on climate and variability of exposure to sunlight. The dietary intake of vitamins A, B_6, C and folacin is below the RDA in most American adolescents. Deficiencies may lead to a decrease in plasma levels or a decrease in the activity of vitamin-dependent enzymes. Vitamin B_6, particularly, is associated with nitrogen metabolism and plays a role in the enzyme systems. The effect of a deficiency or overabundance of many of these nutrients and micronutrients is not known. For example, a vitamin A deficiency, which is common among adolescents, does not appear to be associated with any functional disability.

Acne and Nutrition

A majority of adolescents develop some degree of acne, with an increased incidence occurring between the ages of 16 and 20. The occurrence of acne raises concerns for the adolescent about appearance and social acceptance. It is now believed that for the normal adolescent, acne is not caused or worsened by eating specific foods; therefore food restrictions have little effect. Good hygiene seems the best advice. In some cases, the use of vitamin A and zinc sulfate may also be recommended.

Oral Contraceptives and Nutrition

Many adolescents begin to use contraceptives during their growth spurt, particularly the oral contraceptive pill (OCP). It is imperative that information regarding nutritional changes related to the use of the oral contraceptive pill be included with other pertinent OCP information.

With the OCP, there are alterations in the metabolism of proteins, carbohydrates, lipids, and some vitamins and minerals; variations which occur regardless of the adequacy of dietary intake. The effect of these changes on the metabolism depends upon the following factors: the age and nutritional status of the user, the type of OCP, and the sensitivity of the user to the OCP.

OCPs may also alter the body composition by increasing body weight due to fluid retention and an increase in lean body tissue. Plasma levels of vitamin A may increase as well, with a concurrent decrease in the circulating levels of other vitamins, such as vitamin C, riboflavin, B_{12}, folacin, and pyridoxine. Serum copper and iron levels are also increased while zinc levels generally decrease. Although less niacin may be required, there is an increased demand for riboflavin, thiamine, calcium and phosphorus. There can also be a decrease in plasma albumin levels while serum triglyceride levels rise. An adolescent with a family history of cardiac and diabetic problems may experience an increase in plasma cholesterol and fasting glucose levels, as well as abnormal glucose tolerance tests. Although OCPs alter folate, B_6, B_{12}, thiamine, riboflavin, and vitamins C, A, E, there are few, if any, clinical manifestations as a result. Vitamin B_6 deficiency, however, may be associated with mental depression. The use of OCPs in some adolescents may add to symptoms of existing depression. In such cases, a supplement of 1.5 mg of B_6 daily or a discontinuation of the OCPs may be considered.

OCP RISKS

Because of the effect of OCPs on lipid metabolism with long-term usage cholesterol and triglyceride levels increase, and there is potential for vascular disease. The degree of fluctuation in these levels appears to be greater in the younger adolescent. In the young adolescent who has a potential for long-term contraceptive usage, and who smokes or has a family history of atherosclerotic disease, the potential benefit of OCP usage must be weighed against the potential risks. The practitioner may consider monitoring lipid levels for those with such risks. As previously noted, the metabolism of practically every nutrient is altered by OCP usage, although there is little evidence that increased intake of these nutrients is needed to prevent deficiencies. Therefore, routine supplementation is not indicated.

Physical Activity and Nutrition

There are over 30 different sports approved for adolescent females in school competitions ranging from interscholastic and team sports to dance, swimming, and gymnastics. Twenty percent to 60 percent of today's females spend some time each day in athletic activity. Exercise promotes self-esteem, security, peer and parental acceptance, and positive personality traits. Physical activity, however, is an area full of misconceptions concerning nutrition for the adolescent. Misinformation regarding nutritional supplements, weight control, and training diets are frequently given. A major misconception is the need for high protein intake with heavy exercise. Some additional protein may be needed for the synthesis of lean body tissue during training, but this can be accommodated by increasing dietary intake of protein-rich foods for the growing athlete. If the diet is well-balanced there is no need to use vitamin and mineral supplementation during training. The use of high doses of vitamins A and D do not enhance performance or endurance and can be toxic.

The problem of dehydration is an area of concern regarding adolescent physical activity. Dehydration causes fatigue, limited work capacity, increase in body temperature, and the possibility of heat stroke. These effects also occur when rapid weight loss is attempted either through severely decreasing water and food intake or by sweat loss. Such weight loss can lead to lean body tissue degradation, electrolyte imbalance, and dehydration, all of which cause a decrease in the reserves of the body for athletic demands and an interference with normal growth. With the depletion of sodium and potassium in heavy physical exercise, it is important to drink electrolyte-rich beverages, or to liberally salt food or include potassium-rich foods, such as bananas, in the diet. Fluid should be replaced through frequent, small quantities of water, and the adolescent should be well-hydrated prior to the athletic event. Salt tablets should never be considered for use with adolescents unless the adolescent is losing more than six pints of water during physical activity. With increased physical activity, there is also the tendency for female adolescents to become iron deficient as a result of inadequate dietary intake, loss with menses, and prevalence of lean tissue. It is recommended that female athletes supplement their diet with 30–60 mg of iron per day.

Female adolescents, being weight conscious, are concerned with their increasing appetites—increases stimulated by their developmental growth and physical activity. With light, regular activity, however, food intake will often decrease and weight stabilization or loss will occur. A sedentary lifestyle, on the other hand, is associated with an increased food intake and excess weight gain. The benefits of physical conditioning for the cardiovascular system, rest, and weight maintenance are significant. Additional benefits can be seen in increased caloric expenditure and the positive effect of hyperinsulinemia. Physical fitness improves posture, decreases the reaction to disease and stress, releases emotional tension, and provides an environment for interpersonal growth.

Obesity and Nutrition

Obesity occurs in up to 30 percent of the adolescent population and is identified by excess body fat in proportion to height and stage of development. Obesity is generally considered to occur when one is 20 percent or more over ideal body weight for height. The usual cause of obesity, or exogeneous obesity, is excessive caloric intake in relation to body energy needs and expenditure. This form of obesity is primarily due to poor eating habits such as skipping meals and night eating. It is also associated with depression and a family history of obesity. Often, there is evidence of a long-standing weight problem in an otherwise normal or advanced growth pattern, as well as an unremarkable medical history and physical examination. Obesity may be a factor in the development of other illnesses such as atherosclerosis, cardiovascular disease, gall bladder disease, pulmonary respiratory diseases, cutaneous manifestations, gout, and endometrial cancer.

Some of the factors associated with obesity are genetic make-up, environment, attitudes and habits toward exercise and eating, body size and composition, sexual maturity, and various psychological and emotional influences. It is now believed that there are critical periods in life where a fixed number of fat cells are obtained or where hypercellularity may develop. These periods occur during intrauterine life, infancy, and puberty.

During the first year of life, overnutrition leading to eventual long-term obesity may begin through excessive calories ingested by bottle-fed babies, early introduction of solid foods containing excess calories and proteins, and the development of food preferences for salt and sugar. The normal increase in body fat during the ages of 10 to 14, when combined with decreased physical activity, can lead to adolescent obesity. The result of overnutrition is an acceleration of linear growth and sexual maturation leading to an earlier menarche. If the adolescent combines excessive calories with a sedentary lifestyle during the normal growth spurt, the weight gained will be disproportionately greater, leading to or accentuating obesity. A majority of obese adolescents will remain obese as adults. Early identification of excess fat, and counseling in dietary controls and increased physical activity are, therefore, important.

Assessment tools, used in the identification of the overweight adolescent, include growth charts, height and weight ratios, and in some cases triceps-skinfold thickness measurements. Treatment modalities differ greatly and may include dieting, exercise, behavior modification, drugs, psychoanalysis, and surgery. Diets vary from low-calorie and protein-sparing to fasting. The benefit of many such diets is short-term weight reduction, and such abstinence often carries the risks of retarded growth, psychological stress, and no long-term improvement of dietary habits and eating behaviors. It is inadvisable, therefore, to restrict the intake of calories below 1200 Kcal per day in the growing adolescent, regardless of the protein intake. The obese adolescent who attempts erratic and unsupervised dieting may also suffer from low serum iron levels.

During early to mid-adolescence, weight counseling should strive for weight stabilization through the moderation of eating habits and an increase of physical activity. After peak height and weight gains have occurred, during mid- to late adolescence, the goal of slow but constant weight loss may be obtained. It must be remembered that the overweight adolescent may actually be eating less than her slim counterpart, but she is less active and expends less energy during activity. Other methods of weight reduction for the adolescent are inappropriate in most cases. Surgical jejunoileal bypass is effective but drastic, and such therapy carries the risks of significant side effects, complications and even mortality. Anorexic and hormonal drugs are also potentially dangerous and carry the risk of drug abuse without the benefit of long-term effectiveness.

Behavioral modification, on the other hand, can have both immediate and long-term success as a weight reduction technique. The methods used in behavior modification are aimed toward changing the act of eating and controlling the pattern of eating; goals and methods for coping with life stresses that are achieved through rewards for altered eating behaviors. The UCLA Adolescent Weight Reduction Program combines many aspects of diet and behavior modification to develop sound eating habits and exercise patterns, and to foster good health and psychological attitudes (17).

The emotional sequelae of adolescent obesity include a passive personality, decreased self-respect, a sense of hopelessness, depression, social isolation, and feelings of rejection. This cycle becomes self-perpetuating through the repetition of rejection, withdrawal, isolation, depression, boredom, inactivity and the recurrent increase in eating which maintains obesity. Obesity is a life-long problem, and the adolescent must be motivated to correct it. Education for the adolescent about calorie-restricted, balanced diets supplemented by physical exercise and psychological support must be made available.

Recommendations for Nutritional Health

The promotion and maintenance of nutritional health for the female adolescent can be accomplished through a number of prophylactic measures. Evaluating food needs, screening for nutritional problems, weight assessment, and counseling for special diets or dietary problems may help to identify potential problems. Nutritional education will rehabilitate nutritionally depleted adolescents, and it will assist others trying to adjust to stable weight levels. Provision of nutritional services such as food assistance and supplements, and evaluations with follow-ups help adolescents develop and maintain proper nutritional habits.

It is no longer sufficient to tell adolescents that they should eat a well-balanced diet of set items from the four food groups. Nor can we simply encourage an increase in fruits, vegetables, and whole grains, and a decrease in sugars and fats. Adolescents need individual assessment and nutritional re-education to meet their growth needs.

Nutritional Management for the Pregnant Adolescent

The need for adequate nutrition during adolescence is greater still when combined with additional physiological stress engendered by pregnancy.

Nutritional requirements during adolescent pregnancy include those of the normal growth as well as the growth and development of maternal and fetal tissues. Nutritional inadequacies are to be expected; the pregnant adolescent often does not fulfill the increased nutritional requirements. Nutritional deficiences already present must be calculated in the assessment of the adolescent's diet. The early detection of undernourishment in the pregnant adolescent may prevent some of the negative effects of inadequate nutrition on the growth and viability of the fetus. Nutritional inadequacies that are not corrected can result in increased neonatal morbidity and mortality. Nutritional inadequacies and the lack of appropriate prenatal care are often more prevalent when the adolescent is from a low income background. A majority of pregnant adolescents are deficient in iron, protein, calcium, and vitamin A, and many may be deficient in vitamin C, niacin, B_6, B_{12}, folate, and thiamine. Complications of pre-eclampsia, anemia, cephalopelvic disproportion (CPD), and low-birthweight infants have been demonstrated in the nonwhite population where poor nutrition and poverty were prevalent (18).

Food intake during pregnancy often varies according to trimester. During the first trimester, appetite and food intake are decreased because of the normal experience of nausea and vomiting. Appetite and therefore food intake are increased during the second trimester when these complaints cease. Both appetite and food intake may decrease during the third trimester when heartburn, constipation, and discomfort caused by the size and position of the baby may be experienced. Another dietary problem throughout pregnancy may be the presence of pica, or the compulsive eating of nonfood substances such as starch or clay, which displaces nutrients and food in the diet. Also many pregnant adolescents are victims of restricted diets either out of concern for fashion and figure or by denial of the pregnancy. Such restricted diets to control weight gain are hazardous as they result in inadequate dietary intake for both adolescent growth and fetal development.

The complications of adolescent pregnancy are seen in pre-eclampsia and hypertensive disorders, premature labors, low-birthweight babies, and anemia. Fortunately, many of these complications can be prevented through adequate nutrition and prenatal care. These complications, however, can be encouraged through poor nutrition, neglect, or by the consumption of alcohol, nicotine, and other substances. Cigarette smoking interferes with metabolic processes and often results in smaller babies. Consuming alcohol alters the appetite, displaces food in the diet, adversely effects the gastrointestinal tract, and may result in neurologic damage to the newborn (fetal alcohol syndrome). Maternal disease may also alter maternal absorption, utilization, and placental transfer of nutrients.

Evidence suggests that the pregnant adolescent should reach a certain critical body weight to provide the fetus with optimal conditions for growth. This critical body weight is a 10 percent excess over ideal body weight by the time of delivery. To reach such a critical weight, the adolescent who begins pregnancy with an adequate weight for height needs to gain a minimum of 25–30 pounds during the pregnancy. If the adolescent is deficient in weight for height at the onset of pregnancy, she must first make up her own deficit in body weight, then begin the additional increase of 25–30 pounds weight gain for the pregnancy. Many adolescents, however, gain fewer than 25 pounds during pregnancy (19).

Inadequate Weight Gain

Inadequate weight gain during pregnancy negatively influences birth-weight; adequate weight gain positively influences it. Other factors influencing birthweight are the prepregnancy weight, the length of gestation, and gynecological age. Ten percent less than the ideal weight for height is considered a low prepregnancy weight, whereas a prepregnancy weight of 20 percent or greater is considered a high pre-pregnancy weight. Inadequate weight gain during pregnancy is considered less than 1 kg (or 2 pounds) weight gain per month after the first trimester. When the prepregnancy weight and weight gain during pregnancy are adequate, the effects are additive, resulting in normal birthweight. If one factor is normal or high and the other is low or inadequate, then the effects are neutralized (19). The incidence of low-birthweight infants born to adolescents is increased if the adolescent has a gynecological age of less than 2 at conception (20). Gynecological age can be calculated either by subtracting the age at menarche from the chronological age or by the length of time between menarche and the last menstrual period. Low-birthweight babies are associated with increased mortality rates and morbidity from mental retardation, physical disabilities and handicaps, and lowered potential. The effects of malnutrition on mental development can be seen up to 60 months of age, and some severe effects may last throughout life. A weight gain of less than 10 pounds during pregnancy increases the risk of mortality and low-birthweight problems. More specifically, if by the 20th week gestation, 10 pounds weight gain has not been achieved, there is also an increased risk of neonatal morbidity and mortality since this a critical time of tissue and organ formation and growth.

Pregnancy is not a time to restrict food intake or attempt to lose weight because this often interferes with the growth of both the adolescent and the fetus. For optimal pregnancy outcome, the obese adolescent must be encouraged to achieve adequate, normal weight gain for herself and her baby while avoiding excessive weight gain.

Exercise in moderation is also an important element in the care of the pregnant adolescent. Regular, nonstressful activity promotes health, a feeling of well-being, and may assimilate the pregnant adolescent into normal peer group activities.

RDAs

The provision of adequate nutrition for the pregnant adolescent in accord with the RDAs is not precise, as previously stated; they are approximations and must be individually applied. RDAs for the pregnant adolescent who has completed the majority of her growth spurt will probably be adequate depending on her activity level. In the young adolescent still in the midst of her own growth spurt, even the RDAs for pregnancy may not be sufficient to meet her nutritional needs. The factors of growth, activity level, physical, and mental health may add and subtract from her nutritional demands. Generally, pregnancy increases the demands for calcium, protein, iron, folic acid and vitamin C, as well as for calories and other vitamins and minerals.

Peak caloric requirements for the adolescent increase with the growth of fetal and maternal tissues during pregnancy. Caloric allowances for the pregnant adolescent vary according to activity level from 2400–2700 Kcal per day for a sedentary schedule up to 45–50 Kcal per kilogram for the active adolescent. During pregnancy, the changing body mass increases the demand for caloric intake. Jobs and exercises requiring significant movement may also add up to 20 percent more energy expenditure. The pregnant adolescent who attends school or who participates in moderate exercise or work may require as much as 50 Kcal per kilogram to meet her energy needs. Because weight gain during pregnancy is thought to be the clinical index of adequate caloric intake, a median weight gain of 24–27.5 pounds is expected in most pregnant adolescents (18).

Adequate protein intake is necessary for normal physical growth as well as for fetal development. A sufficient caloric intake is necessary for optimal protein accessibility to meet maternal and fetal needs and to ensure that the protein is not used for energy supply. For the pregnant adolescent with a well-balanced diet, an increase of 20–30 g of protein per day will probably be adequate. For the adolescent who is protein depleted, however, a protein intake of 75–90 g per day may be indicated during pregnancy. If the dietary protein intake is sufficient to meet the pregnant adolescent's needs, the general diet is probably adequate with the exceptions of iron and folic acid intake.

Currently, there is a question about the need to increase dietary calcium for the pregnant adolescent given the body's ability to adapt at lower intake levels (16). Most sources, however, continue to increase calcium intake for the pregnant adolescent to aid in the mineralization of the fetal skeleton, to meet the needs of the growing adolescent, and to prevent impairment of lactation due to inadequate or marginal intake of calcium during pregnancy. The calcium requirement for the pregnant adolescent may be met by a dietary intake of 1200–1600 mg per day of calcium, depending on the stage of maturation of the adolescent. Phosporous intake coincides with that of calcium. Magnesium, also found in the skeleton and muscles, may be increased to a dietary intake of 400–450 mg per day for the pregnant adolescent.

Iron requirements are determined by body stores, physical growth and maturation, and body losses. Normal dietary intake of iron during adolescence is insufficient in providing adequate iron stores for a full-term pregnancy and delivery. To meet the maternal and fetal iron requirements and to prevent iron-deficiency anemia, the adolescent must often take iron supplements of 30–60 mg daily during the second and third trimesters. Often, however, pregnant adolescents do not like to take pills and feel the iron tablets upset their gastrointestinal tract. It is important, therefore, to encourage the increase of iron intake through iron-rich foods and to advise regular intakes of vitamin C, such as orange juice, along with iron intake to enhance the intestinal absorption of iron.

There is no indication that sodium restriction is necessary in the healthy pregnant adolescent. A daily intake of 2.5–5.0 g is adequate and may be increased during the summer months. If, prior to pregnancy, a disease state exists which indicates sodium restriction, the restriction should be continued through the pregnancy under medical supervision. Iodine replacement is only indicated when salt is restricted or in the presence of endemic goiters.

Zinc levels are reduced during pregnancy by almost 50 percent, therefore a daily supplement of 5 mg of zinc may be recommended for the pregnant adolescent. Hypovitaminosis appears to be common in pregnant adolescents, especially deficiencies in thiamine, folate, nicotinate, and vitamins A, B_6, B_{12}, and C. Vitamin D toxicity, however, has been implicated in a variety of disorders involving the newborn, and intakes should not be increased beyond 400 IU per day except through exposure to sunlight.

The pregnant adolescent should receive 5000 IU per day of vitamin A and an additional 15 mg per day of vitamin C. It is also suggested that vitamin C supplements should be given to pregnant adolescents who are heavy smokers (18). Since pregnant adolescents are prone to folic-acid deficiency, a supplement of 600 mg to 1 g per day is recommended to prevent complications of pregnancy and adverse fetal sequelae. The addition of 1 mg per day of vitamin B_{12} is also indicated for the pregnant adolescent and more may be required if a strict vegetarian diet is followed. During pregnancy, the requirement for vitamin B_6 is greatly increased to prevent atherosclerosis, impairment of the postnatal immunocompetence, and pre-eclampsia. A supplement of 5–20 mg per day of B_6 may be advised. An increase of 0.3 mg per day of thiamine and riboflavin and 2 mg of niacin is also indicated for the pregnant adolescent. Vitamins K and E and pantothenic acid appear to be adequate in a well-balanced diet.

Diet History

Prior to formulating a nutritional program for the pregnant adolescent, a health history is necessary. Such a history should include assessments of previous disorders such as acute infectious diseases or gastrointestinal disorders, previous pregnancies, status of physical growth and maturation, chronological and gynecological age, and an evaluation of physical activity level. The diet history should include both a general evaluation and 24-hour diet recall. It is important also to ascertain the consumption of alcohol, nicotine, and other drugs. The emotional status of the adolescent must also be assessed to evaluate potential compliance with recommended nutritional regimens as well as any evidence of self-destructive tendencies. The rare use of nutritional noncompliance as a weapon cannot be ignored and psychological intervention may be indicated in these cases. The detection of undernutrition or malnutrition, either by physical examination or history, is paramount, as is the identification of signs and symptoms of endocrine or metabolic disorders.

Nutritional Management During Pregnancy

One of the best methods of nutritional management for the pregnant adolescent is the Higgins Intervention Method for Nutritional Rehabilitation During Pregnancy, developed at the Montreal Diet Dispensary. This method determines caloric and protein intake on the basis of ideal weight and individual activity level and establishes normal requirements for the adolescent plus allowances for pregnancy and any nutritional deficiencies (5, 21, 22). Higgins (21) uses the 1958 U. S. RDA nutritional standards that call for a daily intake of 2600 calories and 80 g of protein for age 13–15 and 2400 calories and 75 g of protein for age 16–19. Five hundred calories and 25 g of protein are added daily after 20 weeks gestation to the above figures for the normal pregnancy requirements. To this total are added the following corrective allowances: 1) multiple gestation—500 calories and 25 g of protein daily for each additional fetus; 2) undernutrition—for each gram of deficiency in protein intake, 10 calories are added to the normal pregnancy requirements; 3) underweight (as defined as 5% or more under ideal weight for height)—500 calories and 20 g of protein daily are added for the number of weeks equivalent to the number of pounds deficit at conception (these figures may be doubled to make up this deficit by the delivery date); 4) nutritional stress (e.g., pernicious vomiting, poor obstetric history, failure to gain 10 pounds by 20 weeks gestation, pregnancy spacing less than one year apart, and serious emotional upset or problems—for each stress condition identified, 200 calories and 20 g of protein are added to a maximum allowance of 400 calories and 40 g of protein. In summary, to the nonpregnant requirements are added the pregnancy allowance, undernutrition corrective allowance, underweight corrective allowance, nutritional stress corrective allowance, and a multiple gestation corrective allowance (if indicated) for a total caloric and protein requirement (Table 3.3). This method utilizes a thorough diet history and a 24-hour diet recall at the initial visit as well as at the subsequent visits at 20, 28, and 36 weeks gestation. Milk, peanut butter, cheese, eggs and bread are primary food sources used to make up nutritional deficits (5). In many cases, dietary intake may be effectively increased by advising the consumption of 1 quart milk, 1 egg, and 1 orange per day in addition to the adolescent's normal dietary intake (23).

Nutritional management must consider the adolescent's facilities for food preparation and storage, her use of government aid services, and her and her family's cooperation. The goal of adequate dietary intake and weight gain for the pregnant adolescent can be accomplished through early prenatal care and attention to nutritional needs. Nutritional needs can be met through a dietary intake modeled as closely as possible to the RDA with the allowances outlined above to produce a weight gain of at least 25–30 pounds. A significant increase in the mean infant birthweight occurs in the disadvantaged adolescent population when nutritional supplementation is provided. Also, a decrease in low-birthweight infants occurs with dietary supplementation, and the most marked decrease occurs in the nonsmoking population (24).

In general, the diet normally provided for the hospitalized adolescent has been found to be insufficient to meet daily needs and is inadequate for nutritional repletion. When nutritional support is adequate, medical and surgical outcomes improve, and the length of hospital stays decrease (16).

The postpartum period for adolescents is another time to identify nutritional problems and to initiate appropriate diet therapy. The provision of postpartum nutritional education for the adolescent and her family will assist the adolescent in assuming responsibility for meeting her and her child's nutritional needs. During this period, the nutritionally depleted adolescent may be rehabilitated, iron-deficiency anemia may be corrected, adequate linear growth achieved, breastfeeding successfully initiated, and ideal postpartum weight identified. To support the changes during the postpartum period and to achieve adequate lactation, if desired, the following increased requirements are indicated: 500 calories, and 20 or more grams of protein, an iron supplementation, and a fluid intake of 2–3 quarts per day. Such nutritional support can only be maintained through the involvement of all health care providers, school workers and family members.

Table 3.3. *Nutritional Management*

	Calories	*Grams of Protein*
Nonpregnant allowance	2400–2600	75–80
Corrective allowances for pregnancy		
Pregnancy allowance per fetus	500	25
Underweight	500	20
Undernutritional	10	1
	(maximum: 1000)	(maximum: 40)
Nutritional stress	200	20
	(maximum: 400)	(maximum: 40)
Total maximum additions	2400	125

The Episodic Visit During Puberty

Pain

Adolescents seeking primary care for vague complaints of pain may not have an organic cause for the symptom, but an underlying problem that requires intervention. The complaint of pain may often be the stated reason for the adolescent's visit; the most common complaints are abdominal pain, headache, chest pain, back and neck pain. If the pain is associated with an underlying psychosocial problem, the pain itself may not need treatment. The adolescent, however, may need reassurance and support to work out her problems (25).

Pain must be fully evaluated to ascertain whether it is of a functional or organic basis. The complaint of pain warrants a description of the pain, including onset, perceived cause, type, location and any precipitating factors or associated symptoms. In addition, any factors that relieve or aggravate the pain are noted. Any previous history of the same or of a similar complaint requires investigation, including the diagnosis, therapy, and effectiveness of prescribed treatments or medications. Factors associated with organic pain are recent onset, symptoms at time of health appointment, external factors associated with reported pain, secondary symptoms consistent with clinical entities, and verbal and behavioral clues consistent with pain symptom. Factors associated with functional pain are difficulty in describing onset, location, frequency, quality of pain, and broad time frames used; asymptomatic at time of health appointment; external symptoms not associated with pain occurrence; vague and idiosyncratic secondary symptoms; and verbal and behavioral clues inconsistent or contradictory to clinical entity.

Adolescents with organic pain may appear worried, anxious for relief of symptoms, and may show fear of major illness. They are usually cooperative with treatment modalities and are relieved when serious pathology is not indicated. Adolescents with functional pain may appear passive and unconcerned, expect instant analysis of their complaint and a magical relief of their symptoms. They usually are not relieved when complex testing and serious pathology is not indicated, and may not accept a nonorganic origin for their pain (1, 26).

Adolescents may use the complaint of pain to seek health care for unrelated problems, in which case, the pain may identify the need for care. If the cause of an adolescent's functional pain is unclear, assessment of underlying problems may direct the management of the complaint. Pain can be a sign of emotional distress which may or may not be recognized by the adolescent. Factors associated with functional pain are:

1. death of a parent,
2. separation from significant others,
3. marital discord between parents,
4. family pathology,
5. similar complaints of pain in parents or siblings,
6. difficulties in school (27, 28).

Therefore, in evaluating the adolescent, a psychosocial history is imperative (29). Information about the complaint is necessary and, whenever possible, includes the following:

1. onset,
2. recurrence,
3. relation to time, activity, menses, and bodily functions,
4. relation to recent events, social activity, school/home life.

Adolescents complaining of pain may be experiencing underlying problems related to developmental tasks and psychosocial development. Pointing out the relationship between the functional pain and an underlying problem may prove unproductive. Specialized care is usually unnecessary. The adolescent may need reassurance and support over time to adjust to the developmental demands she is experiencing. In time, the adolescent may turn her attention from the complaint of pain to the problem of the developmental task at hand.

Discharge

Most adolescents develop a physiologic vaginal discharge, usually around six months to one year before menarche. The presence of leukorrhea may be disconcerting to the adolescent who may not understand that this is a normal bodily response to her sexual maturation. Usually, this discharge is copious, clear to yellow in appearance, and composed of desquamated vaginal epithelial cells and endocervical mucus from the endocervical glands. The epithelial cells are all that is seen on a wet mount preparation. This physiologic discharge is asymptomatic and fluctuates with estrogen levels during the menstrual cycle. In addition, during the first trimester of pregnancy, the adolescent may again experience leukorrhea. These thick, profuse vaginal secretions are acidic and protect the mother and fetus against some infections but may also provide a medium for growth of other bacteria. The increased secretions of the cervical glands to form the mucus plug may also add to this physiological discharge as well as the increased conversion of glycogen in the vaginal epithelial cells into lactic acid during pregnancy.

The adolescent needs reassurance of the normalcy of these physiological discharges. Exploration of the adolescent's feelings about leukorrhea will address any questions about something being "wrong" or of feeling "dirty"or "unclean." Comfort measures for the adolescent with leukorrhea include attention to personal hygiene, wearing cotton underwear, and more frequent changes of underwear. The adolescent may be tempted to begin or increase douching practices when complaining of leukorrhea. Instructions are given to abandon douching during this time, as it may increase the amount of physiological discharge. Occasionally, the adolescent may want to wear a thin sanitary pad during the time of increased discharge. Clear information regarding the signs and symptoms of vaginitis will help the adolescent in distinguishing between normal and abnormal bodily processes.

Menstrual Disturbances

Menstruation consists of a periodic bloody vaginal discharge resulting from the shedding of the endometrium following ovulation. The normal interval between menses is 24 to 32 days with an average menses duration of 3 to 7 days. The average amount of blood lost during menses ranges from 30 to 100 ml with 70 percent to 80 percent of the total menstrual blood loss occurring during the first two days of menstruation. There are many individual variations in the onset and tempo of menstruation; variations are influenced by environmental and genetic factors.

The biological process of menstruation occurs within a particular social and cultural setting. The attitude of a society or culture toward menstruation can influence the adolescent's perception of herself as a female and as a sexual being. The critical transition at menarche is a major event in the adolescent's reproductive life. There are often negative social and cultural explanations of menstruation and expectations regarding the adolescent's response to it. Many adolescents receive no prior information about menarche. Those that are prepared often are provided with misconceptions about menstrual taboos. Such taboos begin with the inference that menstruation is not to be discussed as it is "dirty" or shameful. Menstruation may be referred to as a period, curse, plague, misery, or in other cases as a "friend" or "country cousin." These social attitudes may be internalized by the adolescent and thereby affect her feelings toward her own femininity and body image. Such conceptions accompanying menstruation may prompt negative physiologic responses than can be readily observed. Adolescents may come to expect that menstruation occurs for everyone in a regular 28 day cycle lasting 3 to 5 days. This expectation is often perpetuated by practitioners, so that adolescents will report a 28-day cycle when their own cycles vary from that pattern.

The adolescent's degree of vulnerability to the normal biological events of menstruation as well as to common menstrual disturbances will vary depending on her developmental stage. The practitioner who is sympathetic and responsive to the needs of the growing individual can attempt to demystify the menstrual cycle and alleviate any misconceptions. Positive reinforcement may be used to present menstruation as a normal bodily function and to promote a healthy feminine identity. Personal support and educational material and advice help the adolescent to accept a normal female body image and develop a sense of self-appreciation. Multiple approaches are available to adolescents with common menstrual disturbances—methods that promote individuality and self-control. Through an awareness of the adolescent's transitions during menarche, the practitioner may be able to prevent related developmental problems and thus ensure an easier transition to maturity by providing a stable focal point for the adolescent as she develops her female identity.

MITTELSCHMERZ

Mittelschmerz is an intermenstrual pain associated with ovulation and sometimes accompanied by bleeding. Occurring between menses or midcycle, it is a dull, aching pain in one of the lower quadrants of the abdomen. This pain usually lasts anywhere from a few minutes to six to eight hours. Occasionally the pain is severe and cramping may last for two or three days. Vaginal bleeding, ranging from brown spotting to an almost menstrual discharge, may be associated with mittelschmerz.

Treatment usually consists of reassurance as to the benign nature of the pain. The use of a menstrual calendar may also be recommended in order to document the pain with ovulation by charting the basal body temperature and other symptoms. Mild analgesics may be given for pain relief as well as the use of heat via heating pad or warm bath. Other pathology requires exclusion such as: appendectomy, torsion or rupture of ovarian cysts, or ectopic pregnancy. In rare cases, a laparoscopy may be indicated. Information regarding the recurring nature of this menstrual disturbance may be helpful to the adolescent.

PMS

A mild form of premenstrual syndrome (PMS) may occur in virtually all females, with about 50 percent or more affected to a significant degree. PMS symptoms occur prior to the onset of menses and may vary and change over time. PMS occurs most commonly during the postmenarcheal period, when the cycles are anovulatory and there is luteal insufficiency. PMS and dysmenorrhea are usually not concurrent.

The symptoms of PMS differ greatly in variety and intensity. The emotional or psychological effects of PMS include: irritability, depression, crying spells, erratic behavior, anxiety, emotional lability, personality changes, and sleep disturbances such as hypersomnia. Physical effects may include: headache, engorgement of nasal mucous membranes, hoarseness, lower pitched voice, facial pallor and puffiness, and eye reddening. Breast effects may involve such discomfort as breast enlargement, tenderness, and transient breast masses. The gastrointestinal tract is also affected, resulting in increased appetite, cravings for food high in carbohydrates, excessive thirst, nausea, vomiting, and constipation. The extremities may experience edema, particularly of the ankles and fingers and a resulting tightness and itching of the skin. There may also be spontaneous bruising as well as joint and muscle pain. In general, there is a feeling of lethargy, bloatedness, and backache; water is retained, and weight and blood pressure fluctuate. PMS sufferers may also be predisposed to alcohol abuse, asthma, hypoglycemia, migraines, vasomotor rhinitis, urticaria, and epilepsy. School or work absenteeism may be a problem.

There are several theories as to the etiology and symptoms of PMS. In the postmenarcheal anovulatory adolescent, luteal insufficiency may be the predominant factor. Another theory of PMS suggests an increase in aldosterone secretion as a result of decreased progesterone, which results in sodium and water retention and potassium depletion. Others suggest an estrogen/progesterone imbalance related either to excess estrogen in proportion to an insufficient amount of progesterone, which can result in water retention and hypoglycemia or a disturbance in liver function where the autonomic nervous system responds with an inadequate estrogen/progesterone ratio. Still others suggest that PMS involves an altered carbohydrate metabolism or glucose tolerance, or an excess in prolactin or mineralocorticoids. PMS may also be related to anxiety states or psychological abnormalities.

The method of treatment depends on the combined symptoms experienced and may include several approaches, some experimental. Education and reassurance is given for mild, infrequent cases. To determine the most beneficial therapy for moderate to severe cases of PMS, a menstrual calendar should be kept for two to three months to establish the pattern of symptoms, along with daily basal body temperatures.

Often sufferers find relief from many of the more common symptoms by simply practicing mild salt restriction, particularly during the luteal phase of the menstrual cycle. Eliminating sweets and eating small amounts of food frequently (particularly protein and starch snacks) may also be helpful. Skipping meals is to be particularly avoided during the premenstrual period. Pyridoxine or vitamin B_6 in high doses has also been effective in relieving symptoms of PMS. Signs of vitamin B_6 toxicity, however, are similar to symptoms of PMS: nausea, headache and depression; and if observed during the follicular phase, pyridoxine toxicity may be suspected.

On occasion, combined OCPs or the progestin-only pill is an effective treatment. Estrogen sulfate may also be given for one cycle during the luteal phase. For breast tenderness, bromocriptine (Parlodel) may be tried (2.5 mg twice daily during the luteal phase) but such treatment is still experimental. Also, for severe cases of bloating, spironolactone may be given during the luteal phase (25 mg four times daily). For symptoms related to tension, progesterone may be given from midcycle until two days before menses is expected (either suppositories, 200 to 400 mg daily or 100 mg intramuscularly daily). For severe psychiatric symptoms, tranquilizers or sedation may be administered, such as diazepam (Valium) in low doses for short periods, observing for signs of habituation; bellergal; chlordiazepoxide (Librium); or chlorothiazide (Diuril). Bilateral oophorectomy and hysterectomy are not appropriate therapies for the adolescent.

DYSMENORRHEA

Possibly half of all females experience some form of dysmenorrhea or painful menstruation at some point in their reproductive lives. Dysmenorrhea may begin anytime from age 12 to 25, appearing more frequently during mid-adolescence. This common adolescent problem usually does not occur until 6 to 12 months after menarche, at which point painless menses may have been experienced, or it may not occur until menses becomes ovulatory. Often symptoms will decrease with age; however, they can continue through menopause. This pain, which accompanies menstruation, begins prior to menses, usually within a few hours of menstrual flow, and may last 12 to 48 hours. Occasionally the pain may begin a few days prior to menstruation, and then may continue for 2 to 4 days into the menses. Usually, the pain during the first day of menstruation is the most severe with relief of most symptoms occurring at the heaviest flow in the menses.

The characteristic pain of dysmenorrhea is recurrent cramping associated with menstruation, located primarily in the lower abdomen. The pain follows uterine and ovarian nerve distribution pathways to the suprapubic region, back, and inner thighs. The suprapubic cramping can be sharp and colicky, or may feel like a dull ache and heaviness in the abdomen. The pain frequently radiates to the lower sacrum and inner thighs. It is often accompanied by other symptoms: nausea, vomiting, constipation or diarrhea, headache, and muscular cramps. Other symptoms associated with dysmenorrhea are: breast tenderness, mild abdominal distention, water retention, and dizziness. Sometimes there are noticeable emotional changes such as lethargy, irritability, anxiety, inability to concentrate, and depression. Cardiac palpitations and hot flushes or vasomotor instability occur infrequently. Dysmenorrhea has also been the cause of recurrent short-term absenteeism from school and work.

There are several theories of the causes for the dysmenorrhea. The most common contributors are related to ovulation, such as a hormonal imbalance between estrogen and progesterone. An excess of myometrial activity, resulting in uterine ischemia and pain, may be a factor, as are increased sensitivity of the pain receptors to prostaglandins or an excess of prostaglandins. Constitutional conditions making one vulnerable to dysmenorrhea include anemia, voluntary weight loss, diabetes, chronic illness, overwork, and a low pain threshold. Psychogenic factors may also contribute to dysmenorrhea.

Secondary dysmenorrhea may be suspected when there is chronic menstrual pain associated with organic pathology. Such pathology may be in the form of a genital tract obstruction or defect. Occasionally, endometriosis, pelvic inflammatory disease, fibroids, polyps or the presence of an intrauterine contraceptive device (IUD) may be factors.

In the absence of chronic unilateral pelvic pain and pathology on pelvic examination, treatment consists of reassurance, health education and symptomatic relief. The use of menstrual calendars marking ovulation, basal body temperature and symptoms is also encouraged. In rare instances when pelvic pathology is suspected, a laparoscopy, hysteroscopy or ultrasonography may be required for further evaluation prior to treatment.

Nonpharmacological treatment modalities for primary dysmenorrhea vary and are used in various combinations. Heat therapy is often effective in relieving symptoms and may be applied by heating pad, hot bath, shower, or sauna. Bed rest is not usually recommended except when necessary, although positioning in a knee-to-chest posture on either the back or side may prove helpful. In some instances, an increase in the time spent sleeping may also prove effective. Exercise is often advised: regular daily exercises, breathing and muscle toning exercises, the "pelvic rock," swimming, or more vigorous exercise such as running. Good nutrition is accentuated at all times. A decrease in sodium intake during the week prior to menses may also be beneficial. Grapefruit and pineapple have been used as natural diuretics, and an increase in water intake may also help to decrease fluid retention. A diet of small, frequent, high-protein meals is also advisable during this time. B complex vitamins may be suggested as well as dolomite, a calcium-magnesium mineral supplement. Some people find comfort in hot beverages. Others derive some relief from limited alcoholic intake, but care must be taken to prevent habituation to alcohol in association with dysmenorrhea. While pain is experienced, massaging the abdomen, lower back, leg or calf muscles may prove comforting. Often relaxation and relief of symptoms may occur through various practices: orgasm by self-stimulation, Hatha Yoga, progressive relaxation exercises, meditation, and alpha training or biofeedback.

Pharmacological relief from dysmenorrhea occurs primarily through the use of mild analgesics, ovulation blocking agents, and prostaglandin synthetase inhibitors. Mild analgesics such as aspirin or Tylenol may give symptomatic relief. Acetylsalicylic acid (aspirin) is also a known prostaglandin synthetase inhibitor and has been successful in symptomatic relief when begun three days prior to menses in a dose of 300 to 600 mg orally four times daily. If necessary, darvon, empirin with codeine or plain codeine tablets may be prescribed on a limited basis. With severe nausea, compazine may be given at the onset of menses. More commonly, ovulation blocking agents are utilized in the form of the combined oral contraceptive pill, usually a 50 microgram estrogen dosage continued for a three- to six-month period. Progestin-only pills, as well as long-acting progestin injections and the Progestasert-T IUD may also produce symptomatic relief. Prostaglandin synthetase inhibitors may also be used immediately prior to menses and during the first days of menstruation. Some common ones are: indomethacin (Indocin), naproxen (Naprosyn or Anaprox), ibuprofen (Motrin), or mefenamic acid (Ponstel). As previously stated, contraceptive agents may be used in the treatment of dysmenorrhea, although occasionally some contraceptive pills may be, in fact, associated with dysmenorrhea. Similarly, IUDs are often associated with painful menses, and frequently removed for this reason, but IUDs containing progesterone may also prove to be therapeutic. Some women report painful menses with the use of the diaphragm when it is in place during menstruation.

In helping adolescents to cope effectively with dysmenorrhea, examination of the adolescent on the first day of menses may help place the pain in perspective both for the adolescent and the practitioner. The practitioner may also be able to assess more accurately the adolescent's needs in terms of emotional support, reassurance, nonpharmacological and pharmacological therapies. The practitioner may also be aware of the association made by the adolescent of the symptoms of dysmenorrhea and the use of the OCP. The needs of the adolescent must be carefully assessed to prevent dysmenorrhea from being used as an indirect method for obtaining contraceptive methods when only protection against pregnancy is required.

Common Breast Disturbances

Many adolescents are understandably concerned about the development of their breasts. During puberty and adolescence the breasts undergo many changes for which the individual is often ill-prepared. The primary role of the practitioner is to inform the adolescent of the normal physiological changes of the breasts and of the more common disturbances. In this way, education, emotional support and reassurance may assist the adolescent in her developmental tasks.

One of the most common disturbances is breast asymmetry which may vary from mild to moderate differences. The extent of the asymmetry cannot be assessed until breast development is complete. Until maturation occurs, the self-conscious adolescent may choose to use foam inserts or breast pads to equalize any inherent differences.

In rare instances, breast hypertrophy may occur, resulting in back pain and possible kyphosis. Both with breast asymmetry and hypertrophy surgical correction, if indicated, is delayed until after breast development has stabilized.

Accessory nipples or glandular tissue and areola and nipple are found in a small percentage of healthy adolescents, usually along the embryological milk line. During pregnancy and lactation, the accessory breasts may become engorged. No treatment is necessary for accessory nipples or breasts.

Periareolar hair may also be found in the normal adolescent. Treatment is generally not indicated, but some adolescents may prefer cutting or plucking the hairs.

Nipple discharge is rarely noted in the adolescent. A thin, milky discharge or galactorrhea may be observed during the postpartum or postabortion course. Galactorrhea may also be associated with amenorrhea and pituitary tumor, trauma to the chest, certain medications such as oral contraceptive pills, and with some recreational drugs. Any blood-tinged nipple discharge is carefully evaluated for signs of an intraductal papilloma or cancer. There is, however, little incidence of breast cancer during adolescence.

Occasionally, the adolescent may discover a breast mass in association with breast tenderness and enlargement prior to menses. These breast changes are known as fibrocystic disease and are usually in the form of a thickening of the breast tissue. These cysts occur monthly but will vary with regard to site and severity. The cysts are usually soft, mobile, regular in outline, and often in multiple sites. Continued observation of breast changes by the practitioner and adolescent is usually all the treatment that is necessary.

Fibroadenomas occur infrequently and must be distinguished from fibrocystic disease. Fibroadenomas are firm, sometimes rubbery, generally fixed, and may be associated with skin changes. These masses usually remain unchanged throughout the menstrual cycle or may increase in size. Ideally, fibroadenomas are evaluated immediately after menses, before further follow-up and treatment is decided.

In the adolescent, particularly those who are active in sports, the practitioner may occasionally find a tender, poorly defined mass. After taking a careful history, this mass is usually found to be the result of a contusion, and disappears within a few weeks. Scar tissue and fat necrosis may remain, depending on the extent of the trauma.

The importance of an annual breast examination, which includes inspection and palpation, cannot be too highly emphasized. Adolescence is a time for education and preparation for many breast changes which occur during this growth period. It is also a time for continual reassurance as to the normalcy of the changes experienced during this developmental stage. It is the ideal time for teaching the adolescent the importance of regualr breast self-examination. In this way, through knowledge and self discovery, the adolescent will grow to know and understand her body, and learn to appreciate, rather than fear, the ongoing physiological changes.

Infections, Infestations, and Sexually Transmitted Diseases

During puberty, the vaginal epithelium is thin and therefore more susceptible to irritation and infection. Since the onset of sexual activity today occurs at an earlier age, there is more time for sexual exploration and usually an increase in the number of sexual partners during adolescence. These factors, along with the epidemic proportions of gonorrhea and other sexually transmitted diseases, increase the adolescent's need for health education and health care concerning sexually transmitted diseases. Usually, infections, infestation, and sexually transmitted diseases (STD) are fostered by poor hygiene and sexual contact. Some "contact vaginitis," especially in the young adolescent, may be due to irritation from such items as perfumed soaps, powders and colored toilet paper. Often several infections coexist and must be identified and treated consecutively. This repetition of examination and continued treatment is often misunderstood by the adolescent who then may not complete the prescribed course of treatment, resulting in reinfection. Adolescents are counseled to continue the prescribed treatment regimen in spite of relief from symptoms or the occurrence of menses. Usually, sexual partner(s) must be treated as well—simultaneous education and treatment being the best method of preventing reinfection.

When there is a complaint of vaginal discharge, the following assessments may be indicated:

1. history,
2. pelvic examination,

3. lab tests of saline and potassium hydroxide (KOH) wet mount preparations,
4. cultures,
5. Pap,
6. VDRL.

The history includes a complete description of the symptoms such as:

1. quantity, color, odor,
2. time of occurrence in relation to menses,
3. pruritis,
4. any associated rashes, fever, malaise.

Other pertinent areas of information concern:

1. the presence of other illnesses, such as diabetes,
2. recent medications, such as antibiotics or oral contraceptive pills,
3. type of sexual activity, such as multiple partners, oral or anal sexual relations.

After the identification and treatment of infection, follow-up counseling and examination are essential aspects of preventing reinfection and ensuring a "test of cure." In some cases, infections may cause abnormal Pap smear results. A repeat Pap smear may be taken two months after completion of treatment for evaluation.

There are many guidelines available for drug treatment regimens, all of which must meet the individual criteria of risk/benefit and effectiveness. Clear instructions are given to the adolescent and her partner(s) to ensure safe and effective treatment. Examples of such guidelines are:

1. iron, milk and milk products should be avoided two hours before and after ingestion of tetracycline.
2. ampicillin, tetracycline and metronidazole (Flagyl) predispose to yeast infection.
3. podophyllin should be washed off after two to four hours of application.
4. alcohol should not be consumed with metronidazole (Flagyl).

Streptomycin sulfate, sulfadiazine, sulfisoxazole, and tetracycline* hy-

---

*Some forms of Nystatin are combined with tetracycline and therefore the precautions associated with the use of tetracycline should be followed.

drochloride are contraindicated for use during pregnancy. The safety or efficacy in pregnancy of such drugs as ampicillin, erythromycin, clotrimazole, and spectinomycin-hydrochloride has not been proven. Metronidazole (Flagyl) is not to be used during the first trimester of pregnancy and only with caution during the second and third trimesters. In addition, metronidazole is not recommended for use in lactating women. As with all prescribed medications, possible adverse reactions and special precautions are considered. The adolescent needs to be well informed about medications so that she understands dosages and possible side effects (30).

Health information regarding preventive action against sexually transmitted diseases may also help the adolescent reduce her chances of contracting such infections. Preventive measures which are recommended to sexually active adolescents are:

1. cleansing the genitals with soap and warm water before and after sexual activity,
2. inspection of genitals before and after sexual activity,
3. use of condoms and some of the vaginal contraceptive medications,
4. urinating before and after intercourse,
5. regular health examinations.

General hygienic measures may also be taken such as:

1. use of bland soaps,
2. avoidance of perfumed soaps, bubble baths or some laundry detergents,
3. avoidance of vaginal sprays and douching with chemical or perfumed mixtures,
4. cleaning of the perineum from vagina toward anus (front to back),
5. keeping the perineum clean and dry,
6. wearing cotton underwear,
7. avoiding tight clothing,

Once an adolescent contracts an infection, early diagnosis and treatment are essential. Some comfort measures appropriate for use during treatment are:

1. sitz baths or warm baths with or without baking soda, twice a day,
2. careful "pat" drying of the perineum,
3. use of cornstarch or unscented baby powder to the perineum,
4. vinegar and warm water douche (although not during pregnancy),
5. frequent changes of cotton underwear,
6. long-term advice of weight loss in the case of obesity,

With this information in mind, we will look at some of the common infections, infestations and sexually transmitted diseases. In the following descriptions an asterisk (*) indicates treatment recommendations by the Centers for Disease Control (CDC) in Georgia (31, 32).

MONILIA (yeast)
Causative Organism:
   Candida albicans.
Symptoms:
   Cheesy, curdy, yellow-white discharge forming patches on vaginal mucosa and cervix; intense vulvar pruritis, redness and edema, scant discharge with pruritis developing prior to menses, dysuria; dyspareunia.
Diagnosis:
   Wet mount preparation from vagina/cervix with potassium hydroxide (KOH) positive for yeast spores, pseudohyphae and epithelial cells; positive growth in Nickerson's or Sabourand's medium; vaginal pH 4-5.0.
Treatment:
   Mycostatin or Nystatin vaginal suppositories BID for 10-14 days;
   Miconazole nitrate 2% or Monistat vaginal cream at night for 7 days;
   Gentian violet vaginal preparation BID for 14 days;
   Clotrimazole vaginal cream at night for 7 days;
   Nystatin rinse for mouth;
   Mycolog cream for external use;
   Sitz baths or warm baths BID with baking soda;
   Betadine vaginal wash.
Partner/Contacts:
   No treatment usually required; when indicated, treat topically with Mycolog cream.
Special Instructions:
   Treatment may need to be continued through several menstrual cycles, beginning one week prior to menses; gentian violet will stain skin and clothing purple; avoid intercourse or use of condoms for length of treatment; may need to wear thin sanitary pad; wear cotton underwear; increase oral intake of yogurt and cheese products; re-examine for "test of cure" 5-10 days after treatment.
Potential Complications:
   Recurrence; thrush in mouth of newborn, which if lactating, can be transferred to mother's nipples.
Prevention:
   Weight loss, if obese; betadine or vinegar douches; good diet; rest; regular exercise; wear cotton underwear and loose clothing.
Comment:
   Predisposing factors: broad-spectrum antibiotics, diabetes, pregnancy, oral contraceptive pills, heat, humidity, obesity, poor diet, oral/rectal sexual

activity, hypoparathyroidism; testing for diabetes may be indicated with frequent recurrences; some suggest treatment with plain yogurt inserted in vagina, but this method has not been proven to be effective.

Gardnerellae vaginalis (hemophilus, corynebacterium, nonspecific vaginitis).
Causative Organism:
Gardnerellae, small coccobacillary organisms.
Symptoms:
Minimal chalky-white, yellow, green, or gray discharge, sometimes "bubbly"; malodorous with "fishy" smell when in contact with KOH; slight vaginal itching; dysuria; dyspareunia.
Diagnosis:
Wet mount preparation from vagina/cervix with KOH positive for clue cells; epithelial cells with stippled, granular appearence; gram stain positive for short, gram negative bacilli; pap smear may be positive for gram negative rods; vaginal pH 5-6.
Treatment:
   *Metronidazole (Flagyl) 500 mg orally BID for 7 days;
   Sultrin triple sulfa vaginal cream BID for 7-10 days;
   Tetracycline or ampicillin 500 mg orally QID for 7-10 days;
   Vinegar douche;
   Metronidazole (Flagyl) 2 grams orally in a single dose.
Partner/Contacts:
   Treat as indicated.
Special Instructions:
   Avoid intercourse or use condoms for length of treatment; re-examination for "test of cure" 5-10 days posttreatment.
Prevention
   Avoid multiple partners; decrease douching and use of chemical vaginal hygienic products.
Comment:
   Predisposing factors: allergies to soaps, tight clothing, rectal intercourse, poor lubrication during sexual intercourse; recent testing questions the effectiveness of ampicillin, tetracycline and sulfonamides as treatment modalities; current recommendations suggest Flagyl as the preferred treatment at this time.

TRICHOMONIASIS
Causative Organism:
   Trichamonas.
Symptoms:
   Frothy, thin, yellow/green/gray purulent discharge; malodorous; vagina and cervix may be inflamed, "strawberry" or small red dots present; pruritis

and increased discharge occur after menses; vulvar itching may be intense causing vulva to be red, edematous, painful; urinary urgency, frequency or dysuria may occur; dyspareunia usually present; occasionally enlargement of inguinal lymph nodes present.

Diagnosis:

Wet mount prepartion from vagina/cervix with normal saline positive for unicellular, flagellated, motile protozoan or trichomonads; Pap smear positive for polymorphonuclear leukocytes and trichomonads; Pap smear and gram stain may be unreliable; vaginal pH 3.8–4.2.

Treatment:

*Flagyl 2 g orally in a single dose;

Flagyl 250 mg orally;

TID for 7 days or 500 mg orally BID for 5 days;

Clotrimazole vaginal cream 100 mg at night for 7 days, if pregnant;

Aci-Jel, Gyne-Lotrimin or AVC vaginal creams for symptomatic relief.

Partner/Contacts:

Simultaneous treatment with Flagyl recommended.

Special Instructions:

Avoid intercourse or use condoms during treatment; avoid alcoholic beverages during treatment with Flagyl; re-examination in 5–10 days posttreatment; repeat Pap smear 2–3 months posttreatment if initial was abnormal; do not breastfeed while taking Flagyl, pump breasts and discard milk during treatment, supplementing baby's feeds for 24 hours.

Potential Complications:

Nausea, vomiting, diarrhea, dryness of mouth, "metallic taste" may occur with Flagyl; may be more common during pregnancy and in association with vaginitis emphysematoza; trichomoniasis in the newborn leads to fever, irritability, failure to thrive and in females, excessive vaginal discharge.

Prevention:

Avoid multiple partners; use condoms.

Comment:

Flagyl is contraindicated during the first trimester of pregnancy and should be used with caution during the second and third trimesters and during lactation; during pregnancy, use comfort measures and condoms; there are questions concerning the carcinogenic properties of Flagyl found in experiments in mice.

GONORRHEA (NG, GC)

Causative Organism:

Neisseria gonorrhea.

Symptoms:

May be asymptomatic or yellow-green purulent discharge at cervical os; vulvar irritation; red, swollen urethra, dysuria; dysmenorrhea; dyspareunia and postcoital bleeding; tenderness in lymph nodes in groin; lower abdominal pain, low back ache; fever; swollen and painful Bartholin's glands; sore throat and hoarseness with gonococcheal pharyngitis.

Diagnosis:

Wet mount preparation from vagina/cervix/rectum/pharynx positive for polymorphonuclear leukocytes; positive growth in Thayer-Martin or Lester-Martin culture mediums in CO_2 environment; positive gram stain and Pap smear for gram negative intracellular diplococcus.

Treatment:

*Aqueous procaine penicillin G (APPG)

4.8 million units intramuscularly with 1 g probenecid orally;

*Spectinomycin 2 g intramuscularly (particularly after previous treatment failures or if pregnant or allergic to tetracycline);

*Ampicillin 3.5 g orally (or amoxicillin 3.0g) with 1g probenecid orally if pregnant or allergic to penicillin;

*Tetracycline (HCl) 0.5 g orally QID for 7 days, total dose 14.0 g;

*Doxycycline hyclate 100 mg orally BID for 7 days, in substitution for tetracycline.

Erthromycin 1.5 g orally, followed by 0.5 g orally QID for 4 days for a total of 9.5 g;

Cephaloxin 500 mg QID for 4 days; for penicillinase-producing NG,

tetracycline hydrochloride 1.5 g orally stat, then 500 mg QID for 4–5 days.

Partner/Contacts:

Same treatment essential.

Special Instructions:

Abstain from sexual intercourse, particularly avoiding oral/genital sexual activity, or use condoms until negative cultures; test for syphilis with VDRL at time of positive results and again three months after treatment; watch for presence of monilia; report if diarrhea present during treatment; reculture for "test of cure" 7–14days after completion of treatment and again 1–3 months after negative "test of cure."

Potential Complications:

Pelvic inflammatory disease; sterility; ophthalmitis, blindness; arthritis; Bartholin's abscess; gonoccal perihepatitis or Fitz-Hugh-Curtis syndrome; cervicitis; urethritis; pharyngitis; salpingitis; endometritis; carditis; dermatitis; meningitis; gonococcemia; ectopic pregnancy.

Prevention:

Avoid multiple partners; use condoms; avoid oral/genital sexual activity; use of some spermicides may provide some protection.

Comments:

Menses may be a precipitating factor; incubation period may be from 3–5 days up to 30 days; small, red, tender nodules on the trunk or extremities which may disappear quickly or be associated with fever, may be signs of gonococcemia; do not use erythromycin in patients with liver disease; the safety of the fetus has not been established with the use of spectin-omycin.

SYPHILIS (Loues-Treponema Pallidum Infection)
Causative Organism:
   Treponema pallidum.
Symptoms:
   In general: hard, painless lesion or chancre with or without regional adenopathy; rash; condylomas.
   Primary: occurs three weeks after exposure; indurated, painless, red-rimmed sore (chancre) on vagina/cervix/rectum/mouth which appears in 2–6 weeks.
   Secondary: occurs six weeks after healing of primary infection; rash on palms of hands and soles of feet; fever, sore throat, headache, arthralgia, nausea, inflamed eyes may be present; symptoms usually disappear in 2–6 weeks.
Diagnosis:
   Dark field examination from chancre/vagina/cervix/rectum/pharynx positive for treponema; serologic tests for syphilis (STS): Veneral Disease Research Laboratory (VDRL), Fluorescent Treponemal Antibody Absorption (FTA-ABS), Treponema Pallidum Immobilization (TPI).
Treatment
*Benzathine penicillin G. 2.5 million units intramuscularly;
*Tetracycline HCl 500 mg orally QID for 15 days, if allergic to penicillin;
*Erythromycin 500 mg orally QID; for 15 days for a total of 30 g, if unable to take penicillin or tetracycline;
Aqueous procaine penicillin G (APPG) 600,000 units intramuscularly daily for 8 days for a total of 4.8 million units;
For symptomatic relief, wet compresses to chancre followed by drying lotions.
Partner/Contacts:
   Treatment essential.
Special Instructions:
   STS four weeks after treatment and every three months for one year, then annual STS; treatment prior to 10–18 weeks gestation when possible to prevent congenital syphilis; after treatment during pregnancy, monthly FTA-ABS and use of condoms for one month.
Potential Complications
   Brain damage; heart disease; condylomata lata; spinal cord damage; blindness; stillbirth; miscarriage; congenital infection.
Prevention:
   Avoid multiple partners.
Comment:
   Serology may not be positive until two to four weeks after inital infection (chancre), repeat serology in 2–3 months if suspect.

PELVIC INFLAMMATORY DISEASE (PID)

Causative Organism:

N. gonorrhea, C. trachomatis, anaerobic bacteria, facultative gram-negative rods, actinomyces, mycoplasma.

Symptoms:

Profuse cervical discharge; vaginal discharge; pain on cervical movement; rebound tenderness; adnexal tenderness and enlargement; pain in abdomen, back, pelvis or leg; menorrhagia; dyspareunia and postcoital bleeding; dysuria, decreased bowel sounds; fever, chills, vomiting.

Diagnosis:

Gram stain or culture from vagina/cervix/rectum positive for bacterial agent or gonococcus; elevated white blood cell count (WBC's) and erythrocyte sedimentation rate (ESR).

Treatment

*Cefoxitin 2 grams intramuscularly or

APPG 4.8 million units intramuscularly or ampicillin 3.5 g orally or amoxicillin 3 grams orally each with 1 g probenecid orally and followed by doxycycline 100 milligrams orally BID for 10–14 days;

TTC 1.5 g orally followed by 0.5 g orally QID for 10 days;

TTC 500 mg orally QID for 10–14 days;

Flagyl 250 mg orally QID for 10 days;

as indicated: bedrest, intrauterine contraceptive device

(IUD) removal, laparoscopy; hospitalization.

Partner/Contacts:

Test and treat when indicated.

Special Instructions:

Bedrest is essential until pain subsides; avoid sexual intercourse during treatment and for 1–4 weeks after treatment; use condoms until post treatment cultures are negative; repeat cultures 48–72 hours post treatment; watch for monilia; avoid milk products using TTC; removal of IUCD, if present, post treatment.

Potential Complications:

Chronic pain and infection; tubo-ovarian abscess, sepsis; tubal occulsion; peritonitis; pelvic abscess; pelvic blood clots; pelvic adhesions; infertility/sterility; ectopic pregnancy.

Prevention:

Avoid multiple partners, use condoms; avoid IUCD's.

Comment:

Menses may be a precipitating factor.

CHLAMYDIA

Causative Organism:

Chlamydia trachomatis.

Symptoms:

Purulent cervicitis; vaginal discharge and pruritis; dysuria; may have symptoms of PID; involves mucosal surfaces.

Diagnosis:

Serology: chlamydial complement fixation test and microimmunofluro-scence test positive for small obligatory intracellular parasites; associated with cervical dysplasia on Pap smear, IGA antibodies in cervical secretions; culture positive for gram negative intracellular bacteria, must exclude herpes and GC; tissue cultures may be taken.

Treatment:

*Tetracycline HCl 500 milligrams orally QID $\times$ 7 days (at least);

*Doxycycline 100 mg orally BID for 7 days (at least);

Erythromycin 250 mg orally QID for 14 days (at least) if pregnant;

TTC 250 mg orally QID for 14–21 days or 500 mg QID for 7–14 days;

Sulfisoxazole 500 mg orally QID for 7–14 days.

Partner/Contacts:

Treatment important, culture and treat as indicated.

Special Instructions:

In general, increase oral fluid intake; after sexual intercourse, urinate and drink water; use condoms; watch for monilia; avoid milk and milk products as well as large amounts of any food between one hour before and two hours after taking medications; report if diarrhea develops; post treatment cultures are advisable 4–6 weeks after treatment.

Potential Complications:

Lymphogranuloma venerum; urethritis; cervicitis; salpingitis; diarrhea; perihepatitis; arthritis; trachoma; infertility; neonatal conjunctivitis; neonatal pneumonia; neonatal ear infections.

Prevention:

Avoid multiple partners.

Comment

Diagnosis is often one of exclusion as cultures are expensive, testing may take weeks and few laboratory centers are equipped for such evaluation; often associated with salpingitis; ampicillin usually not an effective treatment.

GENITAL HERPES VIRUS (Herpes Genitalis, HSV)

Causative Organism:

Herpes simplex virus (Type II).

Symptoms:

Small, painful fluid-filled lesions which erupt to an open sore becoming less painful for 4–5 days then healing in 10–21 days; lesions usually on labia but may be in vagina or on cervix; may have purulent discharge, vulvar itching, dysuria, dyspareunia, enlarged lymph glands, fever, malaise.

Diagnosis

Pap smear of lesion positive for multinucleated giant cells with ground glass nuclear appearance of acidophilic intranuclear inclusion bodies with irregular chromatin displacement beneath nuclear membrane and intranuclear vacuolization; cervical dysplasia may be seen on Pap smear; culture, in viral media, of base of lesion or vesicle fluid positive as early as 24–48 hours or up to 7 days; wet mount preparation of lesion positive for polymorphonuclear leukocytes.

Treatment

No effective known treatment; antiviral medications and vaccines are being studied*; Acyclovir ointment 5 percent may be used to cover lesions every 3 hours, 6 times a day for 7 days—it has not been tested in pregnant or lactating women. For symptomatic relief: sitz baths or warm baths; cold milk baths; aluminium acetate (Burrow's solution) 1:20 soaks; miconazole nitrate 2 percent vaginal cream; surface antiseptics or anesthetics; local or systemic analgesics; maintain cleanliness; wear loose, cotton underwear or no underwear; pour warm water over urethra and vulva while urinating or urinate while bathing; may need to catheterize for urinary retention; VDRL should also be taken; experimental treatments: lysine 1 gram daily orally; local application of betadine or ether; laser treatments; neutral red dye with fluorescent light which may cause viral mutations and may be carcenogenic, therefore is not recommended; corticosteroids are contraindicated.

Partner/Contacts:

No known effective treatment, symptomatic relief of symptoms.

Special Instructions:

Cleanse genitalia with cool water after urinating; keep vulvar area dry; avoid sexual intercourse or use condoms for six weeks after lesions present; abstain or use condoms to prevent recurrence.

Potential Complications:

Recurrence; kerititis; encephalitis; possible association with cervical cancer; if pregnant and contact herpes in first weeks of pregnancy, there is an increased risk of spontaneous abortion; if contracted after 20 weeks gestation, there is an increased risk of premature labor; if contracted in the third trimester, there is an increased risk of major systemic complications of the newborn including infection, low birthweight or death. Cesarean section is performed if herpes culture is positive at time of delivery.

Prevention:

Good hygiene; avoid oral/genital sexual activity when sores are present.

Comment:

Precipitated by overexposure to sunlight, upper respiratory infection, febrile illnesses, physical or emotional stress, certain foods and drugs; may spread through oral/genital sexual activity; healing occurs spontaneously in

2-4 weeks; Pap smear every six months to one year recommended; viral cultures may be expensive.

CONDYLOMATA (Condylomata Acuminata, Veneral or Genital Warts, Verrucous Lesions)
Causative Organism:
Papillomavirus
Symptoms
Dry, fungating, wart-like growths on vulva/vagina/cervix/rectum; warts may be small, large, single or multiple; may be cauliflower-like in appearance; chronic discharge pruritus; dyspareunia occurs if obstructive; warts may appear one to three months after exposure.
Diagnosis:
By appearance; VDRL and GC should also be taken.
Treatment
*Podophyllin ointment or liquid 10-25 percent applied to warts, avoiding normal tissue and washed off in 1-4 hours; protect surrounding tissue with lubricant jelly or Vaseline; re-examine in one week and repeat treatment weekly or biweekly two times if necessary; do not apply podophyllin to large areas of skin, to lesions with bleeding sites or to recently biopsied areas; treat often coexisting vaginitis; for symptomatic relief keep area dry, may use hair dryer; may use sulfa or AVC vaginal creams; for larger, resistent lesions may use cryosurgery, electrodesiccation; tricholoracetic acid or surgical excision and plastic surgery may be indicated; laser treatments used experimentally; do not treat urethral warts with podophyllin; podophyllin is contraindicated during pregnancy due to possible toxic effects to the fetus.
Partner/Contacts
Treat when warts are present.
Special Instructions:
Thrives in moist areas, keep affected area dry; often takes several treatment sessions, leaving podophyllin on for longer periods; abstain from intercourse during treatment period or use condoms; atypical or persistent warts may require biopsy.
Potential Complications
None, unless podophyllin poisoning occurs or there is fetal exposure to podophyllin with toxic affects; may be linked to cancer.
Prevention
Avoid multiple partners.
Comment
Watch for podophyllin poisoning: nausea, diarrhea, lethargy, paralysis, coma; pregnancy may stimulate luxuriant growth.

LICE (Pubic Lice, Phthirus Pubis, Crabs)
Causative Organism:
Pediculosis pubis.
Symptoms:
Intense itching; lice in pubic hair, scalp or body hair.
Diagnosis:
Appearance of lice/eggs (nits) in pubic hair, scalp or body hair.
Treatment:
*Lindane 1 percent lotion or cream, apply thin layer to infected and adjacent areas, wash off after 8 hours, or Lindane 1 percent shampoo, apply 4 minutes and thoroughly wash off. Not recommended for pregnant or lactating women;
*Pyrethrins and piperonyl, butoxide (nonprescription) apply to infected and adjacent areas and wash off after 10 minutes;
Kwell shampoo, repeat 24–48 hours if necessary.
Partner/Contacts:
Treat if infected.
Special Instructions:
Remove all visible signs of lice and eggs; wash hair and surrounding skin first with soap and water; massage Kwell into hair and leave for four minutes; avoid sexual activity until after treatment; boil wash and machine dry, or dry clean clothing, bed linens, toweling; do not apply Lindane to the eyes.
Potential Complications:
None.
Prevention:
Good hygiene.
Comment:
If one family member is infected, all members are checked and household treated and clothing and linens boiled if household infested.

PINWORMS (Metazoan, Enterobiasis, Enterobius Vermiculars)
Causative Organism:
Pinworm.
Symptoms
Clear to purulent discharge, pruritis, particularly around anus.
Diagnosis
Wet mount preparation from rectum positive for polymorphonuclear leukocytes; "Scotch tape" test positive for pinworms (tape blotted against anus in early morning, tape placed on glass slide and examined for ova).
Treatment
Mebendazole (Vermox) one chewable 100 mg tablet;
Pyrantel pamoate (Antiminth) oral suspension 50 mg ml given at 11 mg

per kg or 1 ml per 10 pounds to a maximum of 20 ml as a single oral dose;

Pyrvinium pamoate (Povan) 5 mg per kg orally as a single dose.

Partner/Contacts:

Treat if infected.

Special Instructions:

None.

Potential Complications:

None.

Prevention:

Good hygiene.

Comment:

Pyrvinium pamoate (Povan) may cause red staining.

TOXIC SHOCK (Toxic Shock Syndrome, TSS)

Causative Organism:

Staphylococcus aureus.

Symptoms

Sudden onset of high fever; vomiting; headache; severe diarrhea; muscle aches; weakness; fatigue; erthematous macular desquamating rash on palms and soles; pustules on lips of vagina; eventual severe, prolonged shock and hypotension.

Diagnosis:

Positive culture from vagina, cervix, blood, urine or stool for Staphylococcus aureus.

Treatment:

Maintain fluid and electrolyte balance; antibiotics sensitive to S. aureus; supportive intervention for shock.

Partner/Contacts:

Not applicable.

Special Instructions:

Avoid tampons.

Potential Complications:

Acute renal failure; diffuse intravascular coagulopathy (DIC); shock; death.

Prevention:

Avoid tampons; or, if tampons must be used, use brand with applicator and change tampon frequently; wash hands carefully before and after insertion of tampon; wear sanitary pad for a few hours during the day and at night, alternate tampons and sanitary pads, keep vulva area clean.

Comment:

Tampons act as a culture media for bacterial growth or may promote the release or absorption of toxin from the vagina into the bloodstream; onset usually occurs during or after menses; women at risk are those who insert tampons with fingers, have had a chronic vaginal discharge for the past year or have had herpes infections. If TSS positive, avoid tampons for at least the next three menses after recovery or entirely.

Contraceptives

Pregnancy risk has increased in the youngest group of single, sexually active females through an increase in frequency of sexual activity and a decrease in initial use of effective contraceptive methods. This pregnancy risk is also disproportionately focused during the beginning of sexual exposure. In one study of single adolescents, 36 percent conceived during the first three months of sexual activity, and 45 percent within the first six months. In this study, for adolescent's who became sexually active before the age of 15, the interval between the first and second intercourse was more than four times longer than for those initiating intercourse at age 17 years or older (33). The increased pregnancy risk during the early coital months, particularly the first month of sexual experience, has been confirmed by others (34). Approximately two-fifths of all 15 year olds (or younger) who are sexually active conceive within six months of their first coitus, as do one-fifth of all sexually active 15 to 19 year olds (35).

It is obvious that the adolescent who seeks contraceptive services for the first time has more than likely already become sexually active (96%). Adolescents may continue this risk through unprotected intercourse during a period of a few months to four years before seeking contraceptive services for the first time. Often, the older the adolescent, the longer she risks pregnancy before seeking contraception. In 50 case studies from a Planned Parenthood clinic, the average 14-year-old waited 4.8 months while the 17-year-old risked 10.4 months of unprotected intercourse (36). The delay from first intercourse to first visit for contraceptive services ranges from seven to 24 months of unprotected intercourse. Adolescents can reduce this delay of contraception before or soon after their initial coitus, by four to five months through outreach and community education programs (37). Fear of parental discovery of contraception and therefore sexuality, is a major reason why adolescents delay seeking contraceptive services until a year or more after sexual intercourse (38).

FACTORS AFFECTING USE

The availabilty of contraceptive services does not alter sexual activity. Usually, the adolescent has already formed a pattern for her social and sexual life before seeking contraceptive services. It is often after the adolescent has made the decision to continue to be sexually active and also that pregnancy is not desired that contraception is sought. Most adolescents (96%) seek contraceptive services to obtain a specific contraceptive method. The majority (88%) will state oral contraceptives as their preference, with a small number (2%) requesting a diaphragm (36).

Choosing a Method
The oral contraceptive pill is more often requested partly because it is more familiar; the adolescent's mother, sisters or friends have probably used "the pill". Also, oral contraceptives are not associated with sexual intercourse. Diaphragms, condoms, spermicides and other barrier methods are commonly described by adolescents as messy and a disturbance to sexual pleasure. For the adolescent, these contraceptive choices are intercourse related; involve carrying the necessary materials; require a comfortableness with one's anatomy and a confidence in one's self and one's partner to override any embarrassment; and an interruption of sexual activity to use them consistently.

The use of contraceptives among adolescents, particularly when unmarried, is influenced by social, psychological, developmental, educational and cultural factors. During adolescence there are many changes, often rapid physical and emotional transitions, which can alter the adolescent's contraceptive needs. There is no perfect or foolproof contraceptive method for adolescents. There is no method available without some risks or inconvenience. Contraception, however, carries a lower potential risk for the adolescent than pregnancy. The benefits for the adolescent of any contraceptive method almost always outweigh the risks, especially when considering the societal and personal costs of an unwanted pregnancy (39). The social outcome of an adolescent pregnancy demonstrates such effects as truncated education; limited opportunity to gain skills, job training or employment; a likelihood of being a single parent living in poverty; lack of economic security; and an inability to improve the quality of her life. The greater health risks of the adolescent mother are seen in an increase risk of morbidity and mortality through pregnancy complications of anemia, preeclampsia, prolonged labor, and cesarean delivery. Health risks for infants include an increased morbidity and mortality rate primarily through the complications of prematurity and low birthweight (35). Most of the serious oral contraceptive and intrauterine device problems can be prevented in adolescents by close attention to the contraindications, use of these methods and the early danger signals of any complications (40).

A contraceptive method needs to fit into the adolescent's personal and reproductive life plan. Such an adaptation is particular to every culture, for both sexes, and in rural or urban areas. The suitability of a contraceptive choice may depend upon such factors as a wish to marry, future childbearing plans, family role models, level of education, age at first intercourse, work or career plans, and religious beliefs. Customs, cultural values and personality factors also affect the contraceptive options which may be appropriate for the individual adolescent and her partner. The health care provider tries to facilitate the contraceptive care of the adolescent by clarifying, supporting, promoting, and providing contraceptive information and services. The adolescent herself is the decision-maker concerning sexual relationships, pregnancy risk, and contraception.

The coital behavior of the average adolescent female is seldom promiscuous. The majority of unmarried female adolescents have a single partner in a monogamous relationship throughout their adolescence; however, serial monogamy is also not uncommon. Few adolescent females have more than two or three partners prior to marriage. In such instances, sexual activity develops from a desire for love, affection and intimacy and is seen as an expression of commitment.

The adolescent who wants to responsibly seek contraceptive services may have difficulty in meeting her needs because of her developmental level. She may psychologically be in an egocentric phase, searching for sexual identity, but her views of sexuality may remain rigid and stereotypic. Her lack of perception or denial of her situation may prevent her from anticipating or appreciating the consequences of her current sexual behavior. Future plans may appear unrealistic or involve few goals. She may feel too guilty or uncomfortable with her new sexuality to plan for or admit her contraceptive needs. Conflicts exist between the adolescent and herself, partner(s), parents, peers and society in acknowledging her sexual activity and her contraceptive responsibility. She may find logical reasoning concerning these values and principles to be difficult.

The capacity to think rationally and realistically and to plan for the future develops in late adolescence along with a more flexible acceptance of alternative views and individual differences. In early and mid-adolescence, cognitive thinking is immature and decision-making skills and abstract thoughts are poorly developed. Often the adolescent's physical development outstrips her psychosocial and cognitive development. Adolescents need assistance in associating abstract ideas with personal, concrete experiences to make them understandable. Also, all adolescents are different. In one study of 87 pregnant adolescents, the majority (63%) were pleased with their pregnancies and were also knowledgeable about contraception (94%) (41). Adolescents can have attitudes and values consistent with responsible sexual conduct but not all adolescents are able to translate these beliefs into their own personal conduct of behavior.

There are several motivational factors which promote contraceptive utilization in adolescents. The availability and knowledge of contraceptive services is a first step as is the developmental stage and maturity of the individual adolescent in accepting herself as sexually active and requiring contraception. Acceptance of sexuality and contraceptive services is also affected by peers, support from significant others and partner involvement and commitment. A pregnancy or pregnancy scare can often trigger the adolescent to seek contraception.

Once the adolescent requests contraception, her choice of contraceptive method is influenced by diverse factors. Patterns of sexual activity are strong elements in a contraceptive decision in such areas as frequency of intercourse, the number of partners, and the cooperation between the adolescent partners. The contraceptive services themselves are also factors in contraceptive choice. Access to contraceptive services, staff attitudes, flexibility of appointment schedules, and contraceptive costs all affect the availability of these services to adolescents. In contraceptive decision-making, adolescents are encouraged to develop their own goals and value systems now and for adulthood, including their reproductive values. By assisting the adolescent in clarifying her values, confusions are aired, bringing thoughts and actions into congruence. Peers also can provide support, guidance and a sense of identification which can improve the adolescent's understanding of the consequences of sexual behavior and increase the awareness and confidence in changing self-images, expectations and new roles.

Factors in Nonuse of Contraceptives
There are, however, many reasons why adolescents choose not to utilize contraception. Some of these reasons lie within the adolescent herself while others are more related to the actual method and services. Initially, the adolescent's developmental tendencies may encourage her to take risks while denying the possibility of pregnancy. The adolescent develops complex personal defense mechanisms whereby she feels immune to pregnancy risks and has erroneous beliefs regarding conception. Insufficient and inaccurate knowledge of pregnancy risks and fertility awareness may delay the adolescent in seeking contraceptive services. Often adolescents state they do not know where or how to obtain contraceptive services and that it is too difficult or expensive. Some adolescents never find time to acquire contraceptives or they feel it is unromantic. Occasionally adolescents do not seek contraceptive services if there is a misunderstanding about the legal aspects of these services to minors. Adolescents with a poor self-image, low evaluation of personal health, or feelings of hopelessness may not seek health care or assistance with their problems. By requesting contraceptive services, the adolescent acknowledges her sexuality despite any ambivalence or embarrassment she may feel. These feelings may heighten her fear of public exposure and possible dissapproval or punishment, especially from her parents and peers. The adolescent may find that her parents or friends disapprove of contraception as a health risk or for personal or religious reasons. Many adolescents feel that contraceptives are dangerous and harmful and have exaggerated fears of side effects and safety. For this age group, the contraceptives may appear difficult or unpleasant to use. Necessary discussions of contraceptive needs between adolescent partners are often delayed or not initiated at all. Partners can be unsupportive, uncommitted or have a negative attitude toward contraception. The partner may object or refuse a con-

traceptive method fearing it may interfere with sexual pleasure and natural-ness. With multiple partners or a lack of shared partner responsibility there follows a low level of mutual confidence and inconsistent or no contracep-tive utilization.

The contraceptive services themselves can also affect the adolescent's ability to utilize contraception. The accessibility and convenience of con-traceptive services to the adolescent population is paramount. Delays in ap-pointments, poor public transportation services, long waiting periods and service expenses are factors which can intimidate the adolescent. Contracep-tive services, whether provided by public clinics or private physicians, may not be attuned to the adolescent's needs. Reassurance of confidentiality and privacy is necessary for the adolescent who may appear sexually sophis-ticated but in reality is self-conscious and embarrassed. Adolescents may have fears regarding the physical examination, particularly the pelvic exam. They may also have fears about being treated impersonally, as a number, or in being lectured. The staff may have a bias against the adolescent's pre-ferred contraceptive method or this method may be unavailable, leaving a minimal or unsuitable selection of possible methods. And, there may be lit-tle structure for psychological support and close monitoring of contracep-tive suitability needed in the adolescent age group.

If the adolescent has little understanding of effective contraceptive methods, then these methods and services will not be used. Contraceptive use during adolescence often follows a similar pattern as that of adolescent sexuality—one that is unpredictable, unplanned and inconsistent. When the adolescent participates in sexual intercourse and does not get pregnant, she feels she can continue without worry, particularly when she is ambivalent about her sexual activity. In this way, the adolescent avoids any unpleasant or demanding contraceptive practices while awaiting the next sporadic or unintended sexual encounter.

The Role of the Adolescent Male

Little is known about the particular sexual attitudes and behaviors of single, male adolescents or their opinions regarding contraception. Often, they are the invisible factor in trying to meet the contraceptive needs of the adoles-cent population. Sexually active male adolescents are difficult to reach in health care settings. Their absence is partly the fault of those health care facilities where their presence has been devalued and their participation ex-cluded. This situation may have developed from the male's influence over contraceptive acceptance and compliance. If the adolescent male feels dis-satisfied or uncomfortable with a contraceptive method, such as feeling an IUD string, awareness of a diaphram, penile irritation with spermicides or decreased sensitivity with condoms, he will often complain or terminate its use. Obviously, it is necessary to actively involve the adolescent male in con-traceptive services for greater success.

In one study of 95 recent, unwed black adolescent first-time fathers who represented three states, the majority opposed or disapproved of abortion, but disagreed with the statement "It's not right to use birth control." Most of the males disagreed with the statement "It is OK to tell a girl that you love her so that you can have sex with her," and they also disagreed with "Getting a girl pregnant proves that you are a man." Of these males, two-thirds were willing to share contraceptive responsibility with females and four-fifths felt "Sex education was not a waste of time" (42).

Most adolescent females will still say that contraception is realistically their responsibility, especially in casual relationships. Some adolescent females would not ask a male to defer intercourse until they are prepared; instead they would take a chance, particularly in a casual relationship. The adolescent females find it difficult to discuss contraception with a new partner. Some do not use contraceptives because they are afraid of "losing the guy." They are also concerned about appearing "immature" if they refuse unprotected intercourse. Some state they do not use contraception for fear of diminishing their partner's sexual pleasure. And others naively trust the partner to take care not to get them pregnant (43).

Male adolescents also report a fear of raising the subject of contraception with a new partner. Many males feel such a discussion might anger or insult their partners and "shut things down." Usually, the males feel more comfortable waiting for their partners to bring up the subject of contraception. Some adolescent males dismiss any need for contraceptive discussion, particularly with a new or casual partner. In a serious relationship, however, there appears to be greater motivation for contraceptive discussion in both partners as a sign of caring and a desire to prevent unwanted pregnancy (43).

Adolescent males are often unaware of their legal responsibilities as fathers both financially and in personal involvement with their offspring. The education of these young men regarding the impact of their actions and future consequences is necessary before such behavior will be modified. Today's adolescent males who find out they are now fathers may become involved in lengthy legal battles. Many adolescent fathers want to keep their children or be involved in their care and life. Other adolescent fathers may feel more pressure from the courts in the form of strengthened sanctions when they decline such obligations. As the legal system continues to adjust to meet the multiple demands of today's society, so we all must accept our responsibility to assist these adolescents in their complex and often bewildering lives.

RECOMMENDATIONS

The benefits of deferred childbearing are evident for the adolescent, her partner and her community. Each adolescent has the right to make her own thoughtful and informed reproductive decisions. The encouragement of the adolescent's feelings of self-worth will enhance her abilities to develop responsible attitudes and decision-making skills. Adolescents need more than reproductive and contraceptive facts. Educational requirements for their rapidly changing lives are best developed in a cooperative and safe environment where both male and female adolescents are active participants in their health care choices and decisions. Contraceptive options are fully discussed before the adolescent and her health care provider choose a method to meet her individual needs and preferences. Through personalized contraceptive services and values-clarification, adolescents can learn to utilize effective and safe contraceptive methods consistently from the onset of their sexual activity.

Contraceptive services are also attempting to meet the needs of the adolescent population. Such services are accessible and available in sufficient numbers to attract the adolescent. Services are better utilized when located within schools or in neighborhoods convenient to adolescents. Flexible scheduling, which includes evening and weekend hours, also appeals to the adolescent. Prompt appointment systems and the availability of walk-in visits will decrease contraceptive delays in this population. Brief admission procedures, minimal waiting periods and a 24-hour "hot line" for questions and problems will lower the adolescent's anxiety and frustration with the health care system. Specialized clinic sessions for adolescents are also popular, as are frequent return visits for monitoring concerns and compliance. The circumstances surrounding the contraceptive services play a critical role in the adolescent's attendance and compliance, particularly staff-client rapport. The adolescent requires a level of control over her health care decisions within a climate of support and trust. The assurance of confidentiality and privacy is essential. This provision is easily seen in the careful handling of records, private interviewing, designated dressing areas, use of gowns or coverings, and doors or barriers closed without interruptions during interviews and examinations. An informal atmosphere where staff attitudes are positive and friendly provides support and encouragement to the adolescent. Female health care providers are also assets in the adolescent age group. Continuity of staff, whether within an office, clinic, or in association with school programs, can enhance the adolescent's confidence in herself and her health care. Also, nominal fees for contraceptive services or free services for adolescents relieve any economic problems in seeking care or in compliance. A "back-up method" with instructions and supplies is another important provision in adolescent contraceptive services.

There are many diverse educational programs for adolescents which can be utilized in any setting. Individual counseling, written materials, audiovisual aids, group sessions, role-playing, rap sessions, and peer counselors all assist the adolescent in her reproductive decisions. Incorporating peer counselors either within school systems or health care facilities can increase positive communication skills between adolescent partners as well as between adolescents and health care providers, all of which can improve contraceptive use and compliance.

Community knowledge and support of contraceptive services is also vital to adolescent health care. Parents and schools can be given materials to encourage communications and provide community resources for the adolescent. Community outreach programs for adolescents need to be visible and innovative. Active relationships can be developed between schools and health care facilities focusing on the adolescent. The support of local churches and youth groups can also be enlisted. Information about the prevention of pregnancy and sexually transmitted diseases, including safe and effective contraception, can be distributed to decrease fears and correct misinformation. Pharmacies can be encouraged to display contraceptives where they can be easily reached for sale to adolescents without restrictions. Media advertisement can also be utilized to promote responsible contraceptive decision-making. At the local, state and national level, promotion of minimal levels of education in reproduction and contraception in all public schools can be mandated.

An ideal contraceptive for the adolescent has been described as 100 percent protective, wholly reversible, medically safe with no health risks, easily obtainable at low cost, and well within a young person's capacity to use properly (44). A discussion of each respective contraceptive method and how its use relates to the adolescent population follows this section. The methods of contraception are the same as for adults, as are their functions, indications, contraindications, risks, benefits and side effects. Only the specifics of each method concerning the adolescent are discussed.

ORAL CONTRACEPTIVES

Oral contraceptives appear to be the most effective, reversible method of contraception. The combination oral contraceptives are the most widely used contraceptive method by adolescents because they offer a high degree of protection, few specific risks for this age group, disassociation from coitus, and a self-reliant method independent of partner participation. Lower dosages such as 30–50 μg of ethinylestradiol and 0.5–1.0 mg of norethisterone, or equivalents, are preferable for adolescents as they are well tolerated with few risks or side effects and offer a high degree of effectiveness. The risk of death among adolescents using oral contraceptives is 1.3 per 100,000 users while the risk of childbirth for this age group is 11.1 deaths per 100,000 live births (45).

Disadvantages
For the adolescent, the disadvantages of oral contraceptive usage begin with an acknowledgement and anticipation of sexual activity. To obtain oral contraceptives, the adolescent is required to have a physical examination, laboratory tests, a prescription, and medical follow-up. Adolescents recog-

nize that oral contraceptives are more difficult to obtain than over-the-counter contraceptives. Adolescents may be unable to afford oral contraception or the medical care involved. Adolescents are also concerned about the confidentiality of their contraceptive care and the possible involvement of their parents. "The pill" must be taken every day, regardless of any changes in sexual activity. Adolescents may frequently forget a daily tablet and consider "doubling-up" of pills as a way to catch up. Method failure and breakthrough-bleeding are more likely when this occurs on low dose pills rather than 50 μg of estrogen. Often, there is little motivation for continued compliance when sexual activity is infrequent; thus, continuation rates are low. Improper use of oral contraceptives and low continuation rates are common in the adolescent population. Individual motivation and maturity as well as the level of sexual activity and the ability to take daily medications are weighed prior to initiation of oral contraceptives. The adolescent may discontinue usage if she terminates a relationship, and she may fail to resume contraception later with a new partner. Some adolescents will discontinue oral contraceptive use when they experience minor side effects which affect their appearance such as acne, weight gain, chloasma or stretch marks. Many adolescents feel confused about oral contraceptives. They receive many contradictory messages and misinformation regarding the use of oral contraceptive pills primarily from their peers and the media. Often, today's adolescents are afraid of the reported side effects and risks of oral contraception.

Risks

A primary concern associated with oral contraception in the early post-menarcheal years of adolescence is the possibility of masking an underlying menstrual dysfunction. Such a risk is avoided when the use of oral contraceptives is deferred until the individual patterns of the menstrual cycle are established and assessed. Oligomenorrhea usually occurs within one to two years of menarche. The probable risk of postpill amenorrhea is widely debated but the general risk is thought to be one per 1000 users, and there is no information that oral contraceptive use during adolescence increases this probability. Normal menses returns for the majority of users within one to three months after discontinuing oral contraception. If amenorrhea does occur, it is usually responsive to treatment.

There is also some concern regarding the growth suppressant effect of estrogen in the adolescent population. There can be a slowing or arrest of skeletal growth with high dosages of estrogen but this is contrary to the clinical use of estrogen in oral contraceptives. These estrogen effects are directly dependent upon dosage and bone age at the time of estrogen administration. Estrogen use in oral contraception occurs after menarche when growth is almost completed. In dosages of 50 μg or less of estrogen in oral contraceptives, the risk of interference with pubertal growth is not anticipated (44).

The cardiovascular complications associated with oral contraceptive usage are the same for adolescents as for adults, although they are lower for adolescents than any other age group. Conditions which predispose cardiovascular disease are contraindications to oral contraception in adolescents as they are in adults, such as hyperlipidemia or hypertension. The consideration of oral contraception in diabetic adolescents, however, remains controversial. The major factor in cardiovascular complications is the estrogen-induced alteration of the blood clotting factors in blood lipid profiles. Plasma lipid changes in adolescents who use oral contraceptives or who smoke are identical to those that occur in adults. These changes are reversible with discontinuation of oral contraception. The greatest risk appears to be the acceleration or atherogenesis, which may restrict the total lifetime use of oral contraception. Such risks of cardiovascular disease are associated with smoking and age. Nonsmoking adolescents have the lowest risk of cardiovascular complications of all. Cardiovascular risks associated with oral contraceptives appear to be dosage-related and may decrease with discontinuation. As a preventive measure, oral contraceptives are discontinued prior to elective surgery and in the case of significant trauma. The duration of oral contraceptive usage in adolescence and the long-term cumulative effects require further research.

The risk of neoplasia associated with oral contraception is also present in the adolescent. There is some concern in the initiation of oral contraception during adolescence with the possibility of increased risks from long-term exposure, cumulative effects and a long-latency period. There appears, however, to be no increased risk of breast cancer associated with oral contraception. In fact, oral contraceptives appear to provide a protective effect against benign breast disorders including fibrocystic breast disease and fibroadenomas. The risk of endometrial cancer associated with oral contraception is not seen with the use of the combination pills where the simultaneous use of estrogen and progesterone protects against the precursor state of endometrial hyperplasia which can be seen when unopposed estrogen is used. The risk of cervical cancer is not solely associated with oral contraception but is correlated with a variety of factors including long-term oral contraception and the predisposing factors of the presence of cervical dysplasia at an early age, early initiation of coitus, and exposure to multiple partners. Hepatocellular adenoma is associated with oral contraception although there have been no reported cases during adolescence to date. The greatest risk of this serious complication appears to be in women who are over 27 years old and have used oral contraceptives for seven or more years at a dosage of 50 μg or more of estrogen. Hepatocellular adenoma is a consideration in any adolescent using oral contraception who presents with symptoms of a right upper quadrant mass, especially when associated with pain and signs of shock (44).

Before prescribing oral contraception to the adolescent, a personal, medical, family and sexual history is carefully taken to avoid contraindications. A complete physical examination and laboratory tests are also taken to ensure eligibility. When an adolescent is sixteen years old or younger, maturation of secondary sexual characteristics and expected stature are evaluated as well as the regularity of ovualtion and the menstrual cycle. This later element may involve assessment of 6–12 regular menses prior to initiation of oral contraception. Also, if the adolescent's body weight is less than normal, the adolescent may be more susceptible to some side effects. In this case, the lowest possible dosage of oral contraception is administered. Often the 28-day regimen provides better compliance in the adolescent population. Since there is no starting or stopping daily pill intake, there is less likelihood of forgetting a pill or taking pills incorrectly. There may be an additional benefit to the 28-day cycle when iron tablets are utilized instead of placebos. Finally, oral contraception affects other aspects of the adolescent's life through alterations in nutrition, drug reactions and laboratory tests.

Advantages
There are many advantages to oral contraception in the adolescent population. Oral contraceptives provide effective and convenient contraception while preserving future reproductive ability. Some of the benefits associated with oral contraception besides the prevention of pregnancy are avoidance of ectopic pregnancy, spontaneous abortion, and the risks of surgical delivery, which are leading causes of morbidity and mortality in this young female population. Other beneficial effects are seen in a decrease in premenstrual symptoms including fluid retention and depression, and the reduction of iron-deficiency anemia associated with menstrual blood loss. The incidence of pelvic inflammatory disease, ovarian cysts, ovarian cancer, uterine fibroids and endometriosis is reduced, protecting the adolescent from complications which can lead to infertility. And, some of the menstrual disorders which are lessened or relieved by oral contraception are dysmenorrhea, menorrhagia, irregular menses, intermenstrual bleeding, premenstrual tension and mittelschmerz. Other associated benefits may occur in cases of acne, duodenal ulcers or rheumatoid arthritis.

There are several types of oral contraceptive pills available today with new forms continuing to be developed. The combination pills provide the same amount and classification of estrogen and progestin. The biphasic combination pill keeps the estrogen dosage and classification constant while progestin level changes midway through the cycle. The newest triphasic combination pills entail three different levels of the progestin during the cycle while the estrogen may remain constant or may also change along with the progestin, producing a more physiologic response. The mini-pill or progestin-only pill is taken daily without interruption. For the adolescent using the mini-pill, there are fewer associated risks and ovulation is not regularly supressed. The mini-pill may also have the beneficial effect of decreasing cramping associated with menses. The disadvantages of the mini-pill are the higher method failure rates and the side effects of breakthrough-bleeding, spotting, and unpredictable menses. These side effects can lead to method dissatisfaction and discontinuation in the adolescent population.

Oral contraception is the most widely used contraceptive method among 15 to 19 year olds. Success in using oral contraceptives is associated with careful screening for contraindications and frequent monitoring to minimize side effects and maximize continuation. There appear to be fewer risks of serious complications and health risks for adolescents using oral contraception than in any other age group.

IUD

The following discussion presents the effectiveness of the intrauterine device as a contraceptive method for teenagers. Since the U.S. Food and Drug Administration (FDA) has removed these devices from the market, they are no longer a feasible option. Many adolescents, however, may still have an IUD in place, and because of this, health care professionals should be informed and capable of IUD management.

The intrauterine device (IUD) provides effective, reversible contraception for many adolescents. Greater success in IUD usage in the adolescent population is seen in the copper-wound or progesterone-impregnated devices, although they usually have 1–3 year replacement periods. Newer devices, such as the T-Cu-380A, have an 8-year life span with low failure and discontinuation rates. The availability of a selection and sizes of devices, optimal timing of insertion, and skillful insertion minimizing discomfort and ensuring proper placement all increase the success rate of the IUD in the adolescent population.

For the adolescent with an IUD there are minimum compliance demands once the device is in place. There are no prescription requirements or chances of discovery by others. Its use is not coitus related and is independent of partner involvement. And, it is immediately reversible upon removal.

One disadvantage of IUD use in the adolescent population is the rate of expulsion, which is most likely to occur during the first six months after insertion and usually during menses. The adolescent is instructed to check for the IUD strings after each menses which requires a comfortableness and a degree of knowledge about her body. Larger devices with greater surface areas have lower expulsion rates and can remain in place indefinitely. The drawback of these larger devices is the associated increase in menstrual pain and bleeding.

Another disadvantage to IUD usage is the discontinuation rate. Continuation rates are low, often with one year use the exception. IUD removals fall into the categories of infection, bleeding, pain, and medical or personal reasons. The adolescent needs to be prepared for such side effects as an increase in menstrual flow and cramping which can lead to method dissatisfaction and removal. In some cases, the use of the Progestasert-T or a smaller device may decrease these side effects. Analgesia also may be provided for menstrual discomfort. The partner may be uncooperative regarding the device and complain of "feeling the strings" which can lead to removal. Compliance requires return appointments for careful monitoring and close supervision as well as continued psychological support.

A primary concern with IUD usage in the adolescent population is the risk of infertility. There appears to be little risk of impaired fertility in adolescents after uncomplicated IUD use, and fertility returns promptly after removal of the device. Pelvic inflammatory disease (PID), and its association with ectopic pregnancy and infertility, however, is significant for the adolescent population and can compromise the widespread use of IUDs in young, unmarried females. Single, sexually active female adolescents using IUDs are 1 to 10 times more likely to develop PID than those using another contraceptive method or no method at all. These same adolescents, however, are particularly at risk for developing PID even in the absence of IUD usage. PID for this population, is associated with such factors as early age at initiation of coitus, multiple partners, frequent coitus and repeated exposure to sexually transmitted diseases. Coital behavior may be a more significant factor in PID occurrence than the presence of an IUD. There is also an increased risk of ectopic pregnancy with an IUD, a risk which is no different for the adolescent than for the older woman.

The use of an IUD is discouraged in an adolescent with multiple partners, limited motivation, impulsive behavior, a history of sexually transmitted disease, frequent vaginal infections or a previous pelvic infection. A history of PID is an absolute contraindication to IUD usage. Adolescents who are aware of the danger signals of infection or ectopic pregnancy can report early signs or suspicious symptoms for prompt recognition and early treatment.

Many adolescents are hesitant about IUD usage out of fear. Often, a friend may have had a bad or painful experience. The fear of pain or having "something inside," or even of "losing" the device inside them is frequently stated. Fear of infection or damage to internal organs may also be present, as well as a fear of problems with future pregnancies. Some of these fears have developed from the risk of perforation of the uterus at the time of insertion. IUDs with withdrawal insertion techniques decrease the risk of perforation as opposed to the push-out methods. The risk of perforation is also decreased with proper insertion techniques such as sounding the uterus for correct sizing, and the use of a tenaculum.

The IUD is an appropriate contraceptive method for the adolescent who is unable to use other methods, particularly if she has already been pregnant or if she has previously had an abortion. It is also an acceptable contraceptive method for nulliparous adolescents who understand and desire this method and who meet the criteria for its use. Smaller devices, such as the Cu7, CuT or Progestasert are often tolerated better and are widely available. For an adolescent in a monogamous or married relationship there are similar considerations of risks and benefits in using an IUD as in an older woman. For the adolescent who only wants to delay childbearing a short time, this may be the least attractive contraceptive option. And although the IUD may increase the chance of developing PID in an individual who is already at risk, there is no evidence of an increase in the severity of the infection or the likelihood of infertility from the infection related to the IUD.

BARRIER METHODS

Barrier methods of contraception including the diaphragm, spermicides, condom, cervical cap and cervical sponge are effective methods of contraception when used consistently and in some cases together. The greater rate of accidental pregnancy is primarily due to inconsistent use or nonuse. Greater effectiveness can be achieved when barrier methods are used as back-up for other contraceptives. Barrier methods are safe and reversible and are easily portable for immediate protection as they are only used when the adolescent is sexually active. Health risks or side effects are rare, and usually seen as a local allergic reaction or sensitivity. Many adolescents, however, may be hesitant to use barrier methods. These methods entail an ability to place the barrier correctly in or on the body, requiring a comfortableness in touching intimate parts of the body. Adolescents also consider the barrier method contraceptive messy or an interruption to the spontaneity of sexual activity.

DIAPHRAGM

The diaphragm provides an effective contraceptive method in motivated individuals, although there is a higher method failure rate than with oral contraceptives or IUDs. There are no adverse side effects, health risks or medical contraindications. Diaphragm failure rates are associated with improper insertion, incorrect fitting, defects in the device, displacement or nonuse. A diaphragm may be a method of choice in instances where sexual intercourse is infrequent or sporadic. It is a safe method only used by those sexually active. *It is also easily portable for spontaneous moments.* The diaphragm does require concurrent use of a spermicidal cream or jelly and consistent use with every intercourse.

The motivated, mature adolescent has a higher compliance rate because she may have a clearer understanding of her anatomy. The adolescent who has previously used tampons without difficulty may be more comfortable with the insertion and removal techniques. Adolescents may request a diaphragm if they are concerned about the side effects or risks of other contraceptive methods, or they may use the diaphragm as a back-up method to other contraceptive methods. The diaphragm also appears to have some protection against sexually transmitted diseases and cervical dysplasia. Occasionally, there may be anatomical abnormalities present which preclude a proper fit. Trained personnel are required to ensure the fit, and to provide an understanding of use and maintenance of supplies.

The young adolescent may find the necessary touching of the genital area for insertion and removal of the device too difficult to master. Some particularly young adolescents may feel uncomfortable when the diaphragm is in place. Adolescents may not want to anticipate their sexual activity or to take steps to be prepared for intercourse each time they go out. Many adolescents fear discovery of their supplies either by parents or peers and hesitate to carry the somewhat bulky case or conspicuous spermicide. Because the use of the diaphragm is coitus related, some adolescents find this method unromantic because it can interrupt sexual activity or the spontaneity of sexual pleasure. This element can be corrected because insertion can be performed hours prior to sexual intercourse or as part of foreplay. Many adolescents lack the confidence to use a diaphragm, believing that it is too messy or that their partner will not like it.

Rarely, there is a local allergic reaction to the rubber or the spermicide which can affect either partner. There is also the remote possibility of toxic shock syndrome (TSS) if the device is left in place for a prolonged period of time (more than 24 hours). To decrease the chance of TSS, use a back-up method instead of the diaphragm during menses, avoid leaving the diaphragm in place for extended periods, and watch and report any danger signs of TSS. Adolescents using a diaphragm are also encouraged to urinate before and after intercourse to prevent any tendencies toward urinary tract infections or cystitis.

SPERMICIDES

Spermicides or vaginal chemical contraceptives consist of vaginal foams, creams, jellies, suppositories, pastes and soluable films. Spermicides are a safe, effective contraceptive method when used consistently and correctly, and higher effectiveness rates are seen when these chemical contraceptives are used in combination with other contraceptive methods, such as condoms or diaphragms. There are no serious risks, side effects or complications with spermicides, except in rare local allergic reactions in either partner. They are used only when sexually active and have no long-term effects. Spermicides are inexpensive and easily obtained. They do not require a medical appointment, examination, consultation or prescription. Spermicides are often given as back-up methods to be available at all times because they are easily carried for instant protection. Spermicides also provide some protection against sexually transmitted diseases. Some vaginal foam has been particularly cited as protective against gonorrhea.

Spermicides are suited to the spontaneous and unpredictable pattern of adolescent coital behaviors, and a method of choice if coitus is infrequent. Low rates of use are seen in the adolescent population although spermicides are becoming more popular today as fears associated with other methods increase. An advantage of spermicides, particularly to sexually inexperienced adolescents, is their functioning as a lubricant which can decrease some sexual discomforts. Adolescents can also be instructed to insert spermicides after oral sex if the taste is offensive.

The disadvantages of spermicides for adolescents are that they are coitus related and considered messy or a "hassle." There has also been some concern and publicity regarding possible teratogenic effects of spermicides on the fetus in case of pregnancy; however, the evidence appears insufficient at this time to cause any alarm. Occasionally, spermicides may increase the symptoms of a concurrent, acute vaginitis. Adolescents using spermicides also must read the package information for usage of each vaginal chemical contraceptive to ensure insertion time requirements prior to intercourse.

CONDOMS

Condoms are widely used by a significant number of adolescents, particularly after release of the movie "Saturday Night Fever" with John Travolta. When consistently and correctly used, condoms provide effective, safe protection without side effects or health risks. It is the only male contraceptive currently available. Rarely, there is a local allergic reaction to the rubber, in which case, sheaths made of animal products may be safely used. Effectiveness increases when condoms are used in combination with other contraceptive methods such as spermicides or diaphragms. The combination of condom and spermicide are commonly provided as a back-up to other contraceptive methods. Condoms are readily available and can be purchased without a prescription, over-the-counter, and at low cost with no need of medical consultation or supervision. The ease of access and carrying convenience is attractive to the adolescent population. Also pleasing is the ability to enjoy spontaneous and sporadic sexual pleasure without delay.

Condoms are the only contraceptive that is widely available to males when the contraceptive responsibility involves the male partner. Condoms can be a method of choice when sexual activity is infrequent or usually unplanned, which is typical in the adolescent population. Condoms may also provide protection against sexually transmitted diseases, especially when there are multiple partners.

Often, adolescents fear an interruption in sexual pleasure or a decrease in sexual sensitivity when using a condom. The fear of reduced penile sensation is less of a problem now with the newer products. One other advantage of condom use during adolescence is the reduction of the common problem of premature ejaculation in adolescent males. In slowing the rate of ejaculation, sexual pleasure can be increased for both adolescent partners. Adolescents can be supplied information regarding the various types and thicknesses of condoms.

Often, the major barrier to the use of the condom is the adolescent male's negative attitude and unwillingness, which are demonstrated as an unacceptance of responsibility for contraception. Both male and female adolescents may feel "insulted" if a condom appears, particularly if the relationship is new or casual. The condom is a sign of preparedness which many young adolescents resist as part of their ambivalent and emerging sexual feelings. Female adolescents may be especially reluctant to ask their partner to use a condom. Occasionally, adolescents may also display an exaggerated fear of the condom breaking and are therefore unable to use this contraceptive method.

CERVICAL CAP

The cervical cap is an old device that has been redesigned and reintroduced as an alternative contraceptive method. It is a thimble-shaped, soft, rubber cap which fits over the cervix and has some of the same advantages as the diaphragm. It is an effective contraceptive which can be left in place from 3 to 5 days to throughout the intermenstrual period. The lower effectiveness rate is associated with inconsistent use and dislodgement, and it often results in a high rate of method dissatisfaction and discontinuation. The cervical cap is not FDA approved and is only available in certain areas where personnel have been trained and granted research status to use the device under specified protocols. The caps themselves are usually imported from England. The cap is a nonhormonal and noninvasive contraceptive. It can be used in instances where there are abnormalities of the vagina when the diaphragm is contraindicated.

For the young adolescent who is not highly motivated, the skills necessary for insertion and removal may prove a difficulty because she must be able and willing to reach her cervix. It may be more difficult to check the placement or remove the cap than a diaphragm. Many health care providers feel it is not a recommended contraceptive method for most adolescents. The cap cannot be fitted if the circumference of the cervix is quite irregular or if the cervix if extremely short or pointed upwards. The cap also requires approximately one half hour to form a strong suction seal before intercourse. Occasionally, there may be discomfort from the pressure of the cap rim on the cervix. And, although there are no reported cases, the potential of toxic shock syndrome is more significant because of the length of time the device can stay in place.

CERVICAL SPONGE

The polyurethane contraceptive sponge impregnated with nonoxynol-9 was approved by the FDA in 1983. It has been made from a variety of sources ranging from natural sea sponges to synthetic sponges such as polyurethane, usually containing one gram of spermicide. The sponge acts as a barrier between the sperm and the cervix; it is an absorbent trap for the sperm within the sponge that releases a spermicide to destroy the sperm. Besides pregnancy prevention, the cervical sponge may provide some protection against sexually transmitted diseases and cervical neoplasia.

The advantages of the cervical sponge are similar to those of the diaphragm. There are no side effects or health risks. Occasionally, a local allergic reaction in either partner may occur. Also, toxic shock syndrome may be a potential risk if the sponge is left in place for prolonged periods. The cervical sponge is not recommended for use in anyone with a history of TSS or where there are anatomical abnormalities which interfere with accurate placement.

The sponge can be purchased over-the-counter at the approximate cost of $1.00 per sponge. It is available in one size only and is disposable. It can be used without medical consultation, examination or prescription. The sponge is inserted into the vagina so that it can cover the cervix. It has a concave "dimple" on one side to fit over the cervix which decreases the possibility of dislodgement during intercourse. The other side has a woven polyester retrieval loop to facilitate removal. Prior to use, the sponge is moistened with tap water and inserted deep into the vagina. Once in place, it provides continuous protection for up to 24 hours and does not require further measures for repeat intercourse within that time period. The sponge should remain in place 6 hours after intercourse. After use, the sponge is thrown away. Young adolescents may have difficulty learning the correct insertion techniques, using the sponge consistently, or touching their genital area.

Natural Family Planning

Natural Family Planning (NFP) uses the methods of a calendar, basal body temperature, and cervical mucous to predict ovulation. It requires an ability to accurately predict the fertile period and to abstain from sexual intercourse during this and the periovulatory periods. Menses needs to be regular and consistent with ovulation occurring on a set and predictable day.

This calendar method requires high motivation and careful instruction which may be difficult for adolescents. Their menses are still irregular and variations in the menstrual pattern are common so that prediction of ovulation is uncertain. Also, symptoms and charts may be difficult or confusing for the adolescent to interpret. False readings may be recorded due to variations in growth and activity levels. NFP demands daily effort to maintain charts, including taking one's temperature immediately upon wakening—before any activity. Because of these reasons, this method may not be suited to the adolescent lifestyle. The pregnancy and discontinuation rates for this method are higher than with other contraceptive methods. These rates are usually associated with poor compliance when periodic abstinence is difficult to maintain, particularly if coitus is infrequent and unplanned. On the positive side, NFP can promote communication between partners and it demonstrates a commitment to responsible contraception. NFP is an educational opportunity regarding reproductive life.

Withdrawal

Many adolescents have unsuccessfully used withdrawal as a method of contraception. It is always available and does not cost any money. There is no need for advance planning, purchase, supplies, medical consultation or supervision. Sexual activity can remain spontaneous and unplanned with no bother with a contraceptive method. The method failure rate, however, is only marginally better than no method at all.

Using withdrawal can be unpleasant and distracting from sexual pleasure when partners worry over the timing of withdrawal. The female has to depend upon her male partner to interrupt intercourse, which can cause anxiety and affect closeness. For the sexually inexperienced male adolescent, it may be difficult to know the proper time for withdrawal and he may easily wait too long. Adolescents need careful instructions regarding withdrawal. Knowledge that semen is produced and released prior to ejaculation is also necessary for adolescents using the withdrawal method. The male can be encouraged to wipe off the penis prior to intercourse to remove any fluid containing semen.

Noncoital Sex/Abstinence

Noncoital sex and abstinence are alternative methods of sexual expression without intercourse. It is a positive choice of sexual expression which involves physical closeness through fondling, kissing, touching and possibly oral or manual stimulation of orgasm. These alternative methods of expressing love or making love can be encouraged or reinforced in a nonjudgmental way for those adolescents who are not ready or willing to participate in sexual intercourse. Adolescents often need assistance when saying "no" to sexual activity and this, too, can be provided by health care facilities and providers. Adolescents especially require reassurance of their normalcy when they choose to defer sexual activities.

Injectable Contraceptives

Injectable contraceptives such as Depo-Provera (Depot medroxyprogesterone acetate or DMPA) are effective, progestin-only contraceptives which last three months. Side effects from injectable contraceptives include menstrual irregularities and amenorrhea. In 1978, the FDA banned the use of Depo-Provera in the United States although it has continued to be used in other countries. The World Health Organization 1981 review of DMPA states no life-threatening side effects and supports its use in adolescence when other methods are contraindicated and where unwanted pregnancy and abortion outweigh reservations. The American Academy of Pediatrics also supports this WHO report. DMPA candidates may also include those mentally handicapped females who are at risk for sexual exploitation and who are unable to comply with other contraceptive methods, or for those with medical conditions which contraindicate other methods. DMPA is not recommended for use, however, during the first two years after menarche as a precaution. Injectable contraceptives may decrease the frequency and seriousness of sickle-cell crises and may prove to be the method of choice for women suffering from sickle-cell disease (46).

Postcoital Contraceptives

Postcoital contraception includes such products as diethylstilbestrol (DES), ethinyl estradiol (EE), conjugated estrogen (CE), ethinyl estradiol-norgestrel combination (EE-N) oral regimens and the Cu7, CuT, Tatum T and Progestasert intrauterine contraceptive devices. FDA approval in 1975 has been withdrawn except in the case of rape, incest or emergency because the use in the first and second trimester is associated with vaginal adenosis and vaginal cancer in daughters, and with reproductive tract malformations in both daughters and sons of users. If pregnancy is not prevented by this treatment method, abortion services are made available.

Postcoital contraception is administered within 72 hours of unprotected intercourse. Marked nausea is a common side effect of DES and EE but is less so with EE-N. Extra tablets or antiemetics may be necessary to combat nausea. Irregular bleeding is also possible following oral treatment regimens. Initiation of treatment within 24 hours of intercourse increases the chance of pregnancy prevention. The intrauterine devices obviously provide longer contraception than the few days of protection of the oral regimen. Postcoital contraception is not a regular contraceptive method and is not casually used in the case of unprotected intercourse. The designated use of postcoital contraception remains for extreme cases only. The consideration of the risks and benefits of this choice is the same for the adolescent as for the older woman.

References

1. Russo JF. The spectrum of outpatient adolescent gynecologic pathology. *J Adolescent Health Care* 1982;3:126–127.
2. Health needs of Adolescents. *World Health Organization Technical Report Series No. 609.* Geneva: WHO, 1977;26–27.
3. Rigg CA. Health care in the modern world. In: *Adolescent Medicine: Present and Future Concepts.* Rigg CA, Shearin RB (eds). Chicago: Yearbook Medical Publishers, 1980;68.
4. Levine SV. The anxieties of adolescents. *J Adolescent Heath Care* 1981;2:133–137.
5. Varney H. *Nurse-Midwifery* Boston: Blackwell Scientific Publications, 1980;125–129.
6. Bates B. *A Guide to Physical Examination.* Philadelphia: JB Lippincott, 1974.
7. Malasanos L, Barkauskas V, Moss M, et al. *Health Assessment.* St. Louis: CV Mosby Co., 1977.
8. Cowell, CA. The gynecological examination of infants, children, and young adolescents. *Pediatr Clin North Am* 1981;28(2):247–266.

9. Marks A. Aspects of biosocial screening and health maintenance in adolescents. *Pediatr Clin North Am* 1980;(27)1:153–161.
10. Keith L, Brittain J. *Sexually Transmitted Diseases*. Aspen, CO: Creative Infomatics, Inc., 1978;59.
11. Sarrell PM. Indications for a first pelvic examination. *J Adolescent Health Care* 1981;2(2):145–146.
12. Kaufman RH, Burmeister RE, Spjut HJ. Cervical cytology in the teen-age patient. *Am J Obstet Gynecol* 1970;108(1):515–519.
13. Kaufman RH, Leeds LJ. Cervical and vaginal cytology in the child and adolescent. *Pediatr Clin North Am* 1972;19(3):547–557.
14. Hein K, Schreiber K, Cohen MI, et al. Cervical cytology: the need for routine screening in the sexually active adolescent. *J Pediatr* 1977;91:123–126.
15. Feldman MJ, Linzey EM, Srebwik E, et al. Abnormal cervical cytology in the teen-ager: a continuing problem. *Am J Obstet Gynecol* 1976;126:418–421.
16. Heald FP, Rosebrough RH, Jacobson MS. Nutrition and the adolescent: an update. *J Adolescent Health Care* 1980;1;142–151.
17. Meyer EE, Neumann CG. Management of the obese adolescent. *Pediatr Clin North Am* 1977;24:123–127.
18. Tyrer LB, Mazlen RG, Bradshaw LE. Meeting the special needs of pregnant teenagers. *Clin Obstet Gynecol* 1978;21:1199–1213.
19. Rosso P, Lederman SA. Nutrition in the pregnant adolescent. In: *Adolescent Nutrition*. Winick M (ed). New York: John Wiley & Sons, 1982:51–52.
20. Zlotnik FJ, Burmeister LF. Low "gynecologic age": an obstetric risk factor. *Am J Obstet Gynecol* 1977;128:183–186.
21. Higgins AC. Nutritional status and the outcome of pregnancy. *J Can Dietetic Assoc* 1976;37:17–35.
22. Corbett MA, Burst HV. Nutritional intervention in pregnancy. *J Nurse-Midwif* 1983;28:23–29.
23. Glass RH. *Office Gynecology* (2nd ed). Baltimore: Williams & Wilkins, 1981;344–350.
24. Paige DM, Cordano A, Mellits ED, Baertl JM, Davis L. Nutritional supplementation of pregnant adolescents. *J Adolescent Health Care* 1981;1:261–267.
25. Oster J. Recurrent abdominal pain, headache and limb pain in children and adolescents. *Pediatrics* 1972;50(3):429–436.
26. McDonough PG, Gambrell RD. The adolescent patient and her problems. *Clin Obstet Gynecol* 1979;22(2):491–507.
27. Caghan SB, McGrath MM, Morrow MG, Pittman LD. When adolescents complain of pain. *Nurse-Practitioner* 1978;July–August:19–22.
28. Stierlin H., Ravenscroft K Jr. Varieties of adolescent "separation conflicts." *Br J Med Psychol* 1972;45(4):299–313.
29. Frank RA, Cohen DJ. Psychosocial concomitants of biological maturation in preadolescence. *Am J Psychiatry* 1979;136(12):1518–1524.
30. Keith L, Brittain J. *Sexually Transmitted Diseases*. Aspen, CO: Creative Infomatics, Inc., 1978:86–87.
31. Centers for Disease Control. Sexually Transmitted Diseases Treatment Guidelines 1982. *Morbidity and Mortality Weekly Report* 1982;31(25).
32. Centers for Disease Control. *Sexually Transmitted Diseases Factsheet* (35th ed). Atlanta: Centers for Disease Control, 1981.

33. Koenig MA, Zelnik M. The risk of premarital first pregnancy among metropolitan-area teenagers: 1976–1979. *Family Planning Perspectives* 1982;14(5):239–247.
34. Zabin LS, Hardy JB, Streett R, et al. A school-, hospital- and university-based adolescent pregnancy prevention program. A cooperative design for service and research. *J Reprod Med* 1984;29(6):421–426.
35. Hofman AD. Contraception in adolescence: a review. Psychosocial aspects. *WHO Bull* 1984;62(1):151–162.
36. Kornfield R. Who's to blame: adolescent sexual activity. *J Adolescence* 1985;8 (1):17–31.
37. Kisker EE. The effectiveness of family planning clinics in serving adolescents. *Family Planning Perspectives* 1984;16(5):212–218.
38. Zabin LA, Clark SD. Why they delay: a study of teenage family planning clinic patients. *Family Planning Perspectives* 1981;13(5):205–217.
39. Digest. Contraception is less risky for teenagers than is pregnancy, worldwide study finds. *Family Planning Perspectives* 1982;14(5):274–276.
40. Hatcher RA, Stewart GK, Stewart FH, et al. *Contraceptive Technology 1984–1985* (12th ed). New York: Irvington Publications, Inc. 1984:9.
41. Ryan GM, Sweeney PJ. Attitudes of adolescents toward pregnancy and contraception. *Am J Obstet Gynecol* 1980;137:358–362.
42. Hendricks LE. Unmarried black adolescent fathers' attitudes toward abortion, contraception, and sexuality: a preliminary report. *J Adolescent Health Care* 1982;2(3):199–203.
43. Kisker EE. Teenagers talk about sex, pregnancy and contraception. *Family Planning Perspectives* 1985;17(2):83–90.
44. Hofman Ad. Contraception in adolescence: a review. Biomedical aspects. *WHO Bull* 1984;62(2):331–344.
45. Hatcher RA, Stewart GK, Stewart FH, et al. *Contraceptive Technology 1984–1985* (12th ed). New York: Irvington Publications, Inc., 1984;16.
46. Issues in contraceptive development. *Population* May 1985;No. 15:1–16.

Bibliography

Advisory on Toxic-Shock Syndrome. *FDA Drug Bulletin* 1980;10:10–11.

Barnes EF. *Ambulatory Maternal Health Care and Family Planning Services.* Washington, DC: American Public Health Association, 1978.

Barnes HV, Berger R. An approach to the obese adolescent. *Med Clin North Am* 1975;59:1507–1516.

Barnes RC, Holmes KK. Epidemiology of gonorrhea: current perspectives. *Epidemiologic Reviews* 1984;6:1–30.

Binkin NJ, Koplan JP, Cates W. Preventing neonatal herpes: the value of weekly viral cultures in pregnant women with recurrent genital herpes. *JAMA* 1984;251 (21):2816–2821.

Brewer GS. *What Every Pregnant Woman Should Know: The Truth About Diets and Drugs in Pregnancy.* New York: Random House, 1977.

Capraro VJ. Gynecologic examination in children and adolescents. *Pediatr Clin North Am* 1972;19(3):511–528.

Carruth BR, Iszler J. Assessment and conservative management of the overfat adolescent. *J Adolescent Health Care* 1981;1:289–299.

Cohen MI. Importance, implementation, and impact of the adolescent medicine components of the task force on pediatric education. *J Adolescent Health Care* 1980;1:1–8.

Cupit LG. Contraception: helping patients choose. *JOGN Nursing*(supplement) 1984;March/April:23s–29s.

Daniel WA. An approach to the adolescent patient. *Med Clin North Am* 1975;59:1281–1287.

Dickey RP. *Managing Contraceptive Pill Patients* (4th ed). Durant OK: Creative Infomatics, Inc., 1984.

Durant RH, Jay MS, Linder CW, et al. Influence of psychosocial factors on adolescent compliance with oral contraceptives. *J Adolescent Health Care* 1984;5(1):1–6.

Dryfoos JG, Heisler T. Contraceptive services for adolescents: an overview. *Family Planning Perspectives* 1978;10(4):223–233.

Ehrenreich B, English D. *Complaints and Disorders: The Sexual Politics of Sickness*. New York: The Feminist Press, 1973.

Emans SJ, Goldstein DP. *Pediatric and Adolescent Gynecology*. Boston: Little, Brown & Co., 1977.

Freeman EW, Rickels K, Huggins GR, et al. Urban black adolescents who obtain contraceptive services before or after their first pregnancy. 1984;5(3):183–190.

Friedman IM, Goldberg E. Reference materials for the practice of adolescent medicine. *Pediatr Clin North Am* 1980;27:193–208.

Furstenburg FF. Contraceptive continuation among adolescents attending family planning clinics. *Family Planning Perspectives* 1983;15(5):211–217.

Gantt PA, McDonough PG. Adolescent dysmenorrhea. *Pediatr Clin North Am* 1981;28(2):389–395.

Gallagher JR, Heald FP, Garell DC (eds). *Medical Care of the Adolescent* (3rd ed). New York: Appleton-Century-Crofts, 1976.

Gazella JG. *Nutrition for the Childbearing Years*. Wayzata, MN: Woodland, 1979.

Goodhart RS, Shils ME. *Modern Nutrition in Health and Disease*. Philadelphia: Lea & Febiger, 1980.

Hammerschlag MK. Sexually transmitted diseases in children and adolescents. *Med Aspects of Human Sexuality* 1984;18(7):77–83.

Hatcher RA, Stewart GK, Stewart FH, et al. *Contraceptive Technology 1980–1981* (10th ed). New York: Irvington Publishers, Inc., 1981.

Hatcher RA, Stewart GK, Stewart FH, et al. *Contraceptive Technology 1982–1983* (11th ed). New York: Irvington Publishers, Inc., 1982.

Hawkins JW, Higgins LP. *Health Care of Women: Gynecological Assessment*. Monterey, CA: Wadsworth Health Sciences Division, 1982.

Heald FP. *Adolescent Nutrition and Growth*. London: Appleton-Century-Crofts, 1969.

Herbst AL, Ulfelder H, Poskanzer DC. Adenocarcinoma of the vagina: association of maternal stilbestrol therapy with tumor appearance in young women. *New Engl J Med* 1971;284:878.

Hoffman PG. Primary dysmenorrhea and the premenstrual syndrome. In: *Office Gynecology* (2nd ed). Glass RH. Baltimore: Williams & Wilkins, 1981.

Hogan DP, Astone NM, Kitagawa EM. Social and environmental factors influencing contraceptive use among black adolescents. *Family Planning Perspectives* 1985;17 (4):165-169.

Huffman JW, Dewhurst Sir J, Capraro VJ (eds). The *Gynecology of Childhood and Adolescence.* Eastbourne: W.B. Saunders Co., 1981.

Hurley LS. *Developmental Nutrition.* Englewood Cliffs, NJ: Prentice-Hall, Inc. 1980.

Jay MS, Durant RH, Shoffitt T, et al. Effect of peer counselors on adolescent compliance in use of oral contraceptives. *Pediatrics* 1984;73(2):126-131.

Jelliffe DB, Jelliffe EF (eds). *Nutrition and Growth.* New York: Plenum Press, 1979.

Jones HW, Jones GS (eds). *Gynecology* (3rd ed). Baltimore: Williams & Wilkins, 1982.

Keen MA. The nurse practitioner in ambulatory gynecologic services. *Clin Obstet Gynecol* 1979;22(2):445-453.

King L. *The Cervical Cap Handbook for Users and Fitters.* Iowa City, IO: Iowa City Women's Press, 1981.

Klein JR. Update: adolescent gynecology. *Pediatr Clin North Am* 1980;27(1):141-152.

Koenig MA, Zelnik M. Repeat pregnancies among metropolitan-area teenagers: 1971-1979. *Family Planning Perspectives* 1982;14(6):341-344.

Kols MA, Rinehart W, Piotrow PT, et al. Oral contraceptives. *Population Reports* Series A 1982;No. 6 May/June.

Kramer DG, Brolon ST. Sexually transmitted diseases and infertility. *Int J Gynecol Obstet* 1984;22:19-27.

Kreuther PA. *Nutrition in Perspective.* Englewood Cliffs, NJ: Prentice-Hall, Inc., 1980.

Kulig JW. Adolescent contraception: an update. *Pediatrics* (suppl) 1985:675-680.

Landsberger BH. Adolescents' health status: sex differences among whites and non-whites. *J Adolescent Health Care* 1981;2(1):9-18.

Lane CL, Kemp J. Family planning needs of adolescents. *JOGN Nursing* (suppl) 1984;March/April:61s-65s.

Leichtman SR, Friedman SB. Social and psychological development of adolescents and the relationship to chronic illness. *Med Clin North Am* 1975;59:1319-1328.

Loevsky J. Menstruation: alternatives to pharmacological therapy for menstrual distress. *J Nurse Midwif* 1978;23:34-43.

Marcy SA, Brown JS, Danielson R. Contraceptive use by adolescent females in relation to knowledge, and to time and method of contraceptive counseling. *Research in Nursing and Health* 1983;6:175-182.

Marino DD, King JC. Nutritional concerns during adolescence. *Pediatr Clin North Am* 1980;27:125-139.

Mitchell GW. The gynecologist and breast disease. *Clin Obstet Gynecol* 1977;20(4):865-880.

Moore KA, Wertheimer RF. Teenage childbearing and welfare: preventive and ameliorative strategies. *Family Planning Perspectives* 1984;16(6):285-289.

Namerow PB, Jones JE. Ethnic variation in adolescent use of a contraceptive service. *J Adolescent Health Care* 1982;3(3):165-172.

Namerow PB, Philliber SG. The effectiveness of contraceptive programs for teenagers. *J Adolescent Health Care* 1982;2:189-198.

Nathanson CA, Becker MH. The influence of client-provider relationships on teenage women's subsequent use of contraception. *Am J Public Health* 1985; 75(1):33–38.

Parlee MB. Social factors in the psychology of menstruation, birth, and menopause. *Primary Care* 1976;3(3):477–483.

Rose SD. The periodic health examination. *Primary Care* 1980;7(4):653–665.

Schrag K. The adolescent's first gynecological exam. *J Nurse Midwif* 1978;23:20–24.

Shen JTY. *The Clinical Practice of Adolescent Medicine*. New York: Appleton-Century-Crofts, 1980.

Special report: the pill after 25 years. *Contraceptive Technology Update* 1985;6(1):1–24.

Strassburg MA, Baker CJ, Minkowski W, Friedlander L. Immunity to vaccine preventable diseases among detainees at a juvenile hall facility. *J Adolescent Health Care* 1982 3(2):91–95.

Strax P. Screening for breast cancer. *Clin Obstet Gynecol* 1977;20(4):781–801.

Taylor D. Contraceptive counseling and care. In: *Perspectives on Adolescent Health Care*. Mercer RT (ed). Philadelphia: J.B. Lippincott Co., 1979.

Tyrer LB. Oral contraception for the adolescent. *J Reprod Med* (suppl) 1984;29(7):551–556.

Tyrer LB, Josimovich J. Contraception in teenagers. *Clin Obstet Gynecol* 1977;20 (3):651–663.

Washington AE. Chlamydia: a major threat to reproductive health. San Francisco: Institute for Health Policy Studies, 1984; 2(1):1–3.

Winick M. *Adolescent Nutrition*. New York: John Wiley & Sons, 1982.

Winick M (ed). *Nutrition: Pre- and Postnatal Development*. New York: Plenum Press, 1979.

Zabin LS, Hirsch MB, Smith EA, et al. Adolescent sexual attitudes and behavior: are they consistent? *Family Planning Perspectives* 1984;16(4):181–185.

Zelnik M, Koenig M, Kim YJ. Sources of prescription contraceptives and subsequent pregnancy among young women. *Family Planning Perspectives* 1984;16(1):6–14.

4 Psychological Aspects of Adolescence

LANE M. HOLLAND, *coauthor*

Overview of Adolescence

Adolescence is the transitional period of human development between childhood and adulthood. This stage of development is the adaptation of identity versus role diffusion followed by the state of intimacy versus isolation (1). Within this developmental progression are the elements of autonomy, cognitive changes, and achievement. This psychological growth process proceeds through emotional separations and attachments. The developmental tasks of adolescence include (2)

1. becoming comfortable with one's own body,
2. striving for independence,
3. building relationships with the same and opposite sexes,
4. seeking economic and social stability,
5. developing a value system,
6. learning to verbalize conceptually.

The adolescent's thought processes change from concrete and egocentric thinking to abstract conceptualization and the ability to appreciate another's perspective. These changes in thought patterns affect feelings, attitudes, judgments, values, and goals. The purpose of this psychological growth is to arrive at a stable sense of self or ego identity, primarily through adaptation and resourcefulness.

During the stages of individuation there is an opportunity to modify or rectify childhood needs. Sexual maturation and physical changes initiate mental changes reflected in all aspects of behavior. Delinquent behavior may result from role diffusion where one's identity is doubtful or unstable. There are various stages of experimentation and rebellion that test and form the identity. A vivid fantasy life precedes role-taking behaviors which evolve into role internalization. Defenses, such as asceticism or intellectualization, are unconscious responses that protect the emerging self. Values are also developed as consciousness matures. This movement from dependent child role to independent adult role is expressed in the attainment of a sense of identity and purpose.

Preadolescence

During preadolescence, from 10 to 12 years of age, many physical and psychological changes occur. Compulsive behaviors, single-mindedness or obsessional thoughts may be seen. Conformity to peer group standards is observed through dressing, looking, and acting alike. A brief homosexual phase may be experienced. Tension outlets such as stomach aches, headaches, nail biting, stuttering and hair twirling are common in this age group.

These behaviors continue during the early adolescent period from 12 to 14 years of age. The renunciation of parents as primary love objects begins with seeking new love objects. The turmoil and conflict between family members commences, especially between the adolescent and her parents. The adolescent vacillates between child-like and adult behaviors. She may criticize her parents or find parental discipline difficult to accept while continuing to seek parental love and the stability of her family life. Close, idealized friendships with the same sex become particularly important. Girlfriends can be used as mother substitutes as the adolescent tries to detach herself from her mother. Time is spent away from the family and more time is devoted to friends. Activities with the same sex or in groups are popular during this period.

The young adolescent is interested in her developing body and is concerned with the changes affecting her appearance. She may be more self-conscious now and have a lower self-esteem because of this unstable self-image. Because early or late physical development may feel threatening the adolescent constantly compares herself to her friends and peers. An increased amount of time is spent in front of mirrors or in the bath in self-exploration and grooming. These physical and psychological changes foster a developing sense of femininity. Narcissism as well as bisexual feelings are common. Fleeting, superficial homosexual contacts may occur but do not signify a permanent sexual preference. A rich fantasy life is present and often results in "crushes."

During early adolescence, cognitive thought is dominated by descriptive comments of current circumstances or literal, "here and now" interpretations. In seeking a self-identity, the early adolescent adopts an egocentric style while reorganizing her emotional life. Social awareness, intellectual interests and athletic activities are aroused. The early adolescent may feel insecure with her newly formed interests and judgments and may seek "mentors" and other outside influences to help her adjust to her changing self-image.

Mid-adolescence

During middle adolescence, ages 15 to 16, the adolescent disengages from her parents as she renounces them as love objects. With this separation, a differentiation of the self occurs. The adolescent searches for other object relations and begins to build new, meaningful relationships with the same and opposite sexes. Narcissistic and bisexual positions are abandoned for interests in heterosexual love. It is usually a time of peak turmoil for families. The adolescent often displays new hostile behaviors, with arguments providing a ground for information gathering and testing new roles. New behaviors are tried and their potential and acceptability are explored. Menarche usually occurs during this stage and may cause the adolescent to identify again with her mother as a reproductive prototype.

Emotions vacillate during this period of heightened self-perception and self-absorption. Reality testing is common and may lead to hypersensitivity. It is often a time when the discovery and appreciation of nature and beauty occurs. During middle adolescence the dramatic and creative aspects of the personality are prevalent. Fantasy, intuition and empathy are demonstrated in the keeping of a diary or journal. During this time of character formation, the adolescent may also choose strict disciplines of self-induced exertion, pain, or exhaustion. Defense mechanisms of asceticism, intellectualization, and uniformity may also be observed. Allegiance to the peer group is signified by tastes in music, clothing and language. During this period adolescents may begin risk-taking behaviors in an effort to prove themselves to their peers. They may also use an "imaginary device" where they believe they are the focus of attention as they develop their sense of self-worth.

Middle adolescence is a time of sexual experimentation. The middle adolescent, in adapting to body changes, will utilize clothing and make-up to develop a satisfactory body image. The sexual identity is beginning to form. Usually, "tender love" will precede a heterosexual experience. Transitory homosexual episodes may also occur.

Changes in cognitive functioning occur during middle adolescence. Instead of concrete thinking, formal operational thought begins. The adolescent starts to reason deductively to solve problems and analyze situations. The sequence of an argument can be logically maintained. The adolescent begins to understand complex symbols, words, and concepts enabling her to speak and think in a more adult fashion. This new cognitive thinking, however, may regress during times of stress.

Late Adolescence

Late adolescence extends generally from age 17 to 21, although the actual endpoint of adolescence is less clearly defined. Earlier conflicts between the adolescent and her parents subside. The late adolescent is able to perceive and evaluate her parents more realistically and a more adult relationship forms between them. During this period, the adolescent usually takes the final step in achieving independence and separation from her parents by moving away from home. The adolescent is now able to maintain stable relationships and attachments. She is more aware of the strengths and weaknesses of others. The peer group loses its importance and often its influence over the adolescent. Individual dating becomes more popular than group activities. Often, the first intimate relationship with the opposite sex develops. The sexual identity is established and is usually irreversible.

With the separation from childhood attachments comes a new concept of self and new commitments or attachments. In late adolescence, there is an appreciation of newly found capabilities, skills and talents. New ideas and ideals are followed by new goals and values as the adolescent assumes responsibility for her own thoughts, work, sexuality and lifestyle. A growing self-respect is seen as well as more predictable, less chaotic behavior. The adolescent is able to make decisions about future educational and career goals as her identity becomes clearer. Late adolescence is characterized by purposeful action, social integration and emotional constancy. Social roles are defined and articulated. Idealism is often expressed during late adolescence. In some cases, such idealism results in the joining of movements, religious groups, causes or cults.

During late adolescence, cognitive thinking continues to develop. The adolescent is able to verbalize conceptually, using more advanced, formal operational thought. This understanding of figurative speech and abstract thought is necessary for further academic education. With stable ego and cognitive functioning, the adolescent can view problems comprehensively, making delay and compromise possible. The assimilation and integration of ideas forms the basis for the identification process. Furthermore, the adolescent is able to develop a philosophy of life by questioning such moral concepts as life, death, war and religion.

Conclusion

Adolescence is a time of forming new, satisfying goals and identifications based on cultural expectations during a period of rapid physical, psychological and social change. Maturity is associated with such factors as achievement of an appropriate degree of independence, sexual identification, a secure identity, a suitable vocation, and a place in society (3). Individual variations seen in adolescence are affected by differences in culture, socioeconomic status, mobility, family unity, media influence and many other factors. These differences are demonstrated in the polarities found in adolescence: submission/rebellion, gregariousness/withdrawal, sensitivity/coarseness, optimism/hopelessness, indulgence/ascetism, exuberance/sluggishness, and dedication/indifference (4).

The adolescent is trying to define who she is not only through her own eyes but also through the eyes of others. The pressures to achieve or conform are weighed against the realities of sociocultural conflicts, educational expectations, unemployment and serious family discord. As childhood ends, the adolescent may feel lonely, confused and isolated. The reality of aging and death can lead to fear or panic. While family ties are being severed, adolescents need human love and understanding to dispel their fears.

Risk-taking behaviors are common and can result in injury or death. These behaviors are often based on "personal fable": a belief that one is in some way special or invincible. This attitude can be seen in such activities as smoking, alcohol or drug abuse, dangerous driving, some sporting activities, promiscuity and some sexual behaviors, preventable accidents, violent behavior or attempted suicide, and running away or dropping out.

If the adolescent feels unprepared to assume responsibility for herself and her independence, instability can result. The impact of this stress on the adolescent is seen in identity diffusion, manic-depressive psychoses, suicidal depression, acting out behaviors, or anorexia nervosa. Warning signs of instability in the adolescent are a decrease in school performance, being a "loner," or continuous somatization.

Normal adolescence involves excitement, disappointment, love, loss, anger, joy and a sense of being alone. When there are no family supports to help the adolescent cope with her changing emotions and contain her distress, the uncertainty can lead to vulnerability and regression. Family support may be unavailable in today's society of self-absorption, mobility and divorce. Encouragement and understanding are missing when the home environment is inconsistent. Parents can contribute to the positive development of the adolescent's identity. Four factors which can lead to mature independence in adolescence are good family communication, enhancing the adolescent's self-image, teaching effective decision-making and effective discipline (5).

It is the responsibility of families, schools and health care providers to assist the adolescent on the difficult road to maturity and adulthood. Our abilities to understand, reassure and set examples are critical in helping the adolescent successfully achieve her goals. Adolescents are a challenge to themselves and society, and yet they are our future and our hope.

Developmental Tasks Related to Adolescent Pregnancy

The developmental tasks of pregnancy have been well documented by Duvall and Rubin. When these tasks are imposed on an adolescent who is at an early point in her psychosocial/cognitive development, the risk that both she and her baby may suffer negative psychosocial repercussions is enhanced.

Acceptance

The initial task for any pregnant adolescent is obvious. She must first recognize and accept the pregnancy. One of the earliest tasks is locating a person in whom the adolescent can confide. Because of possible ambivalence and apprehension, the choice of someone to confide in is a significant choice for her. This is after, or in conjunction with, confirmation of the pregnancy. Missed menstrual periods or physical changes serve as initial clues to possible pregnancy. If she has included her confidant in an earlier discussion of a questionable pregnancy, their joint decision may encourage her to go for a pregnancy test. Once she has overcome this first hurdle she must face the responsibility of telling her parents.

Even though the adolescent may be striving for independence from parental authority, the pregnancy places her in a precarious and needy position that returns her to a level of emotional dependence. The desire for prepared acceptance and concern about parental response, along with other factors such as "denial" of the pregnancy and the existence of poor communication between herself and her parents, may contribute to the initial delay in sharing news of the pregnancy.

With the initial help of a confidant (who may be the father of the baby, a close friend, or a sister) the adolescent may decide to terminate the pregnancy. She may also decide to do it with only the support of the confidant or family member other than her mother or father. Even with this initial resolution, many adolescents will need to inform their parents. How, where and when this occurs is as varied as the adolescent herself.

Family, in whatever form it takes, is important to its members as a supportive and nurturing base. Functions of families are varied and almost unlimited. The ability of the family to define new roles, rights, actions and duties required is considered one of its unique characteristics (6). The family as a fundamental social unit is of major importance in our society. One of its key functions is determining character and structure of society through character building of those individuals entrusted to it.

The family is viewed as an integral subsystem within our larger societal order. Crises and conflicts that develop within this subsystem are usually the end result of changes in environmental, cultural and social conditions (7). As a social system, the family composition includes individuals who are bound together because certain ideologies interact with each other on various level' in an attempt to maintain a constant state of equilibrium (8). One important dimension of this social system is an ability to provide to members and nonmembers of the family unit necessary functions, whether they are expressive, instrumental or both (9). Expressive functions include the ability to establish relationships with family members (i.e., love, friendship and affection), and the subtle yet determined and complex ways that members of families relate to each other, instruct each other and develop or deflate each other's sense of dignity and self worth (10). Instrumental family functions also include those concerned with providing the basic necessities of life: food, clothing, shelter, health care and the acquisition of occupational skills (10).

A study of families has identified several components that address themselves to strengths of the family. These include:

1. a concern for family unity, loyalty, and inter-family cooperation.
2. an ability for self help and the ability to accept help when appropriate.
3. an ability to perform family roles flexibly.
4. an ability to establish and maintain growth producing relationships within and without the family.
5. the ability to provide for the physical, emotional and spiritual needs of a family (11).

The degree to which these strengths are evident and workable on some level within the family must be directly related to how often each one has been needed at some point. Some families may function on a much higher level in relation to some of the strengths than others (10). Looking at how families respond to what is determined by them as a crisis becomes an indicator of the internal dynamics of the unit, but three factors have been identified that would make a person subject to viewing a situation as a crisis (12). One is perception of the event. Based on previous experiences, philosophies and levels of emotional response, what is perceived as traumatic or life-changing to one individual may be considered challenging or completely non-threatening to another. Another is situational supports available to an individual. How a person views herself in relation to her family, peer group or colleagues carries substantial weight in her being able to handle situations that arise. The third factor is the development of coping mechanisms.

Crises that occur as people mature are considered as developmental or maturational crises (13). These are expected as a result of the on-going life process and can occur at various levels or stages of life. There are also anticipated crises identified as unexpected, situational, or accidental. Examples of maturational crises include starting high school or college, reaching adolescence or old age. Examples of accidental crises include loss of a significant other, body part, or job, or an unexpected pregnancy.

Reaching adolescence may, therefore, be viewed as a maturational crisis for both the adolescent and the family. While the adolescent is experiencing changes in sexual identity, establishing values of her own that may be different from those of her parents, learning a vocational goal and developing a sense of responsibility, her preparing for the inevitable physical and emotional separation from their child (14).

The occurrence of an out-of-wedlock pregnancy disrupts the family's usual lifestyle (13). When this occurs, attempts must be made to refocus priorities and adjust to the situation. The unwed adolescent places the family unit in a state of "imbalance." Her mother may feel a variety of emotions including anger that her daughter has been sexually active, failure as a mother, and a possible despondency if she feels the pregnancy will circumvent her goals for her daughter. The adolescent may not have a full understanding of family psychology, but she does understand the possibility of loss or alienation and thus only delays informing the family to avoid this outcome.

The actual task of informing the parent(s) can be accomplished in a variety of ways. The adolescent may tell her mother herself. Her confidant or another family member may fulfill this role for her. The adolescent's mother may be approached by the suspicions of an older sibling or relative, forcing the parent to confront the adolescent. Often parents suspect their daughters' pregnancy but wait for confirmation from the adolescent.

When an adolescent pregnancy occurs in a family it is an interactional event between parent and child. As health care providers, it is impossible to trust our initial perceptions of how an adolescent and her family are responding to the pregnancy. It is many times a private grief that is not publicly displayed.

The task of informing parents is followed by the task of reaching a terminal resolution or an agreement about management of the pregnancy. For many adolescents the decision to continue or terminate the pregnancy is made for them. Moreover, because of religious or strong moral conviction, abortion may not be an option to be considered, and often parents continue to play an authoritarian role even with the advent of a new "mother" in the household.

If the parents and daughter reach agreement about the pregnancy or the decision is made for the adolescent and she accepts that decision, a terminal resolution has been achieved. If an agreement cannot be reached (i.e., daughter desires a therapeutic abortion or to continue pregnancy while parent desires the opposite), there is a state of variance. Unless a compromise or reconciliation can be achieved, this disagreement may result in a physical separation that may extend beyond the therapeutic abortion or delivery. The return to a compatible relationship may take time and intervention by professionals who can provide both support and counseling.

Responsibility

The adolescent years are also viewed as a narcissistic period of life. For the adolescent the world revolves around her and her concerns. She has for the most part been given limited responsibility for others and herself. Throughout the adolescent years her self-concept is developing and ideas for future goals are, at best, limited. If there has been little or no chance to participate in clubs or organizations that foster leadership potential and skills in group dynamics, the adolescent has little to draw from in this area. If she is an older sister she may have an awareness of the responsibility involved in child care resulting from her experience taking care of and overseeing siblings.

By carrying her pregnancy to term, the pregnant adolescent has certain obligations to herself and to her unborn child. The basic and most important obligations are early and consistent prenatal care, adequate nutrition, rest and exercise. Evaluating and screening for problems that present at a certain age or according to race is considered routine procedure at most institutions.

A continual challenge in working with pregnant adolescents is finding ways to encourage early registration for prenatal care. For some adolescents, this care may be their first entry into any type of health care system. In this setting, these adolescents are required to function as adults and are bombarded with interviews, information, and forms to complete. If the adolescent comes to the clinic alone or is dealing with other stresses related to her pregnancy, she may respond minimally to the responsibility of her pregnancy. The adolescent who has accepted her pregnancy can be guided through the use of age-appropriate written material, classes and group discussion. However, even with careful evaluation and management care plans, adolescents will sometimes arrive at the clinic with a soda in one hand and a chocolate cupcake in the other. Accepting some behavior as typically adolescent and not as an acting-out or hostile response to pregnancy will enable the care provider to maintain concern for the population served and remain committed on an individual basis.

Each adolescent must be evaluated individually to determine her ability to accept the responsibilities of her pregnancy. Therefore, visible symptoms of stress and aspects of her personality can be significant indications that she is at risk for limited compliance to prenatal. Other signals seen in later visits may be influenced by religion and culture. The adolescent may be denied her previous family and support systems with the discovery of her pregnancy and thus feel alienated.

The beginning of puberty presents various physiological changes requiring certain psychological adjustments. Depending on the degree of preparation, most adolescents adjust with minimal anxiety; however, most adolescents are overly concerned with the developing shapes and contours of their bodies. They spend inordinate amounts of time in front of mirrors assessing clothing, hairstyles and makeup that will accentuate these changes, and they undertake crash or fad diets. During pregnancy dieting is often disguised as poor appetite. When a girl becomes pregnant, she must abandon normal adolescent behavior in favor of what is considered "positive" by an adult authority figure. In an area where she had some control, she is now dictated to by her body and by adult authority figures from whom she was striving to achieve independence. The explanation that her body will return to its prepregnant state 6 to 8 weeks postpartum means bodily changes for a year that may seem interminable to her. Consequently, if she lacks a support system or method for expressing her emotions, she is at risk for depression and negative compliance.

Older adolescents frequently express fears about sexual intercourse during pregnancy. They fear, as all pregnant women do, that intercourse will harm the fetus. Such concerns signify acceptance of not only their sexuality but also of their pregnancy. The young or mid-adolescent may have difficulty voicing these concerns. When she is silent or denies an interest in sex, it does not necessarily mean that the information is not needed. Consequently, an adolescent often asks questions about sex at a later point in her pregnancy when she has reached a greater comfort level with her care provider.

Adolescence is characterized by identity crises and confrontations over the conflicting pull of peer group authority and parental authority. The need to identify with peers creates anxiety and at times feelings of insecurity. Most adolescents are able to negotiate these sometimes intense experiences and advance to a level of maturity. At a time when the pregnant adolescent seeks independence from her parents and struggles to make decisions on her own, pregnancy forces her to become psychologically dependent, creating conflict.

Some adolescents are subject to temporary dismissal from their homes, denied further contact with their boyfriends, and are repeatedly lectured to on the subject of their pregnancy. Others, because of their pregnancy, are expected to assume an adult role instantly. Such attitudes frequently occur in response to the news that a teenage daughter is pregnant. Unfortunately, these attitudes leave little room for the adolescent to discuss her feelings. Parental threats cause her to behave submissively, which does not do well for the future relationship between her and her family. Although pregnancy is considered a positive influence on mothers and daughters, many adolescents find it stressful to maintain a positive relationship with their mothers throughout pregnancy.

Other factors that affect the interpersonal development between a pregnant adolescent and her parents include her rank in the family hierarchy (only child vs. siblings), the family's socioeconomic status, the family's feelings toward the baby's father, and whether or not this is the first out-of-wedlock pregnancy in the family.

If the adolescent leaves her home and moves in with a relative, that person often becomes the arbitrator between the adolescent and her parents. Negotiations may continue for the length of the pregnancy, with provisions made for the adolescent's return home after the baby is born or for placing the infant for adoption or foster care. Some adolescents leave home because they consider their mother's behavior inhibiting or smothering and express frustration with the mother's attempt to claim the pregnancy for their own.

The strengths required to deal with parents and relatives often depend on the quality of the adolescent's relationship with her boyfriend. When the current boyfriend is the father of the baby and the pregnancy is wanted, the boyfriend's support enables the pregnant adolescent to communicate more effectively. The loss of a boyfriend is the loss of a potential support person.

A pregnant adolescent's continuing relationship with her peer group depends on this group's perception of adolescent pregnancy. In some groups, pregnancy may increase a sense of camaraderie and support. This camaraderie is often demonstrated by attendance at prenatal visits with the pregnant adolescent, purchasing baby gifts or giving baby showers, and even acting as the coach or support person during labor and delivery.

Developing Mothering Behavior

Another task that takes place during pregnancy is the assimilation of mothering behavior. There are a variety of ways this is achieved, one being observation. Watching older family members and participating in the care of siblings provides for exposure to and practice in developing child care skills. Friends who have babies present another practical opportunity for the pregnant adolescent to gain experience in childrearing. Like other pregnant women some adolescents, consciously or subconsciously, tend to put themselves in environments, that provide opportunities for child care practice.

It is not uncommon to rehearse mothering patterns mentally, or confirm them verbally, when other pregnant women or friends are present. Also included in the preparatory process is the acquisition of know-how through magazines, television programs and books on the subject of parenting. Because of our mobile society, family, neighbors, and close friends are often inaccessible as role models.

Age, environment and commitment to the pregnancy affect an adolescent's ability to mother a child successfully. For example, an adolescent must understand that an infant needs more for survival than a layette and a formula supply. The mature adolescent will incorporate information about child care and recognize the need for assistance when indicated. A supportive environment will also encourage her to develop appropriate maternal behaviors. Moreover, commitment to the child will motivate the mature adolescent to find a supportive environment if one is not readily available, and to seek appropriate health care and financial assistance for her baby. Further commitment to the mothering role is evident if she discusses the need to prevent future pregnancies and identifies her intent to remain in school.

It is difficult for the immature pregnant adolescent to focus beyond her own needs to those of her infant. Consequently, her ability to develop mothering skills may be limited and result in relinquishing the care of her own infant to mother. Moreover, the adolescent's own need to be nurtured conflicts with her changing role as the care giver rather than the receiver.

Discussion with the adolescent during her pregnancy about child care will reveal areas that require clarification or specific teaching. Helping her at this point to distinguish between truth and the fiction of old wives tales is part of the constructive education that can occur during pregnancy. However, the most significant teaching will actually begin during the immediate postpartum period when observation of mother-child interactions is possible. Attending classes or watching bedside demonstrations is also a non-threatening way for the postpartal adolescent mother to learn. In such situations she will not feel singled out, can observe other new mothers and recognize that they have some of the same questions and anxieties that she has. If the health care provider has questions or concerns related to the adolescent's interaction with her child, a delay in discharge is indicated to give sufficient time to observe and monitor the behavior and allow for appropriate consultation.

Mothering skills are thought to be based on prior experiences and observations. Theoretically, the longer one has to experience and observe, the more efficient one's mothering skills become. Thus the adolescent mother, especially the young adolescent mother whose experiences and observations may be limited, requires more opportunities to observe mothering skills before she gives birth. Combining community resources and those of health care professionals is an appropriate approach to meet this need, and includes teaching mothering skills in health care institutions and community settings such as schools and public health departments.

It is no surprise that many pregnant adolescents have difficulty communicating their feelings to health care providers who are usually older and have significant control and authority over the adolescent's life and habits for the nine months of her pregnancy. In addition, health care providers are initially strangers who may impart discomfort and sometimes pain, however unintentional, on the fearful adolescent. Fortunately, these adolescents learn largely to trust their care providers and subsequently begin to communicate with them effectively. Adolescents who have been traumatized in some manner either before or after they became pregnant can remain withdrawn or overtly hostile despite attempts at communication. Others may exhibit passive aggressive behavior, which is often a plea for attention.

Attempting to establish a rapport with a reluctant adolescent at her first prenatal visit can be a difficult experience. Adequate explanations and an opportunity to ask questions may reduce or eliminate communication problems.

Options to Consider

Abortion

When a pregnancy occurs because of a contraceptive failure or a failure to use contraceptives, the adolescent is often in a predicament. Consequently, she may deny the pregnancy and delay finding professional help. Additional factors contributing to her behavior may include her financial status, misconceptons about abortion, her moral beliefs or fear of parental reaction.

For many adolescents, the cost of an abortion is a major obstacle and may be the decisive factor in their decision to forgo this choice. The alternative is to request financial aid. Such action requires recognition and acceptance of the pregnancy's reality. This may be too threatening. As a result, the pregnancy is retained through default and there may be a passive acceptance. Passive acceptance is less than a fully endorsed and active choice, and hence may manifest itself in future rejection of the child.

Misconception about an abortion's effect on future fertility is often quoted by adolescents as the reason they retained their pregnancies. Many adolescents believe that an abortion leads to sterility. While there is some truth in this belief, it is dependent on the woman's gravidity, the number of abortions that a woman has had and the type of procedure utilized by the physician. The procedure used in first trimester abortions, suction curettage, is not considered a threat to future fertility. Abortions done later in second trimester require a more extensive dilation of the cervix and sharp curettage. Women who become pregnant after this procedure do run a greater risk of mid-trimester spontaneous abortions and even an increased risk of low-birthweight infants. Because the adolescent tends to delay finding professional help in the first trimester, the result is often a second trimester abortion. Theoretically then, her future fertility could become a problem. This fact underlines the necessity to disperse reliable reproductive information to the adolescent community and correct some of their misconceptions.

Moral beliefs and fear of parental reaction are major concerns which affect not only adolescents but the whole population. Some adolescents have strong beliefs about the right to life for both the embryo and fetus. These adolescents will never consider an abortion. They have made an active and committed choice. Many others are naive and young and have not developed any philosophical beliefs. In fact, many are not matured sufficiently to do so. Without appropriate adult guidance, therefore, the influence of their peers may be the sole factor in their decision. This can limit the quality of that decision and the outcome will affect future generations. This is not meant to reflect on one philosophical belief versus another. It is meant to reflect on the limited and uninformed resources available to most adolescents and the impact that this has for both the adolescent and her future offspring.

Adolescents frequently fear parental reaction to their pregnancies, let alone a request for an abortion. This is natural and, in cases of parental child abuse, appallingly real. Many institutions require parental notification before they will perform an abortion on any minor. The Supreme Court in its 1983 summer opinion decided that mature minors need not obtain parental consent before having an abortion (15). The level of maturity is to be decided by the health professional caring for the adolescent. In the event that the health professional decides the adolescent is mature (i.e., understands the implications of an abortion and appears to have considered other alternatives such as adoption or raising the child herself) she may have an abortion without parental consent. If they determine that the adolescent is too young or immature to make such a decision, then parental permission is required and subsequently involves parental notice. The court's ruling does allow the adolescent an alternative. If the adolescent feels parental notification is totally unacceptable to her, she may seek the court's permission to obtain an abortion. It is hard to imagine that an adolescent who has been defined as immature will have the motivation, maturity and capability to successfully seek out that alternative. In essence, the system may program her into a situation which in effect leaves her little or no choice but to continue with the pregnancy unless, of course, she is willing to obtain her parents' consent. Additionally, to petition the court for permission to abort may require extended periods of time. Since time is vital to this procedure and most adolescents are not registered for abortions until late first or second trimester, it is essential that no additional time constraints be raised. If the court's docket is typical, it could take months to reach the court's attention. This would necessitate planning for an abortion before becoming pregnant! In fairness to the court, family courts do hear cases fairly quickly, but is an issue that bears recognition as a potential problem.

In spite of the obstacles, abortion rates for adolescents remain high. In 1977, it was estimated that 400,000 abortions were obtained by adolescents (16), while in 1982 there were an estimated 443,000 abortions reflecting the termination of approximately 40 percent of all adolescent pregnancies (27). Hence, while many adolescents do elect to have their babies, a fair number decide to have an abortion. Consequently, the health care provider is obligated to determine if a pregnant adolescent has been adequately informed about the options available to her. Obviously, if she does not register until late in pregnancy, she has forfeited any opportunity to have an abortion. On the other hand, if she has registered early enough to consider this, the presence of an option should be presented in a nonjudgmental but caring fashion. It is important that there is no attempt at coercion by the family, her peers or her partner to decide one way or the other for her. Of course this is difficult and may be impossible to control. If there is a suspicion of this coercion, the social worker intervenes. Certainly, few women can make a decision of this magnitude without first discussing it with friends or loved ones, and the adolescent is no exception. Indeed, families should be actively involved but should never become adversarial. Such a position would create more stress and make a difficult decision more complicated.

Klein reports that "adolescents who elect to abort lead a less disruptive life than those who give birth and rear a child" (17). According to Evans et al, adolescents who seek abortion also have personal and future goals superior to those who retain their pregnancies (18). This reflects itself in good performance in school and a tendency to return to school after an abortion. Alternately, Steinhoff states that adolescents who continue pregnancy do so because they have no other personal aspirations. If this is true it effectively eliminates a need to decide about abortion (19). Certainly, we all recognize that there are exceptions to Steinhoff's conclusion, but the widespread generality of truth in his statement must also be recognized.

In some circumstances an adolescent is forced to retain a pregnancy against her will. The repercussions in such a situation are formidable and may result in child abuse. Klein communicates that 58 percent of all abused children in Georgia had parents who began childbearing in their teens (17). This is a great concern when one considers the number of infants born to teenagers in this country, and the fact that most of those were unplanned and initially unwanted pregnancies. Since adoption is rarely selected by these teenage mothers, most babies stay with them and are reared by them. This necessitates close observation by health professionals, especially when the potential for child abuse is present or suspected.

Adolescents who have difficulty relating to and trusting others may have been abused as children, and abused children tend to become child abusers. Such adolescents have a poor self-image, have difficulty making decisions and setting priorities and have little comprehension of the principles concerning the rights of others. They find eye contact difficult, have problems relating to touch and have difficulty recognizing a difference between actions and feelings. Any adolescent who subsequently becomes pregnant to escape abuse herself has become pregnant for the wrong reasons. She has, in fact, been unable to note that unprotected intercourse and subsequent pregnancy are different from the desire to become pregnant, and thus she is expressing through her actions a characteristic of an abused child. If it is true that the abused adolescent has difficulty developing trust, recognizing the rights of others and relating through touch, her ability to become a good mother is seriously limited and the child's psychological growth and development are in jeopardy. Such an adolescent mother will expect unrealistic obedience and what she perceives to be correct responses. If her infant fails to meet her expectations, child abuse may result. This is evidenced by verbal criticism, physical abuse, or psychological and physical neglect of her child. Therefore, while we promote the quality of care for both the mother and baby in pregnancy, we must do likewise after birth. Child abuse is a repugnant reality. We need to make every attempt to identify its presence and, if possible, to do so before it has occurred. The clinician who is aware of an abused child's characteristics can identify their presence in pregnancy. If counseling is immediately begun, future child abuse may be successfully averted.

Adoption

The final option for the pregnant adolescent is adoption, although pregnant adolescents seldom select it. The reason probably reflects the philosophy of the time. Until the recent past, fear of an out-of-wedlock pregnancy was the Damocles sword which maintained a female's virginity until marriage removed its ominous shadow. Of course, now and then, wayward girls experienced its cutting edge and were shut off from society to experience their disgrace in private. Once delivered, a benevolent society adopted their infants and the young women returned to the mainstream of society minus the encumberance of an illegitimate child. While these wayward girls were, in fact, the source of a desired commodity for infertile couples, social manipulation was such that the young women were designated recipients who should express gratitude. Ultimately, the wayward girl removed the Damocles sword by accepting the consequences of lost virginity and a subsequent pregnancy. This had a drastic effect on the availability of children for adoption. It also changed society's attitudes toward out-of-wedlock pregnancy, especially in the urban areas. Thus a single woman with a child no longer experiences the social stigma attached to such a situation just a generation ago, and adoption opportunities have dropped accordingly.

Until 20 years ago, children born out-of-wedlock were often put up for adoption. However, because the process was such a covert one, little was ever done to discover its effects on the single mother. Since adoptions today are few and far between, the opportunity for study remains minimal. Some attempts have been made to identify potential issues. Future parenting is one such issue. Young women who had an out-of-wedlock pregnancy and elected adoption later, reported regret that they had done so. This was the finding of a study done between 1964 and 1980 on secret out-of-wedlock pregnancy (20,21). The subjects in the study were adolescent at the time of the pregnancy. Now older women with teenagers of their own, they find it difficult, if not impossible, to discuss this experience with their sons and daughters. They feel the decision about adoption was the right one but that the mistake occurred when they exposed themselves to the possibility of pregnancy. Hence, they are over-protective of their adolescents and this attitude results in family discord. They report spying on their daughters and express a general suspicion of any dating activity enjoyed by their children.

The same behavior is found in fathers who relinquished their children when they were teenagers and is true whether relinquishment occurred through formal adoption or as an abandonment.

A frequent reaction by their children to such scrutiny is rebellion. The child's rebellious behavior just adds fuel to parental concerns, however, and increases the intensity of their surveillance. Since the parents' reason for surveillance is never shared with their children, discord, distrust and disharmony result. In truth, a child and sibling have been lost by this family, but without acknowledgment, opportunity to express grief is limited and may in fact remain unresolved. Active repression of grief is destined to erupt in overt behaviors which may take their form in negative conduct. The ripple effect is obvious.

The health care provider is in a unique position to prevent this negative outcome. If proper counseling is done with the adolescent when she chooses adoption for her baby, successful relationships with her future children will inevitably result. If she does not learn to "let go" of that first child, "letting go" of future children when they become teenagers may create unnecessary family turmoil. For that mother the concern may not be that she fears her teenage son or daughter will repeat her mistake, but rather that she fears the loss of another child to another human being. If adequately helped at the time that an adoption decision is made, the mother may overcome future parenting problems and successfully "let go" of her newborn. This does not mean that she will forever erase the memory of this child from her emotions and her life's experiences. On the contrary, it means she can recognize the memory of this child, the reality of its existence and its right to a present in which she does not share.

Conclusion

The after-effects of pregnancy for the adolescent mother who keeps her child are well documented throughout this book. The emotional after-effects of abortion are generally considered minimal (22). However, other authors report that teens are more apt than older women to develop "sadness, guilt, anxiety and depression after an induced abortion" (16). The reason for this reaction may be directly related to the degree of support received from significant others in the adolescent's world. If parental or boyfriend support is lacking, anxiety and guilt may result; and if no opportunity for counseling is available, the emotional residue may be permanent. Once again the health care provider has an important role to play. Time and opportunity for discussion is included as part of the abortion decision. Without it the adolescent who lacks family support may be denied sufficient resolution. This outcome could affect her attitude toward future childbearing experiences.

The male partners of pregnant adolescents who elect abortion or adoption generally have little or insignificant follow-up. Consequently, it is difficult to determine what their needs might be. The suspicion is that their needs are similar to their female counterparts. Unhappily, the adolescent father is often hard to identify or slow to respond to communication attempts by health care providers. This is especially true in view of Hendricks' (23) findings. He found that most black adolescent males in his study who were responsible for their girlfriends' pregnancy would not want them to have an abortion. The prevalent reason was "it is wrong." If that is their feeling, and their female partner elects an abortion, it is obvious that they need to discuss these feelings. Yet few ever have this opportunity. It is a flaw in adolescent health care which every attempt should be made to alter.

There is no totally successful option for the pregnant adolescent. All of the options require support from families, significant others, peers and health care personnel. As the adolescent goes through the steps of consideration, resources are made available to allow discussion and resolution when she elects either an abortion or adoption. If she selects pregnancy and parenting, which a substantial number will, she will require counseling and support for an extensive period of time after delivery in order to make a successful transition to parenting. If she chooses an abortion she will require an opportunity both before and after the abortion to discuss her feelings about her decision. If she elects adoption for her newborn, she will need counseling support through the process of "letting go."

Counseling requires commitment, patience and time. It is often difficult to find the required time and the necessary energy to deal with the emotional complexities of these situations. It may be easier to withdraw, especially if the adolescent is reluctant to discuss her feelings. However, at this time the need is greatest and counseling will be the most productive.

Psychological Discomforts of Pregnancy

Certain psychological discomforts are assigned to period of pregnancy and birth which can affect the mother-child relationship. Adolescence itself has psychological tasks pertinent to its successful completion. When adolescence and pregnancy coincide, there can be a risk of a less than optimal outcome for both.

The normal pregnant woman's emotions become quite labile in pregnancy. The first trimester is notorious because of the hormonal impact on mood swings. The result is a female who requires a lot of loving input and support during this critical time. Optimally, she first needs the nurturance of her partner, then her family and her friends. Generally, she experiences a period of ambivalence in the first trimester and feels a natural grieving over the loss of her old lifestyle and the anticipation of the new and unknown role as a parent. The task of ambivalence is thought by most to be resolved by the end of the first trimester or early second trimester. By the end of that period, most women who choose not to have an abortion have accepted their pregnancy and resolved their ambivalence.

The pregnant adolescent, however, may not be so fortunate. She is often caught in a situation that was unintended and unplanned and whose existence is unrecognized by her (24). Confronted with an unintended pregnancy, the adolescent's first defense will be denial springing from the fear of discovery. Unlike her older counterpart who either planned a pregnancy or has accepted an unintended one and has loving support at a crucial time, the adolescent has no one to comfort or nurture her through this frightening phase. Instead, if aware of the pregnancy, she may fear social rejection by her peers, her school and the more threatening fear of familial rejection. Many adolescents hope their boyfriends will remain or become an ally, but for some even that support may be lacking. So, imprisoned by fears of rejection, many adolescents deny their own pregnancy. In doing so, they create time to re-evaluate their situation. The danger here lies in the potential for nonacceptance throughout the entire pregnancy, late or no prenatal care, and lack of choices such as termination of pregnancy. In discussing the psychological discomforts and their implications for the pregnant adolescent, it is recognized that this denial process may become a permanent situation which could eventually lead to child abuse and neglect.

The psychological experience of fear and denial is not a pleasant one. Still, it is a frequent discomfort for many adolescents when they first realize they are pregnant. As already stated, grieving over the lost lifestyle is normal for all pregnant women. Because the adolescent may never again have a chance to return to school, obtain an education and subsequently a job, her grief may go unresolved for a lifetime—a less than optimal outcome.

First Trimester

The talk of acceptance is assigned to the first trimester. Because many adolescents may not realize in the first trimester that they are pregnant or may deny it, they cannot accept this task until later. The adolescent who realizes she is pregnant but denies it out of fear may find herself isolated at a time when she needs support. Denial at this point may also act as a blocking mechanism in other psychological tasks of pregnancy.

If the denial of the pregnancy is a concern, the clinician must be sensitive to the adolescent's feelings. Many clinicians, for instance, use a doptone at the first visit to verify fetal life. When the fetal heart is heard, the mother is usually invited to listen. Listening to the fetal heart focuses acknowledgment of pregnancy and most adolescents will want to listen, but some will not. If the adolescent is still ambivalent about or is denying the pregnancy, the clinician must reassure her that new mothers often have those kinds of feelings about being pregnant and that they are perfectly normal and healthy. If negative feelings are present and remain suppressed, they can cause discomfort and yield a poor outcome for mother and child. Thus, every opportunity must be offered the adolescent to discuss these emotions.

Adolescents are often denied the attributes of loving support during the first trimester when it is so vital. While libido is decreased due to nausea and vomiting, breast tenderness and urinary frequency, the need for love is increased. The quest for loving support from adolescent sexual partners will generally be interpreted as a desire for intercourse, which is less than supportive of the adolescent's current psychological needs. Therefore, when "being loved" cannot be differentiated from "making love," the pregnant adolescent suffers. The fact that she is unable to differentiate her needs by herself will usually result in her capitulation. She may also fear losing the relationship if she tells her sexual partner she is pregnant.

Second Trimester

By mid-second trimester, quickening occurs. The reality of pregnancy can no longer go unrecognized. Women tend to respond positively when they first experience the sensation of fetal movement. Many adolescents do also, even though some may be frightened by this new and unusual feeling. For an unwanted adolescent pregnancy, however, it may be just one more event that reminds her of her pregnant state, the impact of the pregnancy on her life and her subsequent loss of control over her body image.

When quickening occurs she becomes aware of the reality that a baby is "living inside of her" and it is an opportunity to discuss the physiology of pregnancy. When discussions are personalized in this manner, adolescents are usually receptive and may ask innumerable questions. Understanding the physiology of their own bodies during pregnancy may also help them regain a sense of control and strengthen their psychological acceptance of the baby's growth and development in utero. It is also an appropriate time to encourage prenatal bonding with the father of the baby. If at all possible, every attempt needs to be made to include the father of the baby during the prenatal visits.

By mid-second trimester, most women begin to re-evaluate their relationship with their mothers. It is then that the pregnant woman prepares to become the care giver as opposed to being the care receiver. The pregnant adolescent may have difficulty in achieving this goal as she is still at a period in her own life when she is primarily a care receiver. As Varney points out (25), this process enables an understanding and . . .

> an acceptance of the qualities of her own mother which she values and respects. The qualities of her mother which are negative, unwanted and do not engender respect are rejected. This may cause guilt and inner conflict.

Varney suggests that the task of changing one's role from care receiver to care provider may create "a possible conflict over competing with one's own mother" (25). The potential for emotional discomfort for the adolescent is evident. Erikson (1) believes it is not possible to have an intimate relationship with another human being until one has successfully developed a positive sense of identity. To develop this identity, one must become independent. The pregnant adolescent is confronted with the possibility of competition with her own mother. She may still feel the need to be dependent while psychologically maturing towards independence, and may develop a sense of guilt and conflict. Neither of these is a positive emotional experience. Ultimately, a strained relationship between the adolescent and her mother may develop as both the adolescent and her child become the receivers of her mother's care, and she subsequently fails to take on the active role of mothering.

Helene Deutsch (26) reported in the 1960s that she believed "resentments against the mother seem considerably greater than in previous generations." If true for the nonpregnant adolescent, this resentment may increase dramatically in situations of direct conflict with one's mother over the right to mother one's own child. The conflict may be on a conscious or a subconscious level. Its presence, no matter how obscure, presents a threat and the potential for psychological discomfort and even trauma.

Third Trimester

The natural feelings of vulnerability associated with pregnancy, especially in the third trimester, are anathema to the adolescent. Most adolescents conceive of themselves as immortal and are, therefore, unable to deal with any personal concepts that are death related. As a result, it is hard to imagine the dimension of fear they face in anticipation of their labor and delivery experience. Additionally, the recognition that they can no longer control the size and appearance of their bodies heightens their sense of vulnerability and increases the feelings of alienation imposed by their pregnancy. Adolescents often make attempts to retain control over their bodies by trying to maintain a nonpregnant weight level and by wearing restrictive clothing such as tight jeans. This may also be an attempt to avoid negative peer evaluation and to sustain a nonpregnant image. This denial can result in rejection of the entire pregnancy. The pattern of nonacceptance is psychologically uncomfortable because it does not allow for growth and maturation. It further threatens to become a learned behavior and encourages an escapist approach to all of her future problems.

Every woman experiences concerns and fears about surviving the labor and delivery experience. This is especially true for the primagravida. Since most pregnant adolescents are primagravidas, they are naturally prone to this concern. As already stated, they are at an age when recognition of their own mortality is difficult. Some are so caught up in this fear that they are unable to discuss it. This can be remedied by the clinician taking the initiative and introducing the topic. If the adolescent is so distressed that she is incapable of voicing her fears, the clinician can discuss the feelings most women have about labor and delivery. Recognizing the commonality of her emotions may encourage the adolescent to discuss them. In helping the adolescent through this difficult time, the clinician may prevent her labor and delivery from being devastating.

Most adolescents cannot afford to pay for childbirth education classes. If the school curriculum does not include information about the physiology of labor and delivery, its health care facility is a reliable source. Understanding the physiology of labor will help the adolescent adjust her fears and concepts of pain for her own and for her baby's well-being during pregnancy and delivery. This learning cannot be overemphasized: it should be a service offered in any prenatal clinic dealing with adolescents.

Although psychological discomforts are common to all pregnant women, the implications for the adolescent are somewhat different. If the health care provider recognizes this and creates opportunities for the adolescent to explore her emotional reactions to pregnancy and birth, this care provider may remove these discomforts blocking the adolescent's ability to parent her child and cope realistically with future pregnancies.

References

1. Erikson EH. *Childhood and Society.* New York: WW Norton & Co., 1950;234.
2. Adams BN. Adolescent health care: needs, priorities and services. *Nurs Clin NA* 1983;18(2):237–248.
3. Bennett DL. Worldwide problems in the delivery of adolescent health care. *Public Health* 1982;96:334–340.
4. Blos P. *On Adolescence.* New York: The Free Press of Glencoe, Inc., 1962;74.
5. Leiman AH, Strasburger VC. Counseling parents of adolescents. *Pediatrics* 1985;76(4-II):664–667.
6. Zimmerman CC. The future of the family in America. *Journal of Marriage and the Family* 1972;34:323–333.
7. Smoyak SA. Symposium of parenting ... introduction. *Nurs Clin NA* 1977; 12:447–455.
8. Bryan-Logan BN, Dancy BL. Unwed adolescents: Their mothers' dilemma. *Nurs Clin NA* 1974;9(1):57–68.
9. Parsons T. *The Social System.* New York: The Free Press, 1951.
10. Billingsley A. Family functioning in the low-income black community. *Social Casework* 1969:563–572.
11. Otto H. What is a strong family? *Marriage and Family Living* 1962;24:72–80.
12. Aquilera DC, Messick JM, Farrell MS. *Crisis Intervention Theory and Methodology.* St Louis: CV Mosby Co., 1970.
13. Barrell L. Crisis intervention partnership in problem solving. *Nurs Clin NA* 1974;9:5–16.
14. Schertz FH. The crisis of adolescence in family life. *Social Casework* 1967: XLVIII(4):209–215.
15. HL. v. Matheson, Governor of Utah et al. 101 S. Ct. 1164(1981).
16. Cates W. Adolescent abortion in the United States. *Family Planning Perspectives* 1981;13(3):18–25.
17. Klein L. Antecedents of teenage pregnancy. *J Clin Ob/Gyn* 1978;2(4):1151–1154.

18. Evans J, Selstad G, Welcer W. Teenagers: Fertility control behavior and attitudes before and after abortion, childbearing or negative pregnancy test. *Family Planning Perspectives* 1976;8(4):192–200.
19. Steinhoff PA. Premarital pregnancy and first birth. In: Miller WB, Newman LF (eds). *The First Child and Family Formation.* Chapel Hill, North Carolina: Carolina Population Center, 1978;180–208.
20. Faizel H. Late social and psychological after effect of pregnancy in adolescence. *Journal of Adolescent Health Care* 1982;2(3):209–212.
21. Dey Kin E, Campbell L, Patti P. Post adoption experience of surrendering parents. *Am J Orthopsychiatry* 1984;54(2):271–281.
22. David H, Rasmussen N, Holst E. Postpartum and postabortion psychotic reactions. *Family Planning Perspectives* 1982;13(2):88–92.
23. Hendricks L. Unmarried black adolescent fathers' attitudes toward abortion, conception and sexuality: a preliminary report. *Journal of Adolescent Health Care* 1982;3(2):199–203.
24. *Teenage Pregnancy: The Problem That Hasn't Gone Away.* New York: The Alan Guttmacher Institute, 1981;16.
25. Varney H. *Nurse-Midwifery.* Boston: Blackwell Scientific Publications, 1980;82.
26. Deutsch H. *Selected Problems of Adolescence.* New York: International Universities Press, 1967.
27. National Research Council. Hayes CD, ed. *Risking the Future: Adolescent Sexuality, Pregnancy, and Childbearing.* Washington, DC: National Academy Press, 1987.

Bibliography

Adams BN. Adolescent health care: needs, priorities and services. *Nurs Clin NA* 1983;18(2):237–248.

Adams GR. Family correlates of female adolescents' ego-identity development. *J Adolescence* 1985;8(1):69–82.

Blos P. *The Adolescent Passage.* New York: International Universities Press, 1979.

Bowlby J. *Attachment.* New York: Basic Books, 1969.

Dashef SS. Aspects of identification and growth during late adolescence and young adulthood. *Am J Psychotherapy* 1984;38(2):239–247.

Erikson EH. *Identity, Youth and Crisis.* New York: WW Norton & Co., 1968.

Felice ME, Friedman SB. Behavioral considerations in the health care of adolescents. *Pediatr Clin North Am* 1982;29(2):399–413.

Hamburg BA. Early adolescence. *Postgrad Med* 1985;78(1):158–167.

Henshaw S, Binkio N, Blaine E, Smith J. A portrait of American women who obtain abortions. *Family Planning Perspectives* 1985;17(2):90–96.

Kreipe RE. Normal adolescent development. *NY State J Med* 1985;May:214–217.

Labarre H. Emotional crises of school-age girls during pregnancy and early motherhood. *J Am Academy Child Psychiatry* 1972;11(3):537–557.

Mercer R. A theoretical framework for studying factors that impact on the maternal role. *Nurs Res* 1981;30(2):73–77.

Mercer RT. *Perspectives on Adolescent Health Care.* Philadelphia: J.B. Lippincott Co., 1979.

Muuss RE. *Theories of Adolescence.* New York: Random House, 1975.

Piaget J, Inhelder B. *The Psychology of the Child.* New York: Basic Books, 1969.

Rogers D. *Issues in Adolescent Psychology.* New York: Appleton-Century-Crofts, 1969.

Schaffer C, Pine F. Pregnancy, abortion and the developmental tasks of adolescence. *J Am Academy Child Psychiatry* 1972;11(3): 511–536.

Shen JTY. Coping in adolescence. *Postgrad Med* 1985;78(1):153–157.

5 Sexuality

Introduction

During adolescence, adult sexual functions emerge and are developed. Psychologically, the development task for the adolescent entails the formation of an identity and the emergence of a mature capacity for intimacy. Physiologically, the adjustment is not as far-reaching because the capacity for sexual arousal and orgasm usually precedes puberty. Generally speaking, adolescents may be seen to evolve through four basic stages (1): awakening of sexuality (age 11–13), practicing social behavior or role modeling (age 14–17), developing sexual roles and a sense of identity (up to 18), and continuing past adolescence toward forming permanent relationships (age 18–25).

The female adolescent is faced with the task of finding her own gender identity and sex role. In doing this, she observes cultural traditions, attitudes and expectations that influence her emerging pattern of sexual functioning. As the adolescent experiments with or searches for her identity, she also tries to find herself in and through others. Her interpersonal relationships mature as she is able to form a personal identity that will, in turn, enhance her new self-image and self-esteem.

By the end of adolescence, the majority of females have experienced sexual intercourse. Many of these females also will give birth, have miscarriages or stillbirths, or obtain abortions. For these sexually active adolescents, some facts are now known. Most initial sexual encounters occur in the home of the girl or her partner. The partner is usually someone she has known for a while. For the adolescent female, the age of initial intercourse appears to be decreasing while the number of sexual partners is increasing. The most frequent season for the initiation of sexual intercourse is during the summer months. And there is usually a gap of a year or more between the time of first intercourse and the initiation of a contraceptive method, a period of high risk of pregnancy for the adolescent.

Role of Sexuality in Adolescence

There are many healthy, happy adolescents who enjoy an active sexual life and are responsible and aware of the implications of their sexual expression.

For many other adolescents, their performance in school or sports remains of greater interest and importance than sexual activity. There are others within the adolescent population, however, who are confused and unsure about their emerging sexuality. For many female adolescents, an awareness of their changing bodies remains mysterious and often frightening. It is during this period that the adolescent is involved in separation from her parents and she may feel alone in the midst of the myths and fears that surround her emerging sexuality. Often, frank discussions of sexual issues are not a part of normal family communications. While the adolescent is struggling with the formation of self-identity, and the concurrent withdrawal from parental guidance, the knowledge of what is normal physically and emotionally during this period may be unknown to her. Although adolescents may be trying to display their independence from familial ties, they may not be ready to accept completely the knowledge and advice of their peer group, especially in the area of sexuality. Thus they may become totally cut off from any avenue of sexual information with regard to the stages of normal development.

Adolescents are preoccupied with their bodily changes and demonstrate marked anxiety toward their new sexual feelings and interests. Many experience feelings of guilt, shame or embarrassment about their sexual activities. Adolescents may struggle with feelings of internal disorganization and inadequacy during this period. They often look to each other for support by sharing their sexual needs and behaviors as they experiment with adult roles and relationships. Through peer comparisons, the adolescent begins to develop a capacity for self-evaluation from which internal values develop.

The stages of sexual maturation during adolescence vary according to the individual but usually follow a tripartite pattern. During early puberty, the home remains the center of life, and friends belong to monosexual groups. The normal changes in physical and sexual growth create a period of anxiety and confusion. During this time, adolescents need explanations regarding these biological changes and reassurance of their normalcy. At mid-adolescence, home-centered life is disrupted as the influence of the peer group increases. It is a time when conformity is the norm. Decisions facing the adolescent during this period cause considerable stress as their capabilities for reasoning are tested and pushed beyond previous experiences. Mood swings are frequently present. The adolescent may have difficulties dealing with authority figures, often challenging the knowledge presented by adults. At such times, in light of the influence of peers, group discussions may be a more effective form of communication. During this period, the adolescent is trying to integrate herself into society at a new level of independence and responsibility. By late adolescence, the ego identity is stabilizing along with the formation of a value structure. The ability to relate to others and to achieve a level of intimacy with another person is also maturing. During this period, the adolescent is beginning to assimilate health information into a developing value system and is more receptive to preventive health care (2).

Adolescent Needs

The common concerns of adolescents during this period of change are not limited to the biological aspects of sexual development. Adolescents express anxiety and confusion regarding sexual behaviors, sexual values and sexual adequacy. In one study of adolescents aged 14–15, 75 percent or more expressed concerns about 1) what intercourse was like; 2) the meaning of slang terms; 3) whether someone loves you; and 4) embarrassment when sex is discussed (3).

Many adolescents need basic information about their bodies, their sexual structures and how they function. As the adolescent incorporates this information, there is a developing awareness of becoming a sexual being. Adolescents who have begun to explore their bodies may need to discuss what masturbation is and how they feel about it. Reassurance of being normal and alleviation of embarrassment and guilt are necessary at this time. Information about what orgasm is and when and how it occurs is also needed. Many adolescents may be sexually active but nonorgasmic out of fear, guilt or simply ignorance. Adolescence may be a time when there is some confusion over sexual preference. Frank discussions about homosexuality and feelings toward members of the same sex may prove very helpful. In addition, adolescents want the facts about sexually transmitted diseases, including the source, treatment and prevention. They also need to be informed of other consequences of their sexual activity, such as the potential for pregnancy. Of course, accurate knowledge about sexual functioning and contraception is best utilized prior to actively engaging in sexual activity.

Some adolescents during this period of maturation may ask for support in saying "no" to sexual activity. Adolescents need reassurance in their desire to reserve intercourse for a later time. Adolescents who want to abstain from sexual intercourse may need to ventilate their feelings toward society's expectations and double standards. They may express the feeling of being trapped or forced into undesired encounters. Adolescents may also want information about those sexual activities exclusive of intercourse. The adolescent, who desires affection and intimacy but wishes to maintain sexual limits, is looking for appropriate counseling to meet her special needs. For many adolescents involved in fragile or transitory relationships, sexual activity, such as touching and caressing without intercourse, may provide an acceptable level of sexual expression and pleasure. Adolescents wishing to defer sexual intercourse often seek reassurance of their normalcy and support in their decisions. Adolescents engaged in sexual activity without intercourse avoid the risks of pregnancy and the stress of contraceptive compliance.

Other adolescents may seek advice in order to say "yes" to sexual activity. Adolescents are permitted to express and enjoy their sexuality in many ways, such as in clothing, appearance and pride in a healthy body. Sexual activity may be natural and normal but it is usually not automatic and is learned through experimentation. Adolescents, like everyone else, discover their own likes and dislikes and also must learn to protect themselves against pain, infection, and undesired pregnancy. Sarrel and Sarrel have developed the concept of "sexual unfolding," a process of growth occurring during adolescence. During sexual unfolding, capacity for sexual response is realized, sexual preferences are recognized, and the capacity for sharing sexual pleasure in a loving relationship is developed. Within the concept of sexual unfolding, nine processes have been identified:

1. an evolving sense of the body which is gender specific.
2. the ability to overcome or modulate feelings of guilt, shame or fear associated with sexual thoughts or behavior.
3. a gradual loosening of primary emotional ties toward siblings and parents.
4. learning to recognize and communicate what is erotically pleasing and displeasing.
5. resolution of confusion and conflict about sexual orientation.
6. a sexual life, free of compulsion or dysfunction.
7. a growing awareness of the place and value of sex in one's life and of being a sexual person.
8. becoming responsible about oneself, one's partner and society.
9. a gradual fusion of sex and love, sex as one aspect of intimacy with another person (4).

In all cases, a trusting relationship based on confidentiality and respect is a prerequisite.

Adolescents often need assistance in controlling where, how and with whom sexual activity occurs. Many adolescents may not enjoy sexual activity because intercourse may be painful. Discussing how the adolescent feels about her sexual activity, as well as the mechanics of that activity, will help her to resolve some common sexual problems experienced by adolescents. If the adolescent is still physically immature, dysparunia may be related to the stretching of the hymenal ring or the vagina itself. Painful intercourse may also occur from pressure on the cervix, inadequate lubrication or a lack of knowledge about sexual response. After ruling out any pathology, information about adequate stimulation, use of lubricants and varied positions for intercourse may increase the pleasure of sexual activity for the adolescent. Anxiety, depression, guilt and other emotional reactions may inhibit sexual participation and satisfaction and may lead to dysparunia or orgasmic dysfunction. The feeling of heaviness or pelvic congestion may occur in the sexually active adolescent and is usually related to being nonorgasmic. This vasocongestion is part of the normal sexual response and is relieved by orgasm. Again, exploration of the adolescent's feelings about her sexuality, discussion of the sexual activity itself, and the encouragement of communication between herself and her partner are all essential in helping the adolescent to cope with her changing world. In adolescence, when close relationships are beginning to develop, sensitivity to the needs and comfort of each partner in sexual and nonsexual encounters is a basic learning objective. Early identification of sexual problems during adolescence, when sexual activity is beginning, may well prevent the later development of sexual dysfunctions or recurring problems with maintaining intimate relationship.

Sexual Preparation and Decision-Making

Making decisions about sexuality is a very difficult task for the adolescent. Often, the first sexual experience is over before thoughtful consideration and evaluation occur. Adolescents feel the pressure of sexuality from all aspects of society, including parents, peers and the media. These pressures often lead the adolescent to react in extremes, by either suppressing her evolving sexuality or by indiscriminately expressing it. Both the attempts by parents to control the adolescent's sexual behavior and the influence of peers to express it, may force the adolescent into decisions she is ill-prepared to make. Yet each adolescent must find her own personal resolutions to her sexual needs and conflicts. The adolescent's ability to establish sexual values and responsible sexual behavior, however, may not develop without advice from appropriate health care providers through sex education.

In today's world of casual or recreational sex, it is difficult for the adolescent to decide what it is she wants. It also demands a heightened level of honesty in communicating those values to others. The integration of the adolescent's sexual expression into her normal pattern of life affects other areas of life choices as well, such as social behavior and career goals. The decision to be physically intimate may also involve the decision of contraception, including issues of method, access and finances as well as the public expression of a sexual relationship. Sexual activity increases the adolescent's responsibility by increasing the social and financial demands which also affect her future.

The desire to be loved or to love someone may be a factor which results in the decision to be sexually intimate. The acceptance of physical intimacy and the responsibility it entails for the adolescent and her partner will lead many adolescents to seek guidance about their relationships, including contraceptive information. The adolescent's decision to use contraception may be influenced by her partner's knowledge and feelings about sexuality, contraception, and pregnancy. If the male partner is uninformed about such issues, the decision to use contraception may be denied out of ignorance or fear. The decision of the sexually active adolescent to use contraception represents an acceptance of the desire to experience sexual activity. By not using contraception, the sexually active adolescent may not be admitting or accepting the possibility of sexual functioning as a normal part of her life.

To help the adolescent understand her own emotional and physical changes, health care providers need to first accept their own sexuality and be aware of their personal attitudes and biases. Many examining practitioners do not elicit sexual histories or assess for sexual problems in the adolescent. Closed rather than open-ended questions are used to preclude any discussion of adolescent sexuality. The sexual history should not be any different from a routine medical history. A nonjudgmental approach is necessary to gather an accurate sexual history of the initial sexual activity, the frequency and type of current sexual activity, sexual preferences, sexual problems, and knowledge of reproduction and contraception.

Often, it is the adolescent who seeks out the practitioner for help with an identified problem. This adolescent is interested in education about herself and her sexuality and is responsive to appropriate information and advice. A pretext, however, is used to enable the adolescent to make an appointment; a pretext which is suddenly forgotten or ignored. The adolescent may be looking for an opportunity to express her concerns and discuss her questions about herself and her sexual functioning. Some adolescents will seek guidance when contemplating sexual activity but fears or embarrassment may prevent them from discussing the issues that actually concern them. Many adolescents do not have accurate information regarding such basic information as the time of greatest fertility within the menstrual cycle. The focus of this interview may be to establish what the adolescent knows, what she wants to know, and how she feels about her emerging sexuality.

The practitioner often begins by reassuring the adolescent of the normalcy of her feelings and experiences. This reassurance includes the subjects of body image, sexuality, menstrual characteristics, and contraception. The adolescent may prefer to be seen alone or with a "significant other," such as mother, sister, boyfriend or girlfriend. If possible, the sexual partner should be included in the interview and decision-making activities. Otherwise, an opportunity for education and communication is missed.

Sexual education attempts to help the adolescent incorporate sexuality into her life in a meaningful way. It includes information about pregnancy, contraception, sexually transmitted diseases, abortion, and rape. In particular, education in sexuality necessarily encompasses the early signs and symptoms of pregnancy, how to get a pregnancy test, alternatives to delivery, possibilities of miscarriage, childcare, education and job counseling, and medical and economic assistance available to the adolescent in case of pregnancy. The contraceptive methods available and how they are applied is an essential element of any program in sexuality. Throughout such education, there is a separation of fact from myth, and correction of misconceptions about sexual functioning, menstrual disturbances, infections, conception and contraception.

The practitioner can be sympathetic and responsive to the needs of the changing adolescent by providing a broad range of critical information. It is an extremely vulnerable time for the adolescent, which makes the task of expressing her feelings and describing her situation a particularly difficult one. The adolescent needs someone who will give her accurate and complete information, enabling her to make a thoughtful and informed decision about her sexual life. This person also needs to maintain and assure confidentiality. To meet the adolescent on this very personal level, the practitioner demonstrates availability and an interest in being flexible in scheduling, to prevent any conflict with the adolescent's school or work activities.

By assisting the adolescent in becoming a responsive and responsible sexual person, the health care provider becomes an advocate for the adolescent. In a supportive family environment, the practitioner may also be a source of support for the parents as they watch their child grow and mature. If parents wish to be involved in this aspect of the adolescent's health care, they can be counseled in a way that recognizes their need for support without betraying the confidentiality of the adolescent. Parents may also need re-education regarding sexuality, and correction of misconceptions they may have passed on to their children. When the parents are inflexible toward the adolescent's sexual behavior, or even confused about such sexual issues, communications may break down and professional help may be advised. The ability of the health care provider to listen and respond in an objective, nonjudgmental manner may be regarded as a role model for the parents (5).

Sexual counseling may occur on several different levels: validation, education, suggestion and therapy (6). Many practitioners feel that sexual counseling "never comes up" in routine office visits. In such cases, the practitioner may not inquire about sexuality, especially when seeing an adolescent; an inquiry which would open the door for discussion of sexual issues. Adolescents require clearly stated questions about their sexual activity and use of contraception in order to be able to respond appropriately. If it is the first health visit, the adolescent may not feel comfortable in discussing her sexual life, but knowing that such discussions are acceptable may set the tone for preventive health care. It takes time to find out if an adolescent's sexual experiences are mutually satisfying and healthy. First of all, the adolescent may not know what her sexual life is "supposed to be like" and may be wondering whether or not she is normal. Also, she may not know the correct terminology to describe her feelings or experiences. Providing understandable information and explanations of technical terminology, as well as the meaning of certain slang words, may be an appropriate beginning for conversations about sexuality between the adolescent and practitioner. When discussing her sexual activity, the adolescent will be more comfortable if she is fully dressed and seated in a chair as opposed to partially draped and lying on an examining table. Barriers such as white coats and large desks often inhibit the adolescent from discussing her feelings and elicit the statement that "everything is fine" instead of an outpouring of doubts and worries. Even the most basic information regarding personal hygiene may be overlooked at the expense of the adolescent's health. Most adolescents do not stop before sexual activities to consider clean hands and genitalia or urinating before and after sexual activity, much less the prevention of sexually transmitted diseases or pregnancy.

Many adolescents have received their sexual education through family, peers and the media. That education may well be inaccurate, unreliable, incomplete or erroneous. The adolescent needs the opportunity to discuss her sexual feelings and activities with her health care provider in an atmosphere of respect and understanding. In this way, the different levels of sexual awareness, in spite of differences in chronological age, can be met with appropriate education and information.

Sexuality and the Media

For many adolescents, questions about sexuality arise from the constant barrage of sexual material that surrounds them. In school, in magazines, on television, in movies—people are constantly interrelating for better or for worse. These sources of sexual information, channeled through spoken lines, displayed gestures, jokes, or a pan to fireworks, all give rise to thoughts, questions, anxieties and fantasies about sexuality. Adolescents are looking for a guideline for their developing sexual behaviors, a point of reference which they can either accept or reject. Parents are primary models for sexual behavior in the way they show affection, respect, and love for each other. Many adolescents, however, live in broken or unhappy homes where there are only negative influences. Adolescents may find it difficult to accept their parents as sexual beings and may look to other adults as role models. Adolescents are keen observers of adult behavior. By watching adults, in real life, on a screen or in pictures, the adolescent learns to mimic adult behavior. When the adolescent is primarily exposed to the unreality of film and television, this illusion becomes the standard which the adolescent tries to imitate. What the adolescent sees in such presentations is far more convincing than what she may hear about how people are supposed to act toward one another. The adolescent's efforts to integrate herself into today's society are often met by a sensorial flood that is confusing and possibly harmful. Adolescents need guidance in finding some resolutions to these conflicts, and accurate information to help correct the fantasies about sexual behavior which are presented to them daily. They need to discuss the realistic expectations of their unfolding sexuality and the normalcy of their feelings and behaviors. The mystery of sex, as well as its reputation for evil and wickedness, can be dispelled through appropriate information. The adolescent is aware that she must choose her own mode of behavior and she can do so by relying on her personal feelings, values and common sense. She seeks verification of these choices through exchange with the responsible adults in her life, those whom she can respect and trust.

Sexuality During Pregnancy

It must be remembered that although the pregnant adolescent has had one or more sexual experiences, she may have little knowledge of reproduction, sexual functioning or understanding of her own sexuality. Her sexual encounters may have been pleasurable experiences in an intimate relationship or they may have been painful and frightening events. Her encounter with and understanding of sexuality is likely to be the same as that of her nonpregnant counterpart. The pregnant adolescent, therefore, needs the same information, discussion and approach to sexuality as any other adolescent. In some cases, it may be even more important to help the pregnant adolescent understand her sexual feelings and behaviors in order to enable her to accept more readily the additional changes of pregnancy. The adolescent first needs to understand her own normal sexuality before the practitioner can explain the demands of pregnancy on her sexual behavior. Pregnancy is a time of confusion and fear concerning sexual activity, particularly for the pregnant adolescent. Sexual feelings do not stop when conception occurs. The pregnant adolescent may become anxious about what to expect during pregnancy and how to adapt to her changing body and feelings.

In the first months of pregnancy, there are many emotional and physical changes occurring simultaneously. Ambivalence toward the pregnancy or denial of the pregnancy may initially cause emotional conflict. As with older women, pregnant adolescents often become introverted and distanced from their sexual partners, who may not understand that this is a normal stage in accepting the pregnancy. Some pregnant adolescents may look to other females for comfort and support rather than to the father of the baby. On the other hand, others may feel more womanly and want to give and receive physical affection. Pregnant adolescents, as well as nonpregnant adolescents, experience mood swings. Childishness may give way to exaggerated seriousness which may, in turn, give way to fears of being out of control.

Often during the early months of pregnancy, sexual activity will decrease, even if the adolescent is normally sexually active. The common complaints of early pregnancy such as fatigue, nausea and vomiting, heartburn, breast tenderness, and increased vaginal discharge all contribute to a loss of interest in sexual activity. However, sexual interest may increase during mid-pregnancy. By this time, the pregnancy has been incorporated into the adolescent's life and the earlier physical complaints have been resolved. The adolescent normally feels well and is able to carry out regular school or work activities. Because of the normal increase of breasts and hips during pregnancy, many adolescents feel more attractive. Although the breasts are enlarged during mid-pregnancy, they are usually nontender and the abdomen is not large enough to discourage normal sexual activity. During the final months of pregnancy, the adolescent again becomes more concerned with the discomforts of pregnancy and less interested in sexual activity. She may feel "too big," unattractive, or she might think that the baby is more promi- nent than she is. Her thoughts may be concentrated on the forthcoming labor and delivery experience. Her breasts may begin to leak toward the end of pregnancy which necessitates some adjustments during sexual activity. The size of her abdomen and the weight and position of the baby may also be obstacles to satisfying sexual activity at this time. Alternative positions for sexual activity, which allow for the increased size of the abdomen, may pro- vide more comfort and pleasure as may other factors such as allowing more time for stimulation prior to intercourse.

For most adolescents, however, pregnancy is a time of abstinence from all sexual activity. Many adolescents are not familiar with sexual activity which does not involve intercourse. Other ways of being physically close and ex- pressing intimacy may not be known. Also, many pregnant adolescents and their partners do not understand the physical changes of pregnancy and are afraid of hurting both baby and mother. Often, sexuality is not discussed during the prenatal visits when so many other subjects need to be discussed in a short time. Yet, pregnancy can be an important opportunity for sexual education and may well provide the necessary incentives to prevent future pregnancies. It is a time when the pregnant adolescent can be sexually active and may be able to develop a sense of intimacy within a relationship which was previously dominated by sexual concerns. A sexual history and an oc- casional discussion about changing sexual behaviors during pregnancy are a necessary component of prenatal care. The few contraindications to sexual activity need to be discussed with the pregnant adolescent to elicit her un- derstanding and compliance. Some of these contraindications are vaginal spotting or bleeding, abdominal or perineal pain, and rupture of the mem- branes.

While the adolescent is on the postpartum unit, learning about her baby, she also needs time to learn about herself and the physical and emotional changes to expect after having a baby. As previously stated, the adolescent's sexual experience may have been limited, misunderstood, or negative. The adolescent's feelings toward her sexuality can be redirected in a positive way. Knowledge of reproduction and sexual functioning is assessed as well as her current feelings toward sexuality. Information regarding resumption of sex- ual activity is also discussed with the postpartum adolescent. Usually, postpartum bleeding stops in 10–14 days and episiotomies are healed in ap- proximately the same amount of time. After this two-week period, depend- ing on the adolescent's desire and comfort, normal sexual activity may resume. A method of birth control can be issued prior to hospital discharge, including foam and condoms, until the six-week postpartum visit. Many adolescents will have fears that their vagina will now be too tight or too big, or their breasts and abdomen unattractive. These fears and feelings need to be articulated and misconceptions corrected. Adolescents can be advised that a relaxed atmosphere and the possible use of lubrication will help in resuming sexual intercourse. Also, if the adolescent is lactating, wearing a bra may prevent any discomfort due to leaking breasts. The postpartum adolescent, who is returning to school and arranging child care, may find herself too tired or without enough privacy to be interested in resuming sexual activities. On the other hand, she may want to reassert herself as an individual, apart from the baby. She may need the closeness and reassurance of physical intimacy while the baby is the focus of attention in the home. The adolescent seeks reassurance, therefore, that it is acceptable for her to want a sexual relationship with another person and that she is not evil or wicked because of her desires. She also needs satisfactory contraceptive support to accept her decision to be a sexually active person.

Conclusion

Adolescents are seeking reliable information about their sexuality. They are confused by their exposure to the various conceptions of sexuality presented to them through ethnic tradition, society and the media. Learning how to communicate intimately with others will allow honest discussions between adolescents about their feelings and sexuality. To learn mature behaviors, adolescents need information about their bodies and how they function. The fully informed adolescent can make thoughtful and responsible decisions about her sexual life. The educational role of sexual information will affect the life time health of the adolescent. Simply making information available to the adolescent is not enough. It is the task of the health care provider to create an environment where questions and concerns can be related easily, and where the adolescent will be encouraged to apply those decisions which she has accepted on the basis of her own reasoning. Health care providers need to be comfortable with their own sexuality and to be able to talk in a way which does not alienate the adolescent. Parents and practitioners help in answering the adolescent's questions with facts and without simply biased and personal opinions. Adolescents want to know about the joys and complexities that are involved in mature and responsible emotional and sexual relationships. They need to be aware of such issues so that they will be able to make thoughtful and responsible decisions about their own sexual needs and role in intimate relationships. Adolescents are capable of developing trusting and loving relationships. Adults frequently ignore or deny the depths of the adolescent's emotional and sexual attachments and may not offer the help and support the adolescent's needs during this period of radical change and adjustment.

Our challenge is to be both a source of support and education. We cannot sit in judgement upon feelings and relationships which we may regard as unethical or irresponsible. To adopt such a stance would be to alienate completely the very person we are seeking to serve, an alienation which would successfully obstruct any constructive or educational communication. At the same time, we must never become insensitive to the need to educate the adolescent by teaching her the necessity of viewing sexuality within the context of intimacy and caring, and to approach it with appropriate sensitivity and responsibility. This responsibility extends to the potential unborn child, the family and the community.

For the adolescent, sexuality can too often be regarded as a weapon, a tool by which to strike out against parental, social or even intellectual expectations. The task of the practitioner is to provide an environment where such issues can be discovered, discussed and addressed, and where the adolescent can be brought to a more mature understanding of human sexuality through sensitive listening and a thoughtful and sympathetic response.

Sexual Abuse During Puberty

Extent of the Problem

One of the recently defined health problems in the United States is the physical and sexual abuse of adolescents. The sexual assault of minors has been reported throughout history but current statistics are now demonstrating an increasing incident of such crimes. Adolescents are frequently victims of sexual offences. Adolescent females are twice as likely to be physically and sexually abused as their male counterparts. One in four adolescent females is sexually abused before reaching adulthood, by either molestation, incest or rape. Of these sexual offences, less than 50 percent are reported, either to health care providers or agents of the legal services (7). Criminal sexual conduct involves subjecting a minor to sexual acts or taking indecent liberties, which may be manual, oral or genital contact by the offender with the genitalia of the victim without the victim's consent. Molestation is a noncoital form of sexual assault whereas incest and rape involve coitus; incest includes contact between blood relatives. The incidence of sexual abuse usually peaks during mid-adolescence, already a time of emotional turmoil. Incest may be the most common form of sexual abuse during this period. The younger adolescent may also be victim of intrafamilial sexual abuse in the form of molestation.

Often the sexual abuse experienced by adolescents is a continuation of offences begun during childhood. In turn, these adolescent incidents may develop into new or more severe forms of abuse. If the onset of sexual abuse occurs during adolescence, it may arise from situational conflicts within the family and begin as a form of physical abuse frequently justified as disciplinary punishment (8). Current literature emphasizes the problems involved in the long-term sexual abuse of adolescents within the family structure, such as molestation and incest, but more recently we are also seeing more adolescents involved in isolated incidents of sexual abuse committed by nonfamily related males (9).

Most acts of sexual abuse involving the adolescent are crimes of actual or threatened violence. In the latter case, coercion by fear, force or fraud is usually employed. Sexual offences reported range from continued sexual abuse, such as molestation or incest, to acts of brutal assault terminating in mutilation or rape homicide. The victim may be unable to provide either consent or denial either through lack of understanding due to age or retardation, or to debilitation caused by the altering of consciousness by illness, sleep, or drugs, including alcohol.

The perpetrator of the sexual abuse is often found to have some form of psychological disorder such as an inadequate, explosive, or antisocial personality. The offender may be characterized as a "loner," or may have been unsuccessful in mature relationships or lack self-esteem. The assailant may have been a victim of physical or sexual abuse as a child, or may have witnessed violence in his childhood home, particularly an incident involving a female. The offender may also have experienced a form of sexual dysfunction such as premature or retarded ejaculation or impotence.

Often the perpetrator is known to the victim and may even be a member of the victim's family. Normal adolescent behavior consists of mood swings, erratic behaviors, testing limits, and experimenting with new behaviors, particularly those of identity and sexuality. The adolescent may be seen as provocative, full of energy and sexually alive. The offender, on the other hand, may be experiencing a mid-life crisis, depression, or a lack of energy with a loss of sexual vitality. The adolescent may be living within potentially abusive situations and be unable to circumvent the inevitable.

The majority of offenders use force, or the threat of force, to initiate sexual contact. Force may be applied through verbal threats, physical overpowering or the use of weapons. Psychological force may be used through demands of loyalty or obedience to adult authority. Coercion may include threats of position or relationship within the family unit as well as bribery.

The efforts of society to modify the behavior of sexual offenders has not met with great success. Few sexual offenders are ever "cured." The recidivism rate is exceptionally high and far exceeds the number of one-time offenders. Seventy-four percent of the convicted rapists are reincarcerated within 18 months of their release. Eighty-five percent of convicted molesters are under surveillance for suspected pedophilia, sexual love by an adult for a child, within the first year of their release (7).

Adolescent Response to Sexual Assault

The victims of sexual assault face many physical and pyschosocial problems. The major complications of sexual misuse are injuries, infection, pregnancy and long-term psychosocial sequelae. Immediately after the initial assault, the adolescent may feel disgust and anger toward both her assailant and herself. She may blame herself for the incident without reason. Feelings of embarrassment, fear, and helplessness can disrupt all aspects of the victim's life and make normal functioning and activities impossible. Pain and fear of infection or pregnancy may force the adolescent to seek health care services. The adolescent is not only concerned about her safety and physical and emotional integrity but may also fear rejection by her family, peers or others. The health care evaluation and possible police involvement may only add to the victim's concern for her safety and acceptance.

The adolescent may respond to sexual abuse in a variety of ways. There are often disturbances in sleep and eating patterns. Regressive and dependent behavior may frequently be noticed. Feelings of guilt about the incident may require continual reassurance. Numerous fears or phobias may add to the depressed state of the sexually assaulted adolescent. Fear of peer reactions may persuade the adolescent to refrain from participating in normal school activities. Normal peer and adult relationships may be interrupted or avoided, particularly those involving males. Even if the assault did not involve family members, there is usually family conflict as a reaction to the sexual abuse. The adolescent may turn away from her family and look for new avenues of support. New coping mechanisms may consist of negative aspects such as delinquency, running away, chemical dependence, or prostitution. The adolescent may act out through aggression and anger or by withdrawal in response to fear. Seductive or fearful behavior toward males may be noticed as well as a certain pseudomaturity on the part of the victim. If the sexual abuse continues over time, the adolescent may not be able to escape or separate herself from the abusive situation, particularly if it means disruption of family life. The adolescent may experience ambivalent feelings towards an abusive relative, and be incapable of reporting the incidence to anyone.

The reaction of the family to sexual misuse of the adolescent varies in accordance with a number of factors. First of all, if the offender is a member of the family system, the relationship of the victim to the offender will affect parental loyalties. If the perpetrator is the father/step-father, the awareness of the mother will also affect the ability of the adolescent and her family to cope with the incident. Whether or not the family is able to help the adolescent victim may depend upon the family's previous ability to provide support to family members in a crisis. Also, the existence of other family problems may override the events of sexual abuse (10). In many instances, the parents appear to be more traumatized than the adolescent victim. Overreaction by parents to the sexual misuse of their children often leads to inattention and lack of support for the victim. Parental anger may be diverted toward the perpetrator but when poor judgment in terms of supervision leads to the placing of the adolescent in potentially abusive situations, this anger may be focused on the adolescent.

Identifying Sexual Abuse

Often it is difficult to identify the sexual abuse of adolescents when it occurs within the family system. Determining what behavior between family members is culturally appropriate and socially acceptable may vary radically, as well as the type and extent of discipline which may be employed within the family unit. Confusion may stem from the perceived rights of parents as to what constitutes abuse versus disciplinary punishment. In addition, differences in abuse of adolescents versus children, and inattention to the individual interactions between the adolescent and her family may also cause confusion (8).

Reports of sexual abuse involving adolescents are often delayed and sometimes are not made at all. The adolescent may be too embarrassed or afraid, or may anticipate disapproval if exposure of a family member is necessary. The victim of sexual abuse may fear further verbal and physical abuse when being "processed" by the medical and legal systems. The adolescent may also fear retaliation, exposure or exploitation. Quite often the adolescent finds it difficult to report a crime of sexual abuse through ignorance or inability to use the vocabulary necessary to describe the assault. Even when using the slang terms, the adolescent may have difficulty expressing herself. The adolescent may resist reporting the incident to avoid further stigma and humiliation. She may not want to risk being blamed for the abuse or disrupt the family. Often there may be precipitating factors which cause the adolescent to report sexual misuse, particularly if it has occurred repeatedly. Such precipitating factors may include a severe injury or involvement of other siblings.

As mentioned earlier, the adolescent may refuse to report the sexual abuse out of fear of the medical examination and the legal processes which are involved. The adolescent may feel a loss of control over her life and may see the medical/legal systems as a continuation of the assault involving further humiliation and loss of control. She may fear the investigative process which will invade her privacy and disrupt her family and may also affect attitudes toward her at school or work. The adolescent may also want to put an end to the event, particularly if it is a single incident of abuse. The thought of the legal proceedings continuing for six months or longer may increase the trauma instead of reducing it. In some areas, such as New York City, there are sexual abuse departments in the legal systems which provide legal aide and support, and attempt to bring the matter to trial within a few days of the crime whenever possible.

Each state has criminal laws governing the reporting of certain offences to the law enforcement authorities. Health care professionals are usually considered "mandated reporters" and need to be aware of the legal requirements and facilities within their own jurisdiction. In some areas, the expense incurred in collecting samples and testing materials in criminal cases can be born by the police department, or the victim can be otherwise compensated. Other modifications in the legal system have been made to ease prosecution in the case of sexual abuse. These modifications consist of relaxation of proof requirements, elimination of corroboration and witness requirements, waving of cautionary instruction of testimony relative to privacy of the victim's personal life, and restriction of admissibility of testimony relative to poor sexual conduct (11).

The purpose of the medical examination required when the adolescent is a victim of sexual abuse is to identify correctly the abuse, provide appropriate treatment for the abuse, and accurately report the incident of sexual abuse. This medical examination is carried out in a nontraumatic, emphathetic and nonjudgmental fashion. A caring, supportive female, who can be the adolescent's advocate, is extremely helpful throughout the medical/legal process. Careful assessment of the adolescent's physical and psychological status is necessary, as well as an evaluation of protection against sexually transmitted diseases and pregnancy. Accurate collection of medical data confirming the assault is vital to the legal process. The medical/legal examination consists of informed consent for examination, samples, photographs, collection of pertinent history, general physical examination with developmental rating, detailed genital tract examination, collection of laboratory samples as evidence, and appropriate medical and psychological treatment and referral. The importance of successfully completing the medical/legal proceedings is necessary to protect both the victim and the community from the offender. The reporting process also provides an opportunity for individual and family therapy.

Molestation

Molestation is defined as a noncoital form of sexual assault where genital fondling, manipulation, the viewing of genitalia, or oral-genital stimulation are carried out without the victim's consent. This may include a variety of sexual acts performed on or with the body of a child or adolescent. Most victims of molestation are within their premenarcheal years. More commonly, the initial molestation occurs between the ages of four and eight years and continues over weeks or years. Intrafamilial molestation if frequently observed where the biological father is the perpetrator, or occasionally an older sibling. The majority of offenders are known to the adolescent or her family as baby-sitters, neighbors, pseudo-relatives, friends, or possibly shopkeepers. Often the offenders are under 35 years of age (7). Molestation is usually recurring and nonviolent, often establishing a relationship between the victim and the assailant; a relationship which frequently hampers the ability of the victim to report and prosecute the perpetrator. Such sustained relationships may require long-term psychiatric intervention to assist the victim in re-establishing a healthy perspective toward intimacy. Long-term family therapy may also be necessary in cases where the mother is aware, consciously or unconsciously, of the abuse of her daughter by her spouse. In such cases, the adolescent may feel "singled out" for such activities.

There are many physical, psychological and social reactions felt by the adolescent when molestation occurs. Physically, there may be a change in weight, either through gain or loss. There may be injuries sustained such as perineal contusions and anal fissures. Insomnia also occurs frequently. Psychologically, there may be a noticeable decrease in academic performance and an inability to concentrate in classroom activities. Usually, the adolescent will display signs of anxiety as well as depression. Socially, molestation often results in a loss of self-esteem which complicates the adolescent's need for acceptance by peers. The adolescent may withdraw and become socially isolated or she may display delinquent behaviors for the first time. The adolescent may separate herself from other males, especially any who may be well known to her and important in her life. In some cases, signs of overt fears or phobias may also be observed and conversion hysteria can be seen as well. Not infrequently, the adolescent will attempt to run away from the situation. She may also try to escape the trauma of molestation through attempted or successful suicide.

Incest

Incest is considered to be sexual intercourse between persons who are too closely related to be able to legally marry. Because of the nature of this abuse among familial members, incest is often underreported and difficult to complete legal proceedings and prosecution. Usually, incest is a nonviolent form of sexual abuse. It may frequently involve the use of drugs, such as alcohol. One analysis of adolescent sexual abuse, however, suggests that in 19 percent of the intrafamilial abuse cases there were occurrences of the rape/trauma syndrome, and that in 30 percent, injuries were involved. These findings would seem to provide a necessary corrective to the misconception that incest is a noninjurous, mutual or loving relationship (10).

The victim's age generally ranges from 8 to 16 years. In many instances, the victim is the first female child of the family. When the victim reaches menarche, the incestuous relationship is often terminated and the adult's attention may be diverted to the next female child. The most frequently reported offenders are father substitutes, such as stepfathers or boyfriends of the mother of the adolescent, with the biological father being the second most frequent offender. In a review of the literature, however, incestuous relationships between siblings were found to occur at a rate five times greater than the rate between fathers and daughters (8). Underreporting of these facts may be related to such factors as the longer persistence of father/daughter incest and the stronger connotations of pathology and social unacceptability involved. As in the case of molestation, the mother of the adolescent may often be aware of the incestuous relationship. The adolescent may demonstrate hostile behavior toward her mother rather than the offender, feeling that her mother allowed the incestuous relationship to develop.

The adolescent's reactions to incest may be similar to those experienced in response to molestation. There may be weight gain or loss. Academic performance may also be adversely affected. When involved in an incestuous relationship, the adolescent may feel a loss of self-esteem and may prefer social isolation and separation from males who would normally be involved in her life. Incestuous relationships usually begin during the time of identity formation and increased sexual awareness in the adolescent. The combination of these factors may lead to promiscuous behavior (by the adolescent) in response to the incestuous attention. More commonly, the adolescent will show signs of anxiety and depression. These feelings may be accompanied by neurotic or psychotic behaviors such as fears, phobias or conversion hysteria. The adolescent may resort to running away from the family situation or may attempt or succeed in suicide. Because of the nature of incest, it is a family dysfunction requiring family therapy.

Rape

Rape is the act of sexual intercourse without the consent of the victim by compulsion through force, fear or fraudulent means. The Latin word for rape means "to seize" and reflects etymologically the violent nature of the crime. The crime of rape has been reported since the dawn of history, and, despite the modern methods of prevention, the incidence of reported rape in contemporary society continues to increase. A United States 1978 governmental report showed a higher than average occurrence of rape in August, a lower than average occurrence of rape in February, and an annual median rate in the months of May and October. The report also stated a higher incidence of rape in lower socioeconomic groups and in the more highly populated Southern states (11).

Fifty to 60 percent of all rape victims are under 19 years of age and are most commonly between the ages of 10 and 17. Almost 10 percent, however, are victims under the age of 10 years (7). More frequently, the victims are postpubertal. Rape is one of the least reported crimes and the majority of the offenders are known by the adolescent or her family. The familiarity of the rapist to the adolescent or her family is one of many reasons cited for failure to report the crime. Victims may also be afraid of complying with the demands of the health care system, or they may distrust the legal system. Some victims experience trauma when confronted with the demands of the criminal court system. Societal attitudes, anticipation of further humiliation for herself and her family, anxiety about an additional violation of privacy, and fear of retaliation by the rapist, all keep the victim from reporting the crime.

The extent of the physical and psychosocial damage may depend in part on the type of force used and the injury sustained during the rape. Injuries resulting from rape may range from minor bruising and abrasions to major genital and nongenital injury, and may occasionally result in death. The most common injuries from rape include bodily trauma and in particular, perineal injuries. Physical trauma to the body consists of abrasions and lacerations of the head, face, neck, chest and extremities. Perineal injuries include primarily perihymenal abrasions and contusions and vaginal lacerations. Usually, the greater the physical trauma experienced, the more significant is the genital injury sustained.

Rape/Trauma Syndrome

The rape/trauma syndrome has been identified as a set of reactions which take place immediately after sexual assault and which then may continue over time. The rape/trauma syndrome frequently occurs in the adolescent, who is the unfortunate victim of forceful rape or sexual assault. In discussing the rape/trauma syndrome, there are some variations which are peculiar to the female adolescent, variations which will be individually identified.

Immediately after a rape, the predominate reaction by the adolescent is fear of life and safety. Such fears are usually followed by feelings of embarrassment and self-blame. Emotions involving shame, guilt and anger usually occur later. The physical and psychological reactions of the adolescent during and after the rape may become intense and bewildering. The behavior of the victim may become inappropriate or "flat" due to the overwhelming emotions she is experiencing.

In general, the rape/trauma syndrome consists of two phases: the acute phase of disorganization and the long-term phase of reorganization. During the acute phase, the adolescent may experience somatic reactions such as headache, diarrhea, musculoskeletal tension, anorexia, dysmenorrhea amenorrhea and vaginitis. Psychological reactions can be reflected in complaints of insomnia, nightmares, depression, and anxiety. The adolescent may become apprehensive, with frequent sudden and startled responses, or she may show signs of intense and irrational fear. Emotional responses may contribute feelings of humiliation, self-depreciation, guilt or revenge. Social interrruptions may occur in the form of changes in interpersonal relationships, a fear of intimacy, a general distrust of men, or sexual dysfunction. During the long-term phase of reorganization, there are often patterns of increased motor activity. The adolescent may seek to change her telephone number, residence, school or place of work. Daily routines are often altered, especially pathways of access to and from the home. The adolescent may experience an increase in nightmares or complain of a repetitive nightmare. The adolescent may also experience persistent depression. During this phase of reorganization, the adolescent may have fears of bodily damage, including a fear of infertility. The reorganizational process involves the somatic, psychological and emotional reactions of both the acute and long-term phases.

While the adolescent is attempting to cope with the physical and psychologial trauma of rape, she is also contending with her parents' reactions to the assualt. Parents often overreact, becoming angry with the victim as well as with the offender and also with the various health and legal authorities. Often the parents respond to the situation by becoming overprotective and restrictive. Communication problems between the adolescent and her parents can increase after a rape experience. The adolescent may feel rejected by her parents or blamed by them for the assault. The parents may want retaliation and counseling time may be spent meeting the parents' needs instead of the victim's. The parents may raise concerns about venereal disease, pregnancy and future sexual functioning which may not coincide with the concerns of the adolescent. Often, members of the health care and legal professions identify with the needs of parents instead of the victim. When this occurs, little attention may be given to the emotional needs of the adolescent. Often, subtle fears regarding bodily damage may be overlooked or ignored. One study demonstrated that the health care professionals judged the parents to be more supportive of the victims than did the victims themselves (9). The acceptance of treatment and recovery from the sexual assault may be dependent upon the parents' support of the adolescent and cooperation with the medical/legal system.

Treatment and Management

Rape crises or sexual assault centers are nationally and internationally based facilities which seek to ensure the integration of health care and legal services for the victims of sexual abuse. Such centers are frequently based within emergency rooms, but maintain an independent and specially-trained staff, who are available for victims of rape and sexual assault. The staff of rape crises centers have been trained in the skills of sensitive interviewing, particularly with regard to the adolescent. They have also received training in coping with the common stresses resulting from a rape experience. The major function of these counselors is to be the adolescent's advocate during the medical/legal procedures. Often they are skilled in identifying and treating both the physical and psychological trauma of sexual abuse. Many emergency rooms, with or without rape crises centers, have developed protocols for the sexually abused victim to ensure minimal trauma during evaluation, treatment and follow-up, as well as integrity of care for medical/legal purposes. Therefore, these sexual assault centers provide acute crisis intervention and on-going counseling, as well as medical care and legal advocacy.

Often, there are volunteers who are trained to provide supportive care of the rape victim within these advocacy programs. The presence of a caring female to guide the victim through the medical and legal procedures and who will concentrate on the victim's needs is proven an invaluable aid to the victim's ability to reorganize her life after a sexual assault. Many centers have well-organized groups of experienced women who volunteer their services to sexually abused victims. Two such national organizations are Women Organized Against Rape (WOAR) and Women Against Rape (WAR).

Crisis centers are also associated with governmental health and welfare organizations as well as local self-help associations. There are often regional referral centers for such organizations as the Children's Protective Services and the Parents United and Shelter organizations. The assault centers are active in community health care systems and programs, increasing the community's awareness of the problem of sexual abuse, and educating health care professionals to meet the specific needs of victims. Often, counselors are involved with the criminal justice department and may participate in the rehabilitation programs for offenders.

Rape crisis or sexual assault centers coordinate the medical, legal and community services for the benefit of the victim and community. They provide a procedural protocol for victims of sexual assault, meet legal requirements for prosecution of offenders, participate in community and governmental programs for the sexually abused, and act as a general resource to the community, as a consultant and as an educator.

After such an experience, the adolescent victim of sexual abuse requires a gentle, reassuring approach to ensure a positive experience with the medical/legal evaluation. The trauma involved in the medical/legal evaluation, if not thoughtfully structured, can appear to the adolescent as a continuation of the rape experience. The adolescent, above all, needs reassurance of her normalcy, and, whenever possible, of the absence of serious injury. The assurance of privacy and confidentiality during the evaluation is also a primary goal. If a member of a rape crises team or a women's support group is not available, the presence of a friend or relative may enable the adolescent to be more at ease during the necessary evaluation. The adolescent may refuse medical evaluation and treatment, particularly if approached by male practitioners. Whenever possible, female health care providers must be available to attend to female victims of sexual abuse.

The adolescent may be overwhelmed with feelings of fear and horror, helplessness and loss of control over her life. It is helpful to encourage the adolescent to re-establish control by providing her with opportunities to make decisions about her evaluation and treatment. The adolescent can decide whether or not to participate in a legal investigation, whether or not to inform relatives and friends,or whether to permit collection of specimens for evidence and to accept protection against sexually transmitted diseases or pregnancy. By participating in these decisions concerning her health and legal care, the adolescent may be more responsive and less fearful during the evaluation.

Prior to beginning the physical evaluation of the assault victim, both the adolescent and her parents are separately interviewed in order to identify specific concerns regarding the rape experience. When these identified concerns differ, or are in conflict, the parents are counseled to accept and support the adolescent through the medical/legal experience. Questions concerning health, safety, legal actions, and interactions of family and friends are directly approached. Assessment of the family, including reactions to the victim and capacity to be supportive to the victim, is a valuable step in establishing and directing treatment goals.

Consents for investigation and examination are a legal requirement. Written consents, appropriately witnessed, must be received for the medical examination, collection of evidence, photography (if necessary) , and prosecution procedures. If the victim is a minor, the consents are signed, with the adolescent's permission, by the parent or legal guardian. In cases where the victim is a minor whose injuries require immediate medical attention, documented telephone consent for treatment by the parent or guardian is acceptable. When photography is indicated, the victim can be assured that photographs can be taken without revealing her identity. Legal procedures for the corroboration of the chain of evidence is followed according to State law. In severe cases of trauma, both physical and psychological, the medical/legal examination may proceed only after consent is obtained for anesthesia.

The initial task in the medical/legal evaluation is to obtain a thorough and descriptive history. The account of the sexual assault is written in the victim's own words. Details of all forms of sexual activity are documented including all areas of the body involved in physical or sexual contact, and the time, place and order of the sexual acts. Any identifying remarks regarding the assailant are also noted. The circumstances of the assault are described, including acts or threats of force, signs of resistance, and the presence of others during the assault. The use of drugs, such as alcohol, by the assailant or victim, is also recorded. Description of any post-assault hygenic measures taken is also documented, such as bathing, douching, urinating, defecating, brushing teeth or changing of clothing. Recording of the victim's emotional status during and after the assault, including any stated anxiety or fears, is also necessary. The date and type of the most recent voluntary sexual activity are stated as well as a thorough menstrual and contraceptive history.

During the taking of this history, the health care provider gathers data to be used in detection of injury or indication for treatment as well as for use as evidence. The practitioner also offers emotional support and reassurance. The professionals involved in the medical/legal evaluation remain objective, refraining from value judgments or feelings or anger or disgust. Such reactions only cause the adolescent to feel further alienation and may make her unwilling to discuss openly the assault experience. The adolescent may also sense the anger or horror felt by the practitioner and direct these feelings toward herself instead of the perpetrator.

The physical examination includes a thorough investigation of all injuries and the collection and preservation of laboratory specimens for use as evidence. The evaluation begins with a general description of the victim's appearance, emotional state, and condition of clothing. Observations are made for extrapelvic injuries such as choke marks, bites, scratches, abrasions, grip marks, or lacerations. Care is taken to describe the site, color, and size of any lacerations. Other signs of blunt trauma such as pain, tenderness, contusions, ecchymosis, or hematomas may take 24 hours to become visible. Victims of trauma with no physical evidence are to return 24 to 48 hours after the sexual assault for further evaluation. If there has been delay in reporting the sexual assault, signs of blunt trauma may have resolved and observation may not be possible. A developmental rating (described in Chapter 2) should be performed on adolescent victims of assault to document their maturity at the time of the offense; prosecution may be delayed for six months to a year and further developmental changes may occur.

The pelvic examination involves a careful and detailed inspection externally and internally for signs of recent sexual activity. Before beginning, the pubic hair is combed for other hair and debris and appropiately labeled. Often, hair from the scalp and pubes are plucked and labeled for identification. Fingernails and occasionally toenails are also trimmed and collected for examination of debris. All findings of hair, fibers, soil, blood or secretions are carefully identified and labeled.

The pelvic examination includes a careful inspection of the genitalia, comprising the mons, clitoris, urinary meatus, vulva, hymen, perineum, vagina, cervix and rectum as well as the buttocks and thighs. Injuries found in the vaginal introitus occurring clockwise between nine o'clock and three o'clock are usually from noncoital trauma whereas injuries found clockwise in between three o'clock and nine o'clock are primarily from coital trauma (7). Also, the use of ultraviolet or Wood's light may be necessary to localize semen deposits.

The adolescent victim is informed of the type of samples needed for the medical/legal evaluation and must give her consent for their collection and use as evidence. Established laboratory protocols for criminal evidence is followed in conjunction with identification, labeling, and sealing, to meet the unbroken chain of evidence regulations. If clothing is collected and sealed, replacement clothing should be readily available. Samples which are usually necessary in a sexual assault comprise swabs from any suspicious areas of the vulva, vagina, rectum or pharynx in order to test for the presence and motility of sperm or red blood cells. Saliva and vaginal pool samples are also tested for acid phosphatase and blood group antigens. A Pap smear and cultures are taken for identification of gonorrhea and other sexually transmitted diseases. Blood specimens are sent for tests of syphilis, pregnancy, complete blood count, and if indicated, to detect drug usage. Urine specimens are sent for urinalysis and culture. Often the police will supply kits containing all the necessary containers and labels to collect specimens for a sexual assault case. In some areas, the police department or other agencies are billed for the expense of collecting and testing the specimens. The victim is informed of such policies or other means of reimbursement.

Prophylactic treatment against sexually transmitted diseases is recommended after discussion with the adolescent of the risks involved. Aqueous procaine penicillin G., tetracycline, spectinomycin, erythromycin or ampicillin may be advisable as prescribed drugs. According to the guidelines of the Food and Drug Administration (FDA), the only approved method for the prevention of pregnancy is the use of diethylstilbestrol (DES), 25 mg orally twice a day for five days. DES treatment must be initiated within 72 hours of unprotected intercourse. The adolescent is advised of the risks and benefits involved. Pregnancy is prevented in the majority of cases, however, there is a risk of adenosis and adenocarcinoma in the offspring if pregnancy is not prevented. If pregnancy occurs after DES exposure, the adolescent may wish to consider a termination of pregnancy. Although not officially approved, conjugated estrogen (Premarin) may be prescribed either in a single intravenous dosage or 25 mg orally twice a day for five days. Ethinyl estradiol (Estinyl) 2 milligrams orally twice a day for five days may also be advised. As with DES, the estrogen treatments are associated with side effects of nausea and vomiting frequently requiring the use of antiemetics. Other side effects may occur with pregnancy prevention treatment such as fluid retention, headache, dizziness, menstrual irregularities, breast soreness as well as failure. The insertion of an intrauterine contraceptive device (IUD) is also an option for pregnancy prevention after unprotected intercourse in sexual assault. Termination of pregnancy may be indicated in sexual abuse cases.

In one week, the pelvic examination may be repeated in order to evaluate the healing of injuries. Pregnancy tests may be repeated weekly until positive, or until the onset of menses. Four to six weeks after the assault, the initial tests for gonorrhea and syphilis may also be repeated.

Counseling

The availability of counseling for the sexually abused adolescent and her family is stressed during the initial medical/legal evaluation. Female adolescents tend to respond less favorably to rape/trauma counseling than do adults. The involvement of a relative or friend whom the victim views as supportive of her needs may be helpful in maintaining long-term follow-up and long-term counseling. The adolescent is informed of counseling goals which not only include acute crises intervention but also prevention of long-term psychosocial sequelae often involved in sexual abuse. The length of counseling may extend anywhere from immediate medical/legal evaluation to six weeks, six months or longer, and often involves both individual and family therapy. Individual and group sessions with other victims may also be available to the sexually abused adolescent, including psychiatric referral.

During the early counseling sessions, the adolescent's strengths in coping with a crisis are evaluated. Family interactions and support systems are also assessed. Initially the adolescent may seek permission to talk about her experience, or to raise questions about what actually happened. She may need to talk repeatedly about her experience in order to correctly interpret what happened and to understand her reactions to the incident. The adolescent may need to role play or re-enact the experience in order to understand it objectively. The counselor provides support, objectivity and education during these sessions. Ideally, the same counselor who was available at the time the assault was reported continues to maintain contact with the adolescent through telephone and office visits. Through this continuity of care, the adolescent may form a trusting relationship with a caring professional, who will become her advocate. Gradually, the adolescent can be reassured of her normalcy, femininity and sexuality.

The adolescent will experience several phases of emotional adjustment to the experience of sexual abuse. Initially, there may be an outpouring of emotion, characterized by shock, fear and anxiety. Once the initial adjustment is made, the adolescent will return to normal daily activities. Later, the adolescent may withdraw from counseling efforts, denying or repressing the abusive experience. In time, attempts to resolve the experience may result in continued depression, and counseling may have to be discontinued if it is a painful reminder of the rape/trauma experience.

In some cases, the sexual assault may be the first sexual experience of the adolescent. The rape or sexual abuse may be interpreted as a sexual act instead of a crime of violence. In such cases, questions concerning sexual values, adequacy, and normal sexual behaviors need to be discussed. Decisions regarding future sexual activities, including the adolescent's prerogative to choose time, place and partner are emphasized. Psychotherapy may be indicated depending on the extent and impact of the sexual abuse.

The adolescent may seek help in maintaining her family structure in spite of an abusive situation. When questions of home safety are raised, the counselor or police may provide protection for the adolescent through temporary shelter. Abuse often occurs in stressful family situations. Counseling may enable the adolescent and her family to maintain open lines of communication and avoid destructive interactional situations. By reporting and seeking assistance for abusive family situations, the adolescent receives help for herself and for her family. The cycle of abused children becoming abusing parents may then be halted. Counseling can often help the adolescent regain the independence she may have temporarily lost. The ability to consider the consequences of her actions or inactions may be sharpened. After the assault, the adolescent may become acutely aware of potentially abusive situations and learn how to evade them. The adolescent can be educated regarding preventive measures which may be taken to avoid sexual assault. The adolescent victim of sexual assault needs time, encouragement and support in order to understand her experiences and regain her equilibrium. She requires tremendous support so that her body and mind may continue to grow and develop on her path to maturity.

References

1. Rigg CA, Shearin RB. Adolescent sexuality. *Adolescent Medicine: Present and Future Concepts.* Chicago: Year Book Medical Publishers, 1980;147–151.
2. McDonough PC, Gambrell RD. The adolescent gynecological patient and her problems. *Clin Obstet Gynecol* 1979;22 (2):491-507.
3. Parcel GS, Finkelstein J, Luttman D, Nadar PR. Sex concerns of young adolescents. *Birth Fam J* 1979;6(1):43–47.
4. Sarrell LJ, Sarrell PM. Sexual unfolding. *J Adolescent Health Care* 1981;2:93–99.
5. Masland RP. Sex education. In: *Pediatric and Adolescent Gynecology.* Emans SJ, Goldstein DP (eds). Boston: Little, Brown & Co., 1977:173–179.
6. Spence AK, Mann J. Office sex counseling. In: *Office Gynecology* (2nd ed). Glass RH (ed). Baltimore: Williams & Wilkins, 1981;177–211.
7. Woodling BA, Kossoris PD. Sexual misuse: rape, molestation and incest. *Pediatr Clin North Am* 1981;28 (2):481-499
8. Blum RW, Runyan C. Adolescent abuse. *J Adolescent Health Care* 1980;1 (2):121-126
9. Mann EM. Self-reported stresses of adolescent rape victims. *J Adolescent Health Care* 1981;2(1):29–33.
10. Bach CM, Anderson SC. Adolescent sexual abuse and assault. In: *Adolescent Medicine: Present and Future Concepts.* Rigg CA, Shearin RB (eds). Chicago: Year Book Medical Publishers, 1980;103–112.
11. Breen JL, Greenwood E. Rape. In: *Office Gynecology* (2nd ed). Glass RH (ed). Baltimore: Williams & Wilkins, 1981;212-225.

Bibliography

Akpom CA, Akpom KL, Davis M. Prior sexual behavior of teenagers attending rap sessions for the first time. *Family Planning Perspectives* 1976;8 (4) :203–208
Ambrose L. Misinforming pregnant teenagers. *Family Planning Perspectives* 1978; 10(1):51–57.
Burgess A, Holmstrom L. Sexual assault: signs and symptoms. *J Emergency Nursing* 1975;1(2):10–15.
Burgess A, Holmstrom L. Sexual trauma of children and adolescents. *Nurs Clin NA* 1975;10(3):551–563.
Cates W, Blackmore CA. Sexual assault and sexually transmitted diseases. In: *Sexually*

Transmitted Diseases. Holmes KK, Mardh P, Sparling PF, Wiesner PJ. New York: McGraw-Hill, 1982:119–125.

Crist T, Gray MJ. Sex counseling for the single young woman. *Interact* 1978;2(1): 1–13.

Davidson EC. An analysis of adolescent health care and the role of the obstetrician/ gynecologist. *Am J Obstet Gynecol* 1981;139(7):845–851.

Evans JR, Selstad G, Welcher WH. Teenagers: fertility control behavior and attitudes before and after abortion, childbearing, and negative pregnancy test. *Family Planning Perspectives* 1976;8(4):192–200.

Felice M, Grant J, Reynolds B, et al. Follow-up observations of adolescent rape victims. *Clin Pediatr* 1978;17(4):311–315.

Hammerschlag MR. Sexually transmitted diseases in children and adolescents. *Medical Aspects of Human Sexuality* 1984;18(7):77–83.

Hawkins JW, Higgins LP. *Health Care of Women: Gynecological Assessment.* Monterey, CA: Wadsworth Health Sciences Division, 1982.

Katchadourian H. Adolescent sexuality. *Pediatr Clin North Am* 1980;27(1):17–27.

Keen MA. The nurse practitioner in ambulatory gynecology services. *Clin Obstet Gynecol* 1979;22(2):445–453.

Kisker EE. Teenagers talk about sex, pregnancy, and contraception. *Family Planning Perspectives* 1985;17(2):83–90.

Kornfield R. Who's to blame: adolescent sexual activity. *J Adolescence* 1985;8(1):17–31.

Leichtman SR, Friedman SB. Social and psychological development of adolescence. *Med Clin North Am* 1975;59(6):1319–1328.

Lief HI. *Medical Aspects of Human Sexuality.* Baltimore: Williams & Wilkins, 1975.

Malinowski JS. Sex during pregnancy: What can you say? *RN* 1978;41(11):48–51.

Mosher DL. Three dimensions of depth of involvement in human sexual response. *J Sex Research* 1980;16(1):1–42.

Munt LC. Sexual abuse of children and adolescents. In: *Adolescent Medicine: Present and Future Concepts.* Rigg CA, Shearin RB, eds. Chicago: Year Book Medical Publishers, 1980;275–284.

Parcel GS, Finkelstein J, Luttman D, Nadar PR. Sex concerns of young adolescents. *Birth and the Family Journal* 1979;6(1):43–47.

Rosenthal MB. Sexual counseling and interviewing of adolescents. *Primary Care* 1977;4(2):291–300.

Sladkin KR. Counseling the sexually active teenager: reflections from pediatric practice. *Pediatrics* 1985;76:681–684.

Thornton A, Freedman D. Changing attitudes toward marriage and single life. *Family Planning Perspectives* 1982;14(6):297–303.

Zelnik M, Kantner JF. Sexual and contraceptive experience of young unmarried women in the United States: 1976 and 1977. *Family Planning Perspectives* 1977; 9(2):55–71.

Zelnik M, Kantner JF. Contraceptive patterns and premarital pregnancy among women aged 15–19 in 1976. *Family Planning Perspectives* 1978;10(3):135–142.

Zelnik M, Kantner JF. Sexual activity, contraceptive use, and pregnancy among metropolitan-area teenagers: 1971–1979. *Family Planning Perspectives* 1980;12(5): 230–237.

6 Common Complications Associated with Adolescent Pregnancy

The pregnant adolescent is often described as a high-risk obstetric patient because, according to statistics, she is predisposed to: 1) higher maternal and infant mortality rates, 2) anemia, 3) pre-eclampsia, 4) low-birthweight babies, 5) sizing and dating problems, and 6) multiple socioeconomic complications.

Maternal Mortality

From 1972 to 1975, the U.S. maternal mortality rate for adolescents who continued their pregnancies was 9.5 per 100,000 live births (1). In 1981, the Alan Guttmacher Institute reported that the maternal mortality rate for adolescents under age 15 is 2.5 times that for pregnant women age 20–24 (2). Reasons for these outcomes are difficult to pinpoint. However, documented statistics suggest that pregnant adolescents run a significant risk of developing prenatal complications. This fact, coupled with the adolescent's frequent poor eating patterns, poor prenatal health habits, and poor compliance with prenatal management of care or failure to seek early prenatal care, increases the maternal death risk.

Maternal mortality can be eradicated simply by preventing pregnancy. Appropriate sex education about human reproduction is a preliminary step. Although skeptics say sex education for teenagers is a waste of time and energy, teenagers deserve the chance to learn about the their physiology, the reproductive process, and risks of pregnancy at an early age. If caring adults present these facts to teenagers in an interesting way and in an environment that is psychologically comfortable, the response is likely to be positive. For many adolescents, accurate information and subsequent awareness will result in the effective use of contraceptives.

Even if pregnancy occurs, prevention is still the key to reducing the threat of maternal mortality. Accordingly, the pregnant adolescent must be carefully monitored for complications throughout her pregnancy. This surveillance will require more accumulated prenatal clinic visits than are necessary for the average pregnant woman. Such attention may increase the care cost for the pregnant teenager, but Medicaid costs will decrease when a healthy mother and baby result.

The Compliance Factor

Compliance with clinical management is a significant factor in a successful outcome for the pregnant teenager. Without it, all risk factors multiply. A factor in an adolescent's compliance frequently lies with the clinician. When the clinician is truly committed to the adolescent and this commitment is apparent, the adolescent generally complies. If there is no compliance, the clinician should investigate the reasons in a nonpunitive way. Threats such as "Do you want the baby to die?" do not work and create a communication barrier between care provider and teenager. It is far more productive to search out the root of the problem. Such routine factors as the cost of transportation, motion sickness when riding the bus, having to wait long periods in the clinic, meeting different clinicians at every prenatal visit, and simply having more exciting things to do are common reasons for poor clinic attendance. The last excuse is often a seasonal one and becomes a particular problem during the summer and at school vacation time.

Home situations may also affect compliance. These often include nonsupportive family members who ridicule and contradict the prescribed prenatal management or impose family responsibilities such as child care on the adolescent. Interference of this nature may affect the teenager's capability to comply with prenatal instructions and management or to get to the clinic for her appointments.

Coping with the adolescent's family situation requires substantial fortitude on the part of the clinician. If the adolescent agrees that nonsupportive family members are a problem, a family conference with the care provider may help reduce some of the obstacles to compliance. Such a conference enables the family to discuss its feelings about the teenager's pregnancy in a safe environment. Expressing these feelings may help reduce the family's anxieties about the pregnancy or turn its ambivalence into a positive force, which ultimately improves the adolescent's compliance with prenatal management. Occasionally, a short note to the parent(s) or guardian may be sufficient to obtain family support. Contact with the family by whatever means is worthwhile when trying to rectify compliance problems.

Adolescent complaints about the clinic may prove difficult to correct. Most adolescents find themselves in high-volume clinics where there are too many patients to be seen by too few care providers. It would seem easy to eliminate these problems by cutting down on volume, sticking to the appointment schedule, and reducing the number and variety of health care providers, but this is usually not feasible. Clinics have no choice but to accept an assigned volume, and thus enlist a variety of care providers to serve the clientele. This large staff of clinicians reduces the waiting period for the teenager but often demands that she expend more emotional energy in adapting to a new care provider at each visit. It is easy to see why this discourages clinic attendance.

If the number of teenage pregnancies is reduced and quality prenatal care begins at an early stage in pregnancy, it is hoped that the rate of maternal mortality will decrease for this age group.

Infant Mortality

Data recorded in New York state between 1974 and 1978 showed a higher death rate for the infants of teenagers than for those of older women (3). Many infants in this group suffer from dehydration due to vomiting and diarrhea. The infant's ability to tolerate dehydration is minimal, and it will die quickly if there is no adequate intervention. Vomiting and diarrhea often result from the mother's poor knowledge of hygiene and sanitation. Because most adolescents do not breastfeed, they rely on formula, which may be left sitting in a warm place (sometimes for hours), or the bottle may fall to the floor and its nipple wiped with on dirty clothing or hands and given to the baby. The risk of infection becomes obvious.

Many infants die as a consequence of diarrhea and vomiting because the family lacks knowledge of the clinical severity of these symptoms in the newborn. Home remedies also contribute to morbidity. The family may consider the grandmother in the household an authority on home remedies and child care, which can create a dilemma for the health care provider who is forced to contradict her "authority." The solution lies in helping both the adolescent and her grandmother recognize the signs and symptoms of a serious problem. This information may be contained in the packet of instructional materials given to the adolescent postpartum to be reviewed by her and her family before leaving the hospital. Approved home remedies may also be included in the materials and discussed so that the adolescent can distinguish between appropriate and inappropriate home cures.

Breastfeeding

One obvious correction for problems of poor hygiene and sanitation is to encourage adolescents to breastfeed. Many initially respond negatively to breastfeeding, considering it time-consuming and a practice that adversely affects their breasts (i.e., sagging, leaking). Some teenagers have a negative concept about the breasts and consider breast-feeding "dirty" and, in addition, frequently cite friends who have tried and failed. While the failure rate for breastfeeding adolescents cannot be denied, it is generally owed to the lack of informed, caring individuals on the scene who take the time to help young mothers master the process.

Many of these negative responses toward breastfeeding echo the attitude developed by society in general in the United States. Immediately after World War II, bottle-feeding became the standard feeding method for upper- and middle-class mothers. The poor eventually were able to emulate the habits of higher income groups and discontinued breastfeeding. Consequently, a whole generation lost the opportunity to see and learn from their mothers the skills of breastfeeding. In addition, many adolescent mothers have not yet completed the identity process associated with maturation and are therefore unable to develop the degree of intimacy with another human being required for breastfeeding. Moreover, they are susceptible to peer reaction and negative pressure from their boyfriends. This results in formula-fed babies who must rely on their mothers' good hygiene in preparing and preserving their formula.

Once the adolescent has chosen to bottlefeed her baby, the same support, education, and encouragement offered to breastfeeding mothers is necessary to ensure that she and her family are able to prepare safely and adequately formula feeds with the appropriate equipment. This can be taught during the postnatal stay via demonstrations and practice sessions.

Anemia

Iron-deficiency anemia is a frequent complication in pregnancy. It is a nutritional disease common to males and females alike but occurs most often in reproductive age women. Studies in three Western countries revealed that 8 percent to 10 percent of the women living in those countries had iron-deficiency anemia (4). Additionally, the incidence increases with pregnancy. Adolescents, who are notorious for their poor eating habits , are especially prone to develop iron-deficiency anemia in pregnancy.

The average woman loses approximately 40 to 45 cc of blood during each menses. This is the equivalent of 15 to 20 mg of iron. If she has recently given birth, she has lost an additional 800 mg of iron. Since general absorption of dietary iron is only about 10 percent, the dietary intake of iron must be high enough to compensate effectively. Absorption rates, however, occasionally vary and, to an extent, depend on the body's need for iron. To meet effectively the needs of the average nonpregnant adolescent female, the daily diet should include 18 to 20 mg of iron. The pregnant adolescent is believed to need 3 mg per day of iron (1 mg more than the nonpregnant adolescent), ideally resulting in a daily dietary intake of 30 mg. That amount of iron is difficult to attain on a dietary basis, and most pregnant women are iron deficient as a result.

Although it is believed that only 10 percent of all ingested iron is absorbed, pregnancy enhances the absorption process. Ascorbic acid also increases iron absorption, and for this reason, many clinicians recommend vitamin C during pregnancy. Good dietary sources of iron include meats in general and liver in particular. Liver, however, is not popular with adolescents, and few will eat it. Interestingly, vegetables such as spinach and collard greens are recognized as only fair sources of iron, as are egg yolk and dried fruit. Pinto beans and fortified cereals are excellent iron sources.

Hypervolemia

There is a natural physiological response to pregnancy that results in increased plasma volume. This hypervolemia occurs early in pregnancy and results in a drop in the ratio of red blood cells to the plasma volume. A falling hematocrit will manifest itself until the end of the second trimester, or possibly until 28 to 32 weeks gestation. By this time, the number of red blood cells increases, which begins to offset the increase in plasma volume. By 36 to 38 weeks of gestation, the accumulated hemoglobin is sufficient to stabilize the hematocrit, and by 40 weeks gestation, a slight increase may have occurred. The oxygen requirements of both the fetus and the mother as well as the anticipated maternal blood loss at delivery dictate the increased need for red blood cells during pregnancy. After delivery, the mother's need for iron is facilitated by the breakdown of the surplus erythrocytes that were produced during pregnancy.

Diagnosis

Traditionally, the diagnosis of iron-deficiency anemia is determined by the presence of: 1) microcytic, hypochromic erythrocytes; 2) a serum iron less than 60 mg per ml; 3) an iron binding capacity usually well over 300 mg per ml (this number may vary with the laboratory, however) or a serum iron to iron binding capacity (transferrin saturation) ratio of 15 percent or less; and 4) a positive hematologic reaction to iron therapy (4). The best laboratory method for diagnosing iron-deficiency anemia is a complete blood count (CBC) with indices and reticulocyte percentages. Black adolescents may also require a hemoglobin electrophoresis to rule out hemoglobin S.

The clinician will be aware that the serum iron levels may be skewed if the adolescent has taken supplemental iron for the previous 24 hours. If this is the case, the serum iron level may appear normal when an actual iron-deficiency anemia exists. Therefore, the routine screening for iron-deficiency anemia includes instructions to discontinue supplemental iron intake for 24 hours prior to testing. Unfortunately, clinical urgency does not always allow for this advanced planning.

A good physical (including dietary history) and laboratory data are essential to diagnose an iron deficiency. First, it should be established whether or not the pregnant adolescent is taking her dietary and supplemental iron. Often asking her to describe the color of her stool will give evidence to establish compliance. The color change should be explained to the adolescent; it may frighten her and prompt her to discontinue her iron pills if it is not. She may also experience nausea, vomiting, and constipation, or she may find swallowing the pills difficult, and each of these will discourage compliance. Forgetting to take the pills is another problem. In such cases, clinicians may urge the adolescent to keep the iron pills on the bathroom sink next to her toothbrush as a daily reminder.

Identifying the adolescent's food preferences will help the clinician to recognize iron-fortified areas in the adolescent's diet. Once this is done, the clinician can reinforce the need for those foods and introduce others that may be similar and therefore more acceptable to the adolescent. Most teenagers will eat iron-fortified cereal and meat. Pinto beans are often unknown to adolescents, but those willing to try them should be encouraged to eat them. Although eggs are only considered a fair source of iron, most adolescents like them; eggs can be recommended for both their protein and iron values. Dried fruits with the exception of raisins are usually not popular, and as they are also expensive and only a fair source of iron, recommendation to include them in the adolescent diet is carefully weighed.

The clinician needs to clarify the adolescent's nutritional likes and dislikes before making any recommendations. A simple listing of iron-fortified foods provided by the clinician will ordinarily prove to be a dull and often worthless approach. On the other hand, involving the adolescent in an active exchange regarding her dietary preferences will stimulate interest, and the chance for dietary improvement is correspondingly enhanced. A large clinic volume interferes with an in-depth nutritional approach, but taking the time will promote early identification and successful intervention of problems, and in the long run will reduce the amount of clinic time needed to resolve the problem of anemia related to poor nutritional status.

Pica (Nonfood Cravings)

A dietary history also includes investigating for pica. Ingestion of substances such as starch or clay must be identified. Clinicians disagree as to whether pica causes anemia, but it is known that starch discourages the appetite. Pica also remains in the stomach, therefore serving as a direct impediment to appetite and a nurturing diet, thus possibly contributing to the development of anemia. In addition, McFee (4) reported that clay may impede iron absorption. Moreover, antacids that adolescents take for heartburn may affect iron absorption. Ice chewing—common among adolescents—may be evidence of pica. To identify this habit, the clinician should question the adolescent's family or close friends, as the adolescent herself may find it difficult to be objective about the frequency of the habit.

Iron-Deficiency Anemia Treatment

When an adolescent develops iron-deficiency anemia, the treatment is usually ferrous sulfate (325 mg) three times daily. Ferrous sulfate contains 60 to 65 mg of elemental iron per tablet. Ferrous gluconate (325 mg tablets) taken three times daily is another choice. Ferrous gluconate contains 37 to 39 mg of elemental iron per tablet. Replacing iron in this way will rebuild the body's iron stores, and since both pregnancy and the status of reduced iron stores increase the body's rate of absorption of available iron, it is expected that the iron stores will be regained. If this does not occur, compliance may need to be investigated. If the adolescent is unable to swallow tablets, liquid iron, an alternative, is effective. Both ferrous sulfate and ferrous gluconate can be obtained in liquid form. This is all in addition to a high-iron diet.

Although it may take six weeks for an iron-deficiency to resolve itself, a response to therapy will usually begin in two weeks, and the clinician may order a hemoglobin and hematocrit then. It is noteworthy that some women simply do not appear to respond to iron therapy and will continue to be mildly anemic throughout pregnancy. These individuals are usually more hemodiluted than most. Extended hemodilution causes anxiety for clinicians, and the use of parenteral iron may be substituted for oral tablets. Parenteral iron, however is not absorbed more rapidly than oral iron; so unless the adolescent is unable to take iron orally or simply will not comply, the use of parenteral iron is not indicated. The only outcome of certainty attributable to parenteral iron is the established fact that the adolescent has indeed received her medication.

Ultimately, determining the point at which iron deficiency becomes a diagnosis in pregnancy is difficult. McFee (4) referred to a hematocrit of 33 percent or a hemoglobin of 11 g as diagnostic. Varney (5) cites a generally accepted working definition of anemia as a hemoglobin of less than 12 g in nonpregnant women and less than 10 g in pregnant women.

Of the vast numbers of adolescents cared for in clinical practice, especially in high-volume urban clinics, the adolescent with a hemoglobin of 11 g or more may be rare. Even early in pregnancy, the majority of adolescents tend to have hemoglobins between 10 and 11 g. Thus it is more than apparent that a large portion of adolescents are in a borderline state of anemia when they become pregnant; some may remain so throughout pregnancy while others will develop iron-deficiency anemia.

Folic-Acid Deficiency

Folic-acid deficiency can also lead to anemia. Folic acid is a water-soluble vitamin required for the synthesis of DNA in every cell in the body. By definition it is "a group of biochemically similar compounds found primarily in green leafy vegetables, meats, peanuts, yeasts and organ meats. The name 'folate' refers to these molecules which are all required in the daily diet in microgram amounts" (6).

A folic-acid deficiency in pregnancy that goes unrecognized and subsequently untreated may lead to megaloblastic anemia. This condition is rare, however, and does not manifest itself until late in pregnancy because the demands of folic acid do not reach their maximum until that time.

The presence of macrocytes in the blood is one of the laboratory findings necessary to diagnose folate deficiency. A marked anemia is another indicator of its probable presence. The likelihood of its occurrence is reinforced by a low level of folate in the red blood cells. This test is considered by experts to be the most reliable in determining the presence of folic-acid deficiency in pregnancy. Unfortunately, a drop below 150 mg per ml of folate in the RBC is a late indicator, and, in fact, by that time some degree of macrocytic anemia may already be present. Obtaining a serum folate level is another means of evaluating folic acid stores but is not considered as reliable an indicator as the red blood cell folate level is. Some authorities believe that large amounts of formininoglutamic acid (figlu) in the urine reflects a folic-acid deficiency. Others disagree and claim that this test is unreliable in pregnancy because it may give artificial results.

The astute clinician will also realize that folate and iron deficiencies tend to coexist. When this occurs both deficiencies need to be treated simultaneously. Today, many clinicians routinely give oral folic acid (1 mg daily prenatally) to prevent the development of folic-acid deficiency. One to 2 mg daily is considered adequate treatment if folic-acid deficiency is diagnosed.

The availability of folic acid in the diet is limited. Green leafy vegetables are a common source, but overcooking them in a large amount of water that is later discarded can eliminate a majority of the folic acid content. Folic acid is also present in meat, especially organ meats, as well as in peanuts and yeast. Many adolescents may be unwilling to eat yeast or organ meats, but peanuts are usually acceptable and popular. Boiled, unsalted peanuts in the shell are ideal if available and can be encouraged as they have a double dietary value high in both protein and folic acid.

An association between folic-acid deficiency and low birthweight has been noted by some authorities (7). They found that babies with birthweights below 2500 g tended to have low folate levels as did their mothers. This correlation warrants attention as low birthweight is also a major risk factor in adolescent pregnancy. Consequently, when a size/date discrepancy occurs in adolescent pregnancy and folic acid is not already prescribed, folic acid therapy may be initiated. Finally, folic-acid deficiency is also known to be associated with thrombocytopenia. Therefore, if thrombocytopenia is present, it is not contraindicated to begin a folic-acid regimen in addition, of course, to a regular thrombocytopenia investigation.

Reports and studies suggest a significant relationship between adolescent pregnancy and anemia. Because of the frequent association of anemia and infections, the anemic adolescent may also suffer chronic infections. Adolescents are therefore encouraged to continue taking iron tablets orally for 8 to 10 weeks after delivery so that this risk will be minimized. Because the postnatal period is notorious for leaving the new mother vulnerable to infectious agents, the need to protect her from anemia is doubly urgent.

Hypertensive Disorders of Pregnancy

Pre-eclampsia/eclampsia is predominantly a disease of primigravidae. As the pregnant adolescent is frequently a primigravida, she is a potential candidate for this disease. The fact that she may have had an abortion prior to the current pregnancy does not alter this risk. While the etiology of pre-eclampsia is not known, its symptomatology is well documented and includes subjective complaints, clinical findings, and laboratory data.

The standard definition of pre-eclampsia includes: 1) a 30 mm Hg rise in systolic blood pressure or a 15 mm Hg rise in diastolic blood pressure, or a blood pressure of 140/90 on two or more occasions taken six hours apart; 2) edema in the face and/or fingers that is not relieved by a night's rest; and 3) proteinuria of 2+ in a routine urine specimen. Severe pre-eclampsia is defined (7) as: 1) a blood pressure of 160 systolic or 110 diastolic taken on two occasions six hours apart while resting in bed; 2) proteinuria of 5 g per 24 hours (3+ or 4+ on a random urine sample); 3) urinary output less than 400 ml every 24 hours; 4) cerebral or visual disturbances; and 5) pulmonary edema and cyanosis.

Pregnancy-induced hypertension can include the above clinical symptomatology but does not include the presence of proteinuria or generalized edema to establish the diagnosis. Hypertension, however, must be manifested.

Diagnosis

Frequently, the primary care provider for the pregnant adolescent is a certified nurse-midwife. To her falls the responsibility of determining and identifying the early warning signs that generally occur before the classic symptoms arise. As Chesley (8) stated. "It [prenatal care] does not prevent the hypertensive disorders, rather it serves to detect preeclampsia early and often to prevent its progression." That fact is central to the successful management of pre-eclampsia in pregnancy.

The first step in prenatal management is recognition that the standard definition of prenatal hypertension may not be an appropriate one for the pregnant adolescent. As pointed out by Hellman and Pritchard (6). "In a teenage primigravida such an increase [in blood pressure] is alarming." If not guided by the standard definition, how does one accurately evaluate a rise in an adolescent's blood pressure? The baseline blood pressure is an important tool in this determination. Many adolescents tend to register for prenatal care in the second trimester, which is not an opportune time to obtain a baseline blood pressure. Studies indicate (8) that women with essential hypertension reflect a significant drop in their blood pressures during the second trimester; therefore a baseline obtained then may be misleading and may prompt a clinician to diagnose pregnancy-induced hypertension when a natural rise begins to occur early in the third trimester. Thus the best baseline blood pressure is one that is recorded before pregnancy or in early first trimester. Without the baseline the clinician may diagnose pregnancy-induced hypertension or pre-eclampsia when in reality it does not exist. This will result in unnecessary management restrictions that frustrate the adolescent and may even discourage her from continuing her prenatal care. It is helpful to remember, however, that it is the adult hypertensive woman who has the greatest drop in blood pressure during the second trimester. Consequently, if the clinician does note a rise from the second trimester baseline, he/she may be responding appropriately if pre-eclampsia precautions are begun. Data "supports the hypothesis that gestational hypertension is a sign of latent hypertension unmasked by pregnancy" (9). Recognizing that possibility, the clinician who makes the decision to go ahead with hypertension precautions has probably made a correct decision.

Precautions are certainly indicated whenever the clinician has the slightest suspicion of pre-eclampsia during the prenatal course of the adolescent. The immediate family history may be a helpful and predictive factor. A mother who was pre-eclamptic increases the risk that her daughter will also develop pre-eclampsia during her first pregnancy. While many adolescents do not recognize the term pre-eclampsia, most will know if their mothers currently have high blood pressure. A simple check is to have the adolescent ask her mother whether she had high blood pressure during her first pregnancy. If so, clinical caution and assessment is indicated.

Diagnostic Value of the Diastolic Rise

As stated, the classic definition of hypertension in pregnancy is not an appropriate guideline to evaluate hypertension in the pregnant adolescent. Hughes (10) emphasized the need to monitor changes in blood pressure, "even at levels in the low range of normal," and to consider it a danger signal if a rise developed any time after the 20th week of gestation. Clinical experience has proved that utilizing this criterion is helpful in preventing preeclampsia among adolescents. With this risk in mind, nurse-midwifery precautionary management for adolescents frequently begins if there is a consistent 5 mm Hg rise in the diastolic blood pressure on two prenatal visits scheduled one week apart. The subsequent precautions consist of 1) a rest regime of two hours every afternoon on the left side, 2) nutritional consultation emphasizing a high-protein diet and sufficient caloric intake to protect the protein, and 3) weekly prenatal visits to monitor blood pressure, symptomatology, and compliance.

In a study involving adolescents over a four-year period (11), management in the first two years was not initiated until the diagnosis of pre-eclampsia was actually made based on the standard definition. During those years, 15.3 percent of the population developed pre-eclampsia. In the last two years of the study, however, the precautionary management described above was utilized and only 7.2 percent developed the disease (11). Since the clinic profile did not change during those years, the improved outcome was attributed to the prevention aspects of this management regimen. Factors prompting compliance with management during the four years of the study included an investigation of the adolescent's home situation and her routine daily schedule. This review helped to identify problem areas that might interfere with the teenager's ability to comply. The adolescent was asked to recall her daily activities, beginning with the hour she rose in the morning. The clinician noted if something was obviously omitted, such as mention of school or little or no time spent with friends, but did not interrupt. Once the recall was finished, the clinician shared the noted areas of omission with the adolescent and corrections were made. If the adolescent was confident that she could eliminate the conflicting obstacles, she was trusted to do so. If clinical improvement did not occur, further investigation followed.

Certain essentials for taking blood pressure also merit mention. A cuff that is too small for an obese patient will often give an elevated reading. The arms should be at heart level when the blood pressure is taken and should be free of restrictive clothing for at least five minutes before inflating the cuff. If the adolescent has rushed to the clinic or is anxious, angry, worried, or intimidated by the clinic, her blood pressure may be artificially high. An adolescent anticipating a pelvic examination is going to be apprehensive, and for this reason her blood pressure should be taken after the pelvic examination is complete and the clinic routine understood. Many cases of hypertension will resolve spontaneously once anxiety is reduced. The "roll-over test"—which has been heralded by some clinicians, denounced by others, and still questioned by many—is impractical in a large-volume clinic because of the time it requires. Additionally, false negatives do occur. Because the test cannot predict hypertension before late second trimester or the beginning of third trimester, valuable time may be lost to control the hypertension through preventive management. To date, therefore, careful monitoring of the adolescent's blood pressure throughout pregnancy still remains the prime factor in determining the potential for pregnancy-induced hypertension or pre-eclampsia.

Edema

Over the years many clinicians have considered edema of the face and hands an early symptom of pre-eclampsia. Yet, many women have edema of the face and fingers and never develop hypertension in pregnancy. In other words, this finding is common in normal pregnancy. While marked edema usually accompanies pre-eclampsia, exceptions do occur. Occasionally, pre-eclampsia exists without any visible edema. Therefore, the clinician cannot depend on the presence or absence of edema in making the diagnosis of pre-eclampsia. Alternately, the pattern of weight gain may be more indicative of fulminating pre-eclampsia, but this, too, can be benign. A sudden excessive weight gain in the later part of pregnancy, however, is generally accepted as a precursor of pre-eclampsia. Chesley (8) believes the weight gain associated with pre-eclampsia is primarily fluid retention and not related to caloric intake. For that reason, he warns that attempts to control weight through caloric restriction will not reduce the incidence of pre-eclampsia. In the absence of an increase in blood pressure, a sudden excessive weight gain first calls for discussion and clarification about eating patterns with the adolescent. This initial step solicits the adolescent's opinion about this occurrence, and she may contribute invaluable information to clarify the clinical picture. Holidays and family occasions or a simple eating binge are commonly given as reasons. Obviously, dependent edema in the summer heat will increase weight, as will additional clothing in the winter. Each of these situations requires individual attention and must be evaluated appropriately. Consistency in removing shoes, boots, and coats in the winter months before weighing the adolescent are routine clinical procedures. Human error is more apt to occur in weighing adolescents in rushed, crowded clinics where a mistake in reading the scale or in recording the correct weight on the right chart can occur.

Left-sided rest is indicated if edema is responsible for the weight gain. The adolescent must be told why this resting position is preferred; otherwise the adolescent's mother may consider it a strange request and question whether her daughter correctly understood the clinician's instructions—she may even show up at the clinic to find out why the left-sided rest was prescribed. Unfortunately, most mothers do not exhibit this degree of commitment, and because most adolescents do not have the sophistication or experience to ask appropriate questions when confused, they tend to go home and question a parent or adult who may not know either. The adult's disinterest in determining the reason for left-sided rest may subsequently reduce the adolescent's compliance. Therefore an explanation to the adolescent that left-sided rest displaces the enlarged uterus to the left, thereby decreasing compression of the inferior vena cava and enhancing venous return from the lower extremities to the heart and kidneys, will expedite matters.

Proteinuria

While edema is considered an early symptom of pre-eclampsia, proteinuria is considered a late one. When protein is detected in the adolescent's urine, determining whether or not the procedure for obtaining the specimen was followed correctly can be a problem. Specimen contamination is a frequent cause of proteinuria, and it may be difficult for the adolescent to appreciate her role in preventing it. Although time consuming, teaching an adolescent the correct procedure for obtaining a midstream specimen will prevent the need for expensive testing and encourage her to accept responsibility for good hygiene. If the health care provider has reservations about the adolescent's ability to follow instructions, he/she may prepare the adolescent and stay with her while she collects the specimen. A clean specimen is necessary if protein levels of 1+ or higher are detected.

Proteinuria may be caused by 1) pre-eclampsia, 2) urinary tract infection, 3) contamination from vaginal infection, and 4) poor hygiene. The adolescent is evaluated for each of these problems before proteinuria is finally diagnosed. If hypertension is identified, the presence of proteinuria is ominous.

Hyperreflexia

Every adolescent requires assessment for hyperreflexia during the first prenatal visit. This baseline is used for comparison if hyperreflexia develops later in pregnancy. When present with hypertension, hyperreflexia can be a late sign of pre-eclampsia and an indication of the disease's severity. Occasionally, hypertension and hyperreflexia may be the only two symptoms of pre-eclampsia noted by the clinician, but the fact that neither edema nor proteinuria is present does not change the diagnosis.

Subjective complaints such as visual disturbances and headaches are frequently, although not always, present in pre-eclampsia. Some sight problems are thought to be caused by retinal arteriolar spasm, ischemia, and edema. Severe headaches and visual disturbances associated with hypertension, however, are an indication of pre-eclampsia. These headaches—generally frontal but occasionally occipital—do not respond to routine medication as a rule and may owe to cerebral edema.

Hemoconcentration

Hemoconcentration is also a symptom of pre-eclampsia. It appears to reflect a restricted intravascular volume that is underfilled due to vasospasm. The plasma volume expands routinely in the beginning of pregnancy but then changes prior to the onset of hypertension. Peck and Arias (12) believe that a close association exists between physical activity and blood volume. They claim that people who are generally inactive have a lower blood volume than do more active people (12). Therefore, if the adolescent is physically inactive she may also have a low blood volume, and such a phenomenon may increase her risk of developing pre-eclampsia when pregnant. Further study is indicated, however, before conclusions can be drawn, but the implications are worthy of investigation.

Regardless of its cause, the incidence of pre-eclampsia is high in many prenatal clinics treating adolescents. In a review of 884 adolescents under age 18, Chanis (13) and others found the incidence of mild pre-eclampsia to be as high as 87 percent and severe pre-eclampsia/eclampsia to be 14.4 percent. The Guttmacher Institute (2) reported that adolescents are 15 percent more likely to develop pre-eclampsia/eclampsia than their older counterparts are. The disorder's frequent occurrence in this age group jeopardizes both mother and baby, and for this reason careful monitoring is indicated.

Prevention of hypertension in pregnancy is primarily achieved through quality prenatal care and careful monitoring of the diastolic pressure. As

Pritchard et al. (14) state, "The diastolic pressure is probably a more reliable prognostic sign than is the systolic." Therefore when subtle changes occur, a daily schedule of two hours of left-sided bed rest, a high-protein diet, and weekly or more frequent visits for blood pressure monitoring are recommended for safe management.

Low Birthweight

One significant reason for the alarming frequency of low-birthweight babies born to adolescents may be the mothers' tendency to obtain little or no prenatal care. Stickle (15) reported a low-birthweight incidence of 26.4 percent in adolescents who did not receive prenatal care. He also noted that while frequent prenatal visits (13 or more) and registration in the first trimester appear to be factors in favorable birthweight, the adolescent population that complies with such a schedule is still at a greater risk to have a low-birthweight baby than are their older counterparts who obtain adequate obstetric care. Studies (15) reported that the incidence of low-birthweight babies being born to teenagers who received adequate prenatal care was only 5.3 percent, while that for teenagers who did not was 26.4 percent.

In 1978 the National Center for Health Statistics (NCHS) collected data from 44 states and Washington, D.C., on when pregnant adolescents registered for prenatal care. The NCHS found that only 33.3 percent of the sample under age 15 registered in the first trimester. Ironically, this age group runs the greatest risk of all age women of giving birth to a low-birthweight baby and would thus benefit most from early prenatal care (15). Whether early and comprehensive prenatal care removes the threat of low birthweight for infants born to adolescent mothers is difficult to answer, but it apparently makes a substantial difference.

In general, factors contributing to a good birthweight include 1) compliance with prenatal care, 2) a satisfactory maternal weight gain (16), and 3) the gynecological age of the mother—the age of the mother at pregnancy minus the number of years since menses began. Hence, a female pregnant at age 15 with a menarche at age 13 has a gynecological age of 2 years. Studies of gynecological age suggest a correlation between low birthweight and a gynecological age of less than 4 years (17). When the gynecologically young mother's diet is supplemented with additional protein, however, the birthweight of her offspring improves (18). This outcome reinforces the need for consistent nutritional counseling and evaluation for this age group throughout pregnancy. On the other hand, this does not mean that the nutritional patterns of adolescents over 15 years of age or of those with an extended gynecological age are ignored. This group is also vulnerable to low-birthweight babies and will require almost as much attention in this area as their younger sisters do.

Jacobson (19) found that pregnant teenagers in America have the same type of diet as their nonpregnant peers. Such a finding further confirms the need for increased nutritional counseling throughout pregnancy for all teenagers. The RDAs for those aged 11 to 14 is 2700 calories per day. The daily allowance for nonpregnant adolescents over 14 is 2100 calories. In pregnancy, an extra 300 calories per day is recommended (19). Moreover,

---

NORMAL REQUIREMENTS
The normal caloric and protein requirements for mothers 20 years of age or more are determined on the basis of ideal body weight, physical activity, and week of gestation, according to the recommendations in the Dietary Standard for Canada (1948) prepared by the Canadian Council on Nutrition. For mothers 19 years of age or less, we use Recommended Dietary Allowances (1958) prepared by the Food and Nutrition Board, National Research Council, United States. For all mothers we add 500 calories and 25 g of protein after 20 weeks of gestation as recommended in the Canadian standard.

ADDITIONAL CORRECTIVE ALLOWANCES
Corrective caloric and protein allowances are given in addition to the normal requirements according to the degree of UNDER-NUTRITION, UNDER-WEIGHT, or for special high risk conditions which may be indicative of NUTRITIONAL STRESS. A mother may have none or one or more of these conditions.

UNDER-NUTRITION ASSESSMENT AND REHABILITATION
UNDER-NUTRITION is determined if a protein deficit is found between actual dietary intake and requirement.

The method used is a 24-hour recall diet history, cross-checked with a food list and family market order compared with the appropriate standard.

UNDER-NUTRITION CORRECTION is equal to the amount of protein deficit allowing 10 calories for each gram of protein added to normal pregnancy requirements.

UNDER-WEIGHT ASSESSMENT AND REHABILITATION
UNDER-WEIGHT status is determined if the mother's pregravid weight is 5% or more under the weight recommended in the Table of Desirable Weights, prepared by the Metropolitan Life Insurance Company.

UNDER-WEIGHT CORRECTION should provide sufficient additional calories and protein to ensure that the mother gains during pregnancy the number of pounds she was underweight prior to conception. We allow 20 g of protein and 200 calories a day added to normal pregnancy requirements to permit a gain of one pound per week. Since 1971 the calorie correction has been changed from 200 to 500 calories.

NUTRITIONAL STRESS ASSESSMENT AND REHABILITATION
NUTRITIONAL STRESS is determined if any one of the following maternal conditions is present: pernicious vomiting, pregnancies spaced less than one year apart, previous poor obstetrical history, failure to gain 10 pounds by 20th week, serious emotion'

NUTRITIONAL STRESS CORRECTION provides for the addition of 20 g 200 calories for each stress condition added to normal pregnancy require

---

Figure 6.1   The Higgins intervention method for nutritional rehabilitation durir Procedure for estimation of caloric and protein requirements developed at the N Dispensary (20).

Higgins (20) recommends an additional 500 calories per day and 20 g of protein after the 20th week gestation (see Fig. 5.1).

The Division of Vital Statistics of the U.S. government (21) reported that adolescents age 12 to 19 ingested an average of only 1900 calories a day. Additionally, it found the amount ingested for those age 15 to 17 to be only 1750 calories daily. The discrepancy between the above figures and the RDAs is conspicuous. Consequently, if as Jacobson says, pregnant teenagers have the same types of diet as nonpregnant teenagers, the former need to add approximately 700 to 1000 calories daily to supplement their diets.

In the pregnant adolescent, inadequate caloric intake may result in the use of maternal protein, thereby depriving the growing fetus. Since it is known that protein is vital for fetal growth and development and that the caloric intake for the average adolescent is generally below the recommended levels, the impact on the birthweight of her offspring is clearly evident. Therefore, *both* an adequate caloric and protein intake is necessary if the adolescent is to maintain a positive nitrogen balance and, hence, a nurturing and supportive environment for her maturing fetus.

High-volume clinics give little opportunity for an intensive investigation of an individual adolescent's diet. Unfortunately, the availability of a nutritionist in the clinic does not necessarily alleviate the problem. Many nutritionists are overextended and subsequently only see the patients on a scheduled basis. As a result, nutritional problems that develop as the pregnancy progresses are frequently first identified by the clinician providing prenatal care. Redirecting the dietary problem to the nutritionist at that point may substantially reduce the adolescent's compliance with recommended management. This is true because the nutritionist may or may not be present at the clinic, or her/his schedule may require the adolescent to wait for a prolonged period. Many adolescents consider routine nutritional counseling dull and repetitive and the waiting intolerable. This frustrates them into no longer listening. However, the adolescent's awareness of a dietary problem will increase if the clinician who identifies the problem discusses it immediately. The clinician can later inform the nutritionist of the problem and refer the adolescent for further assessment.

One approach to nutritional counseling that has been used effectively is a separate appointment for individual nutritional evaluation for adolescents at 24 weeks gestation who exhibit a poor weight gain. Prior to this appointment (which does not include an obstetric examination) the adolescent is asked to record and bring to the interview a seven-day diet history. Her dietary history, food preferences, activity level, and her family's nutritional habits are discussed at the interview. The clinician expresses enthusiasm about the recorded diet, carefully avoiding punitive comments about undesirable items (i.e., potato chips). In fact, the clinician may empathize with uch preferences and note her own preference for them. This exchange encourages the adolescent to trust the clinician and to be honest in her dietary profile. Adolescents are invited to bring their partners, mothers, or persons who are important to them to these appointments. The presence of a support person often helps the adolescent describe her diet more clearly and helps her relax and carry on a more interesting exchange. The presence of a family member may, on occasion, threaten the adolescent. If this is the case, the clinician should discuss her perception of the interaction with the social worker to determine the need for family counseling.

Exercise/activity habits are also discussed during the nutritional interview to evaluate the need for a caloric intake higher than that recommended for the adolescent's pregnancy age. Personal stress is another factor to consider in the interview. Some adolescents openly admit to stressful family situations or relationships but are reluctant to discuss them, especially if their mothers are present. Once these situations are acknowledged, however, the social worker can intervene and is often able to alleviate the source of the stress. Higgins (20) identified stress as a factor in poor weight gain and subsequently in low birthweight. She recommends 200 extra calories and 20 g of protein a day to compensate for each known stress factor, up to a total of 400 calories and 40 g of protein per 24 hours. If the dietary history indicates a caloric and protein intake below the recommended levels, the diet is adjusted accordingly. In addition, an adjustment is made for the pregnancy: an extra 500 calories and 25 g of protein a day. This allowance follows Higgins's standard (20).

The nutritional supplement most appealing to adolescents is generally a milk shake containing ice cream. This food, of course, also increases the caloric and protein intake. The simple recipe calls for milk, ice cream to taste, 1 teaspoon vanilla, 1½ tablespoons sugar, and one egg. Many adolescents will agree to two milk shakes a day in addition to routine meals.

Nutritional management also includes rest to gain weight and preserve caloric and protein intake. Hence, the adolescent is encouraged to discontinue unnecessary activity and return home immediately after school to rest. Such a regime, however, is only advised if the adolescent has had little or no weight gain or has stopped gaining weight for no known reason.

Of 738 12- to 17-year-olds exposed to these techniques in one study (11), the total low-birthweight rate was 9.1 percent, while the incidence for those age 15 and under was 8.8 percent. In a statewide matching population of 2018 adolescents giving birth during the same period but not attending the clinic offering these techniques, the low-birthweight incidence was 9.1 cent for those under age 15 and 12.7 percent for the total pop should be added that the Women's, Infant's and Children's tritional program was available on an equal basis to all pregnant the state during the period covered by the study. These statistics su the additional time and effort devoted to nutritional counseling d difference in birthweight outcome. Additionally, the fact that the study was carried out in a state with one of the highest infant mortality rates in the nation and where low birthweight is an obvious problem increases the significance of the results. Moreover, both the clinic's population and state's population included a significant number of black adolescents—a group that is particularly vulnerable to producing low-birthweight infants.

Worldwide statistics associate low birthweight with a higher rate of morbidity and mortality, cerebral palsy, and mental retardation. If improved birthweight can reduce the frequency of these outcomes, the output in professional commitment and time is well worth the effort. Without this effort, poor nutritional habits are apt to continue throughout the average adolescent's pregnancy; subsequently low birthweight will continue to be a risk.

The average adolescent has a diet deficient in vitamin B_6 and plasma zinc. Such deficiencies have also been identified with a poor pregnancy outcome. Additionally, Kaminetzky et al. (22) reported that B_6 levels were particularly low for teenagers who had low-birthweight babies. If a B_6 deficiency coexists with low-birthweight outcomes (and adolescents in the United States do tend to have low-birthweight babies), then nutritional counseling must include reference to sources of vitamin B_6. Moreover, others (23) have reported a correlation between B_6 deficiency and mental depression. One study (24) found that infants whose mothers' diets contained an adequate amount of B_6 at the first prenatal visit had higher Apgar scores at birth than did those whose mothers had an inadequate B_6 intake. While one study is not sufficient to establish such a relationship, it certainly suggests that further evaluation is needed, as is a diet correction for B_6. Vitamin B_6 is found in meat, poultry, fish, legumes, whole grains, potatoes, sweet potatoes, and bananas.

Plasma zinc has recently been identified as a factor associated with congenital malformation, dysmaturity, and abnormal partuition (25). The RDA of zinc is 20 mg per day, but the average intake is only 10 to 15 mg per day. Furthermore, studies (24) reveal that zinc deficiency is most prevalant during the adolescent's periods of rapid growth and is therefore least available during the years of puberty. Consequently, the adolescent—considering her age and poor dietary habits—probably has levels of zinc that are not sufficient to contribute to a good pregnancy outcome. In addition, a correlation between pre-eclampsia/eclampsia and a lower mean plasma volume of zinc appears to exist (24). The actual reasons for this are unknown, but the correlation is significant and is particularly so for pregnant adolescents. Crosby and others (26) have found an association between fetal growth and low plasma zinc levels. Consequently, a low plasma zinc level prevalent in adolescence may be yet another factor contributing to the poor pregnancy outcome common to this age group. Thus, pregnant adolescents must be encouraged to eat foods high in zinc such as meat, liver, milk, and eggs.

Summary

Factors of concern that may indicate a low-birthweight infant include the adolescent's

1. age (especially if she is under 15 years)
2. prepregnancy weight and weight gain during pregnancy
3. commitment to her nonpregnant image (which may destroy motivation to gain weight in pregnancy)
4. nonacceptance of her pregnancy
5. conception of a small baby as a "cute baby," thereby indicating her preference to keep her baby "small"
6. tendency to eat junk food
7. tendency to be calorically undernourished for her age
8. caloric and protein intake meeting her own growth needs as well as the needs related to her pregnancy
9. gynecological age
10. low levels of zinc that may contribute to poor pregnancy outcome
11. risk of developing pre-eclampsia/eclampsia
12. low vitamin B_6 levels, which may contribute to low birthweight

As already noted, the infant's low birthweight predisposes it to a higher morbidity/mortality rate. One study (16) found birthweight a significant factor in cranial volume and motor development. That study did not find a significant correlation between birthweight and mental development, but it did find one between motor and mental development. Thus, if motor development is significantly related to birthweight, the effect of the latter on mental development, although indirect, cannot be ignored.

Intrauterine Growth Retardation

The effects of intrauterine growth retardation (IUGR) on birthweight are obvious, but determining IUGR's presence is sometimes difficult. IUGR is generally not recognized until the beginning of the third trimester. However, weight gain in pregnancy and birthweight are closely related, and thus any adolescent who has had a poor weight gain must be monitored early for possible IUGR. Moreover, any teenager with hypertension or pre-eclampsia is predisposed to IUGR and prematurity; this teenager will require IUGR monitoring if poor weight gain is documented or if her weight gain owes solely to edema.

Because IUGR may jeopardize the health of the fetus, nonstress tests are often used to monitor the status of the fetus. For this reason, most clinicians evaluate fetal stress with a nonstress test when they suspect IUGR (around 30 to 32 weeks gestation). Lavery (27) concluded that weekly testing is generally sufficient for IUGR unless postdates, diabetes, or Rh isoimmunization are present or suspected. In those cases, the exact frequency with which to perform the nonstress tests is unknown (27). While the prognosis of a reactive test is not affected by prolonging the test over an extended period of time, attention is given to baseline variability. Rochard et al (28) found that serial tracings featuring a progressive loss of baseline variability were consistent in "fetuses destined to die." Thus, the value of information provided by the baseline variability is an essential one.

Some clinicians who fear the fetus is jeopardized may instruct their patients to assess fetal movement on a qualitative level. Such assessment requires objectivity. Subjective impressions of fetal movement are less reliable and are therefore discouraged as the sole indicator of fetal well-being. Maternal impressions are best evaluated when the mother has been taught an effective procedure to count fetal movements. Teaching the adolescent to note the number of fetal movements for two hours after each meal for three days (29) is quite dependable. This method was proved to be more reliable than maternal subjective impressions of fetal activity. The clinician instructing the adolescent needs to be mindful of the teenager's tendency to forget, and her propensity for subjectivity rather than objectivity. Of course, any mother of any age would find it difficult to be objective in her perception of her baby's activity, but the adolescent's perception may be particularly colored in that respect. However, in a clinical setting with no nonstress test facilities, this procedure may be the only alternative available. In situations where a nonstress test is available, maternal monitoring of fetal movement is a valuable reinforcement to the test and may be used in that capacity, but not to the exclusion of the nonstress test.

Cesarean Sections

Because of their youth, pregnant adolescents have been considered prime candidates for a cesarean section throughout the years. Some studies support this concept; others do not. Because adolescents are biologically immature, the concern is that they are predisposed to cephalopelvic disproportion (CPD), which can result in an operative delivery. Many argue therefore that attempts to increase the birthweight of the adolescent's infant will increase her risk for CPD. In a five-year retrospective study of an adolescent population served by nurse-midwives (12), it was found that the numbers of babies weighing ≥3000 g increased by 13 percent, but this increase in birthweight was *not* accompanied by a corresponding increase in cesarean section rates for CPD. While birthweight is obviously a factor in cesarean section rates, it may not be as significant as other factors such as gynecological age, chronological age, and the risk of prematurity associated with this age group. Moerman, in a study conducted on healthy middle-class girls (30), found that those in their early and mid-teens with apparent maturation in height and reproductive system did not necessarily demonstrate a matured "pelvic birth canal." Moreover, he also found that low gynecological age was more significant in younger teenagers. Hence, girls who had a late menarche also had a larger pelvic size because they had had sufficient time for growth and maturation. Whereas those who had an early menarche had not sufficient time for maturation of the vagina and the pelvis, even though their stature and reproductive status would indicate otherwise. Therefore, maturation of the birth canal may proceed at a slower pace than do other maturation processes, including that of growth in stature, and may be a significant factor in the rate of adolescent cesarean sections.

During pregnancy many adolescents will ask about cesarean sections. Most have heard about the procedure and are frightened by its prospect, but few have the courage to express their fears. Consequently, the astute clinician will encourage discussion of this topic. Once the subject is raised adolescents usually become quite verbal about their concerns. Most will want to know who is apt to have a section and why. Understanding the reasons for a cesarean section, anesthesia, and the recovery process may therefore reduce adolescents' anxiety and help them adjust to this possibility.

While a cesarean section is considered a routine surgical procedure, it does increase morbidity and mortality rates for the mother, particularly when general anesthesia is used. Consequently, a reliable history of last food intake is vital. Adolescents in labor having difficulty with labor pains may have a difficult time recalling the hour of their last meal. Subsequently, if aspiration occurs under general anesthesia, the effect can be fatal or severely debilitating. This outcome is considered one of the major risk factors associated with general anesthesia and surgical procedures and, thus, adolescents need to be taught during pregnancy to note the time they last ate when labor starts.

Postoperatively, the adolescent will require special teaching about hygiene. While nutrition, adequate rest, and cleanliness are a routine part of postpartum teaching, adolescents who have had a cesarean section will need additional teaching about care for the incision, lifting, exercise, and infection. After a cesarean, consideration must be given to the needs of mother and baby—their bonding experience and their phase of initial adjustment.

Some women are able to deliver vaginally after a cesarean section, however, the majority still do not. Thus, a previous cesarean may place an adolescent in a high-risk category for the remainder of her childbearing life.

Dating the Last Menstrual Period

Describing the case of "the missing menstrual period" is not an attempt to be facetious; this is a real problem and complication. As most adolescents register after the first trimester, which is the optimal time for uterine sizing, the opportunity to date accurately the pregnancy by uterine size is lost. This loss increases the need to obtain an accurate last menstrual date (LMP). Unfortunately, the adolescent's memory of her last menstrual period is frequently unreliable and, unfortunately, not all clinicians take the time to obtain an accurate last menstrual history.

Most adolescents are aware that they will be asked for this date at their first prenatal visit, thus they rationalize that any date is better than none and arbitrarily select one. While the selected choice may be the accurate month, it may not include the actual days of her period. Such a discrepancy can create havoc when a due date derived from the recorded LMP passes and there are no signs of impending labor. Clinical concerns about postdatism subsequently develop, and nonstress tests are begun. In some institutions amniocentesis may be used to determine the presence of meconium (as well as a total intrauterine volume) to assess reduction in amniotic fluid. Eventually, induction may be selected as the only acceptable means of management of the postdates. Once an induction is begun, a cesarean section may be indicated if fetal distress occurs. To prevent such a scenario, a number of things can be done throughout the pregnancy to attempt to date the pregnancy accurately. These include 1) detecting the date when fetal heart tones are first heard with a fetoscope 2) performing ultrasound mid-second trimester if size differs noticeably from LMP, and 3) evaluating size with current calendar date and LMP.

If careful fetal heart tone monitoring was done in early pregnancy, it is anticipated that a mature fetus will be developed 18 to 20 weeks from the date the fetal heart tones were first heard with a fetoscope. Of course, if the adolescent does not register until late second trimester when fetal heart tones are easily heard with a fetoscope, this means of determining fetal age is lost. However, if she registers early when fetal heart tones can only be heard with a doptone, then it is possible to document the date when fetal heart tones are first heard with a fetoscope. This requires weekly visits around the time the uterine size indicates that fetal heart tones can be heard with a fetoscope—usually 16 to 18 weeks. Once fetal heart tones are heard with the fetoscope, the adolescent can return to a routine prenatal appointment schedule. However, if reliance on fetal heart tones is planned, it should be noted that some authors do not believe that the first audible fetal heart tones are sufficient alone as a means to date the pregnancy. This is especially true if the patients are not seen on a weekly basis. In such cases, the standard deviation ranges up to three weeks (31). Weekly visits are therefore mandated if reliance on fetal heart tones is planned as an aid to determine fetal maturity.

An adolescent who admits she has forgotton the date of her menses is more easily managed than one who either knowingly or unknowingly misleads the clinician. When the LMP is not available, an ultrasound for dating purposes needs to be obtained at a suitable time in pregnancy. However, when a falsified LMP is thought to be reliable by the clinician, the situation becomes more difficult. An ultrasound for dating purposes is considered most accurate between 16 and 24 weeks gestation, but because most size/date discrepancies do not become apparent until the latter part of the second trimester, the ideal time to size by ultrasound is frequently passed before the problem is identified.

To avoid these consequences, the clinician should ask the adolescent why she remembers the particular date that she has given as her LMP. If her reason is reliable it is usually immediate: "I wrote it on the calendar" or "It was my brother's birthday," etc. On the other hand, if she has fantasized a date, the questions may confuse her and result in an admission of her memory loss. If honesty prevails and she simply cannot remember, the clinician may ask her to re-live the menstrual period to the best of her ability. This may help her recall an associated event on a given day. To gain the adolescent's full cooperation in this, it is imperative that she understand the reason for the questions about the accuracy of this date. Otherwise, she may resent the intrusion and consider the process a total waste of time. An earnest effort at the initial prenatal visit to establish a reliable LMP will prove itself invaluable in future management decisions.

A reliable LMP not only reduces risks associated with poor dates, but also decreases the financial cost of personnel and technology required to evaluate the status of a fetus suspected of postdatism. Spotting, which is frequently identified as a last menstrual period, must be differentiated from implantation bleeding. This is a difficult task especially for an adolescent not yet familiar with her own menses schedule. Moreover, she may not yet have developed a normal and regular menstrual flow. In such cases it is necessary to rely on clinical sizing and ultrasound. When doing clinical sizing in any of these situations, it should be remembered that a full bladder can make as much as a 7 cm difference in fundal height (32). It is therefore especially important to ask the adolescent if she has voided prior to her examination.

It is unfortunate that not all clinicians take the time to obtain the best menstrual history. One approach is to have a clinic policy requiring all practitioners to review thoroughly each adolescent's menstrual dates at the initial clinic visit and then appropriately note this procedure on the chart. Such an effort will reduce duplication of clinical effort and time, eliminate frustration for both the adolescent and the clinician, and facilitate and improve prenatal management.

Physiological Discomforts

Anyone who has ever been pregnant, worked with pregnant women, or studied the subject of pregnancy is aware of its associated discomforts. There is certainly nothing exciting or enticing about "morning sickness," constipation, or persistent nonpathological diuresis. These complaints are unappealing and are best described as "the blahs of pregnancy."

The physiological discomforts of pregnancy are no different for the adolescent than they are for women in any age group. The difference lies in their related implications for the adolescent.

Most adolescent pregnancies are unplanned. Lacking knowledge about conception and the physiology of pregnancy, many adolescents are not aware of their pregnancy until confronted with its discomforts during the first or second trimester. While a missed period may seem absurdly obvious as an indicator of pregnancy, a large number of teenagers have no accurate recall of the date of their last menses because their menses may still be irregular. Subsequently they have no concern about pregnancy if a monthly period does not occur.

The result for many adolescents is an unexpected confrontation with nausea and vomiting, fatigue, urinary frequency, breast tenderness, and headaches. Experiencing these first trimester discomforts may be frightening and even overwhelming for the uninformed adolescent. Being in a public place such as a school for six or seven hours each day makes the implication of these discomforts apparent. A system that requires a teacher's permission to leave class to urinate imposes an embarrassing emphasis on the frequency of the need. Peer reaction will be quick and in some instances acutely perceptive and even cruel. Some of the adolescent's more informed peers may suspect her condition before she does herself. In that event it is generally a matter of time before the suspecting classmate will suggest the possibility of pregnancy to the unsuspecting adolescent.

The realization of pregnancy may generate fear of parental and peer reaction, anxiety about where to find help, and concern about confidentiality if the adolescent decides to seek a pregnancy test. In short, experiencing one of the minor discomforts of the first trimester may be the adolescent's introduction to her pregnancy, and this may occur in public in an embarrassing manner. Body image and vulnerability are excessively important during adolescence. This sudden vulnerability of the adolescent's body to a variety of ills can be shocking. Being unaware of why this is occurring enhances the impact of that fear, and hence, fear becomes an added discomfort of the first trimester for these adolescents. Normally, fear as a psychological discomfort is experienced in the third trimester by all primigravidae in relation to the unknowns of labor and delivery and the concern for the safety and well-being of their babies. But for the primigravida adolescent, fear is frequently a psychological discomfort in the first trimester as well.

Gastrointestinal Discomforts

Food cravings that are a form of pica are not unusual in pregnancy. Women are generally able to recognize and control this urge but adolescents may not be. Many adolescents think their craving is funny and, because it often brings attention from others, its popularity may actually increase. With the adolescent's propensity for junk food, there is a greater risk that she will eat what she craves and ignore the need for a well-balanced diet. This increases the clinician's responsibility to review periodically the adolescent's diet, especially when weight gain is poor or excessive. In addition, the clinician needs to be alerted to other cravings such as excessive ice chewing, smoking, and ingesting starch. Each of these, if excessive, can affect the pregnancy outcome. As the adolescent may have difficulty imposing self-discipline, it is doubly important to monitor frequently her addictive habits.

Persistent nausea and vomiting throughout pregnancy require careful evaluation. The immediate diagnosis may be hyperemesis gravidarum—a diagnosis not to be underevaluated. However, a more common cause of nausea and vomiting is the adolescent's subconscious anxieties about herself, her relationships with her family and peers, and a future that includes the unknown of labor, delivery and parenting. On the other hand, if the adolescent gives a history of nausea and vomiting, and is obviously dehydrated, losing weight and spilling ketones in her urine, medication is generally indicated and the physician consulted. However, an attempt should also be made to determine any personal problems or anxieties that are paramount. A quick talk with a clinician the adolescent trusts will often help her identify and discuss suppressed feelings she has been afraid to recognize. Once this is accomplished, the physical symptoms may rapidly subside, and weight gain may begin. Without this opportunity, many will continue to lose weight, complain of nausea and a poor appetite, and gain little relief with either medication or comfort measures.

Recognition must also be given to the few who simply have a chronic problem with nausea and vomiting throughout their pregnancies. In such cases the clinician can only offer caring support and standard comfort measures and monitor the pregnancy's progress carefully. Growth in fundal height consistent with the gestational age determined by LMP or ultrasound is a positive pregnancy indicator even when weight gain is poor. When both fundal height and weight gain lag, IUGR is possible.

The adolescent may also develop vomiting in the third trimester. At that time, the stomach is compressed by the enlarged uterus. The alert clinician will note that the complaint is of vomiting but not of nausea. There is a reason for this distinction. Adolescents with good appetites tend to gorge themselves when hungry. Subsequently, they overfill an already compressed stomach and vomiting results.

Because of junk food preferences, the adolescent's diet frequently consists of greasy fried foods. These foods contribute to an increase in heartburn. Lying down immediately after eating facilitates regurgitation of digestive juices from the stomach to the esophagus through a relaxed cardiac sphincter. Consequently, this too contributes to heartburn, and adolescents need to be instructed accordingly.

Constipation is not uncommon among adolescents, and is a frequent discomfort when they are pregnant. Protinsky et al (33) state that "pregnant girls are inclined to be inactive . . . tend to be loners with few hobbies or recreational interests." This lack of physical activity may be a major factor in compounding constipation problems. The clinician should therefore begin by investigating the adolescent's activity level. As body image is already a sensitive area for the adolescent, most find constipation a difficult topic to discuss. A few may not even recognize the word or are more apt to talk about "straining." Many never complain of it because they either lack the vocabulary to describe the symptoms or find the topic too threatening or repugnant to discuss. Often, the clinician only discovers its presence when attempting to do a pelvic exam—the rectum is so impacted that it is difficult or impossible to insert a speculum and perform a digital rectal exam. In some cases, the only solution may be a mild enema given at the clinic. Patient education consists of preventive measures such as exercise, increased fluid intake and common bulk-builders like whole grain cereals. The condition should be re-evaluated throughout the pregnancy. If the constipation is not resolved, hemorrhoids may result, which will only complicate the problem. Also, iron if taken orally, may have a constipating effect and will turn stool black. Many adolescents may be frightened to discover this change in stool color and some will spontaneously discontinue their iron tablets as a result. Generally, the adolescent will not refer to a change in stool color unless questioned by the care provider. Most adolescents express great relief to discover the cause of this color change, and they will resume their iron if it was discontinued for this reason. If the iron is actually constipating and anemia is not a concern, a high-iron diet may suffice. However, if the adolescent's commitment to maintaining the diet is questioned, the alternative is to try another iron preparation and utilize constipation prevention measures.

Urinary Frequency

Another minor discomfort with special implications for the pregnant adolescent is urinary frequency. As noted, the adolescent may be in a classroom where permission is required to go to the toilet. This is a terrible imposition for someone who is suffering from urinary frequency, and the adolescent may consequently suppress the urge to void. Every attempt must be made to explain to her why this is unadvisable.

Nocturia may occur in the third trimester and results from the shifting of the enlarged uterus off the inferior vena cava when one lies on one's side while sleeping. This facilitates venous return from the lower extremities and a diuresis develops. Frequent trips to the toilet at night disturb sleep and cause fatigue that may affect the adolescent's performance in school by making it difficult for her to concentrate or stay awake during class. Consequently, many health care providers recommend discontinuation of all fluid intake after the evening meal. Reduced fluid intake reduces urinary frequency and subsequently allows more opportunity for uninterrupted sleep. In this case, the adolescent needs to clearly understand that the fluid intake restriction is limited to the evening only.

Round Ligament Pain

The final physiological discomfort with special implications for the pregnant adolescent is round ligament pain, which can be very uncomfortable. Given the adolescent's natural concern about her changing body image, her reaction to this sudden, unexplained pain may be exaggerated and overstated. Thus, adolescents may limp, clutching their sides, completely preoccupied with the pain. Once reassured and instructed in comfort measures (i.e., knee flexion with a pillow to support the knees, warm tub baths and support for the uterus when lying on the side), most teenagers will relax and perceive the pain more realistically. Because round ligament pain often occurs early in pregnancy, it may interfere with sports activities. On the other hand, its occurrence is reason to request dismissal from physical education class if the adolescent is required to attend those classes. At the same time, the adolescent needs to be encouraged to carry on such exercises as walking and swimming or any other sport that she is comfortable performing.

Psychosocial Complications

No discussion of complications associated with adolescent pregnancy is complete without mention of its psychosocial aspects. These vary with each individual and may even change over the years. For some, a pregnancy that began as a negative experience may become one of growth and productivity, while the reverse may be true for others.

In the mid-1970s, studies reported that eight out of 10 adolescents permanently dropped out of school because of their pregnancy. Today, however, statistics on this point are more qualified and report that adolescents who return to live with their families after delivery also return to school, while their counterparts who elect to set up their own housekeeping unit fail to do so (2). Obviously, the adolescent who is nurtured and supported both emotionally and financially by her family has a better chance of a psychosocial survival because she has the opportunity to pursue her own goals in spite of the fact that she has recently had a baby. On the other hand, her counterpart who does not stay with her family is not as fortunate. Generally she lives below the poverty level because her lack of education restricts her job marketability. Deprived of her own potential, she must live on one welfare check to the next because little else is available to her. Some adolescents are, of course, satisfied with this existence, but the majority are not. It is a demeaning existence in a society geared to the success of the individual. Caught as she is, alone and removed from the mainstream of society, she often drifts into another pregnancy. Critics sometimes view this as an attempt to obtain additional money from the government, but the scant financial reimbursement does not compare realistically to the costs of raising another child. It is more probable that a host of unrelated factors contribute to a repeat pregnancy. Loneliness and a poor self-image are two examples. The need to feel self-worth and love are vital to one's emotional well-being. For the adolescent mother who is alone, the search for such emotional needs is natural. Tragically, her psychological needs re-create the obstacle of her initial deprivation. Current statistics indicate 15 percent of adolescents who become pregnant will have a repeat pregnancy within two years (2). In addition, these second pregnancies run even a greater risk of low-birthweight outcome than do those of the adolescent primigravida. Subsequently, the risk of infant morbidity and mortality is also increased. These facts, coupled with an already stressful situation, can further complicate the adolescent's life.

The teenage mother who marries because she is pregnant is predisposed to divorce. Statistics show that approximately half of the marriages made by pregnant adolescents will end in divorce within 15 years. This rate is three times greater than it is for the general public who delay marriage until their 20s (2). As a result, most female adolescents will raise their children alone. Children raised in such an environment have been found to exhibit deficiencies in cognitive development. Baldwin and Cain (34) reported that negative cognitive and social development is apt to occur in settings where the adolescent mother raises her children alone without the help of other adults or the child's father. The final irony lies in the fact that children raised in this environment tend to become adolescent parents themselves. Hence, the tragedy reimposes itself on another generation.

Conclusion

The complications of adolescent pregnancy can be reduced and alleviated. In clinics where individual attention is emphasized and continual care provided by the same care providers, the result is frequently impressive. Preeclampsia, anemia, and the incidence of low birthweight can be changed. To achieve this goal, it is necessary to obtain the adolescent's commitment to her prenatal management. This is a real challenge and may require many hours of patience on the part of the health care provider, but the results are worth the effort. Without that compliance the complications will remain, and the adolescent will continue to be classified as a high-risk obstetric patient. In the end, a key factor to achieve this goal is simply the clinician's love and caring for this special patient.

References

1. Cates W, Tietze C. Standardized mortality rates associated with legal abortion. United States, 1972-1975. *Family Planning Perspectives* 1977;10:109-112.
2. *Teenage Pregnancy: The Problem that Hasn't Gone Away.* New York: Alan Guttmacher Institute, 1981.
3. *Quarterly Vital Statistics Review.* New York: New York State Department of Health, 1980;Table 6.
4. McFee JG. Iron metabolism and iron deficiency during pregnancy. *Clin Obstet Gynecol* 1979;22:799.
5. Varney H. *Nurse-Midwifery* (2nd ed). Boston: Blackwell Scientific Publications, 1984; 173.
6. Hellman LM, Pritchard JA. *Williams Obstetrics* (4th ed). New York: Appleton-Century-Crofts, 1971;761.
7. Kitay DZ. Folic acid and reproduction. *Clin Obstet Gynecol* 1979;22:809.
8. Chesley LC. *Hypertensive Disorders in Pregnancy.* New York: Appleton-Century-Crofts, 1979;10.
9. Kotchen JM, McKean HE, Kotchen TA. Blood pressure of young mothers and their children after hypertension in adolescent pregnancy: Six to nine year follow-up. *Am J Epidemiol* 1982;115(6):861-867.
10. Hughes TD. Ante-natal care and the prevention of eclampsia. *Med J Austr* 1956; 2:48-50.
11. Piechnick S, Corbett MA. Reducing low birthweight among socioeconomically high-risk adolescent pregnancies: Successful intervention with certified nurse-midwife managed care and multidisciplinary team. *J Nurse-Midwif* 1985;30-(2):88.
12. Peck TM, Arias F. Hematologic changes associated with pregnancy. *Clin Obstet Gynecol* 1979;22(4):791.
13. Chanis M, O'Donahue N. Adolescent pregnancy. *J Nurse-Midwif* 1979;24:3-18.
14. Pritchard JA, MacDonald PC, Gant NF. *Williams Obstetrics* (17th ed). Norwalk, CT: Appleton-Century-Crofts, 1985; 540.
15. Stickle G. Overview of adolescent pregnancy and childbearing. *Birth Defects* 1981;17(3):9.
16. Mophissi KS. Maternal nutrition in pregnancy. *Clin Obstet Gynecol* 1978;21(2):279-309.
17. Zlatnik FT, Burmeister LF. Low "gynecological age": An obstetric risk factor. *Am J Obstet Gynecol* 1977;128:183-187.

18. Paige DM, Cordano A, Mellits DE, Barth JM, Davis L. Nutritional supplementation of pregnant adolescents. *J Adolescent Health Care* 1981;1(4):261–267.
19. Jacobson H. Nutritional risk of pregnancy. *Birth Defects* 1981;17(3):69–83.
20. Higgins A. Nutritional status and outcome of pregnancy. *J Can Dietetic Assoc* 1976;37(1):17–35.
21. Carruth BR. Smoking and pregnancy outcome of adolescents. *J Adolescent Health Care* 1981;2:115–120.
22. Kaminetzky HA, Langer A, Baker A, et al. The effect of nutrition in teenage gravidas on pregnancy and status of the neonate. *Am J Obstet Gynecol* 1973; 115:639646.
23. Vitamin B$_6$ status of low income adolescents and adult pregnant women and condition of their infants at birth. *Am J Clin Nutrition* 1981;34:1731–1735.
24. Cherry FF, Bennett EA, Bazzano GS, Johnson LK, Fosmire GJ, Batson HK. Plasma zinc in hypertension/toxemia and other reproductive variables in pregnancy. *Am J Clin Nutrition* 1981;34:2367–2375.
25. Heald FP, Rosenbrough RH, Jacobson MS. Nutrition and the adolescent: An update. *J Adolescent Health Care* 1980;1(2):142–150.
26. Crosby WM, Metcoff J, Coshiloe JP, Mameesh M, et al. Fetal malnutrition: An appraisal of correlated factors. *Am J Obstet Gynecol* 1977;128:22.
27. Lavery JP. Non-stress fetal heart rate and pre-eclampsia testing. *Clin Obstet Gynecol* 1982;25(4):689–703.
28. Rochard F, Schifrin BS, Goupil F, et al. Non-stress fetal heart rate monitoring in the antepartum period. *Am J Obstet Gynecol* 1976;126:699.
29. Sorokin Y, Dieker LJ. Fetal movement. *Clin Obstet Gynecol* 1982;25(4):719–734.
30. Moerman ML. Growth of the birth canal in adolescent girls. *Am J Obstet Gynecol* 1982;143(5):528–532.
31. Nichols C. Postdate pregnancy. Part I: Literature review. *J Nurse-Midwif* 1985; 30(4):222–239.
32. Worthen N, Bustillo M. Effect of urinary bladder fullness on fundal height measurement. *Am J Obstet Gynecol* 1980;138:759.
33. Protinsky H, Sporakowski M, Atkins P. Pregnant and non-pregnant adolescents. *Adolescence* 1982;17(65):73–79.
34. Baldwin W, Cain VS. The children of teenage parents. *Family Planning Perspectives* 1980;12:34–43.

Bibliography

Asmussen I. Ultrasound of the villi and fetal capillaries in placentas from smoking and non-smoking mothers. *Br J Obstet Gynaecol* 1980;87:239–245.
Beschiner GM, Friedman AS. *Youth Drug Abuse: Problems, Issues and Treatment.* Lexington, MA: Lexington Books, 1979.
Gant NF, Worley RJ. *Hypertension in Pregnancy: Concepts and Management.* New York: Appleton-Century-Crofts, 1980.
Gazzella J. *Nutrition for the Childbearing Years.* Wayzata, MN: Woodland Publishing Co., 1979.
Reid C. A comparison of measurements for prediction of pregnancy-induced

hypertension in adolescent primigravidas. Master's thesis (1981): Yale University School of Nursing, New Haven, CT.

Sim J. The role of nutrition in the prevention of toxemia. Master's thesis (1981): Yale University School of Nursing, New Haven, CT.

Stenchever M. The use of tobacco and drugs in pregnancy. *Contemporary Obstet Gynecol* 1976;8(1):133–136.

Tafari N, Naeye RL, Gobezie A. Effects of maternal undernutrition and heavy physical work during pregnancy on birthweight. *Br J Obstet Gynaecol* 1980; 87:222–226.

Zinc, copper supplements needed in pregnancy. *OB/Gyn News* 1986;21(6):25.

7 Drugs in Pregnancy

MARY ALICE JOHNSON

Overview

The use of psychoactive agents is common to virtually every culture and era. Since the early 1960s, however, there has been a dramatic increase in the medical and nonmedical use of psychoactive drugs and substances in the United States. The social upheaval and crises of the 1960s were accompanied by a spread in the use of illicit drugs to youths of all social strata—a trend that reached epidemic proportions in the 1970s. Annual nationwide surveys of high school seniors showed an increase in illicit drug use throughout the 1970s, followed by gradual moderation of use in the 1980s (1,2) (Fig. 7.1). In fact, two-thirds of American teenagers have tried an illicit drug before finishing high school, and one-third have tried an illicit drug other than marijuana. While use of certain illicit drugs has declined, the proportion of high school seniors who have had some illicit drug experience has not changed substantially. Daily use (use on 20 or more occasions in the past 30 days) of marijuana, alcohol, and cigarettes rose dramatically in the 1970s and has gradually declined (Fig. 7.2). Despite moderation of the trends of recent decades, drug use by adolescents continues to be a nationwide problem (Fig. 7.3). One out of every 16 adolescents drinks alcohol daily, and 41 percent of high school seniors reported binge drinking (five or more drinks on one occasion) within a two-week period (1,2). Daily use of marijuana has declined from a peak of 11 percent in 1978 but is still prevalent at just over 6 percent. Thirty percent of students surveyed smoked cigarettes in the prior month (1,2). Substance abuse by American adolescents is widespread, constituting a serious social problem with significant implications for health and health care of adolescents.

Patterns of adolescent drug use are changing as well, with a trend toward experimentation at an earlier age, use of more dangerous substances, and multiple drug use. Involvement with drugs in adolescence generally begins with beer and wine, cigarettes and hard liquor, then marijuana. If drug use progresses, use of stimulants, depressants, and psychedelics follows, then use of opiates. Progressive involvement, while by no means inevitable,

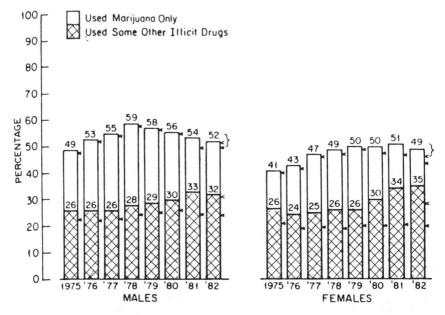

Figure 7.1. Annual prevalence of illicit drug use by sex. The shaded areas include any use of hallucinogens, cocaine, and heroin or any use of opiates, stimulants, sedatives or tranquilizers that is not under a physician's order. The solid arrows indicate the resulting percentage if all stimulants are excluded from the definition of "illicit drugs." The open arrows indicate the resulting percentage if only nonprescription stimulants are excluded. The bracket near the top of the bar indicates the confidence limits (95%). (Reproduced with permission from Johnston JD, Bachman JG, O'Malley PM. *Student Drug Use, Attitudes, and Beliefs: National Trends, 1975–1982.* U.S. Department of Health and Human Services Publication No. (ADM) 83–1260. Washington, DC: U.S. Government Printing Office, 1982.)

begins with occasional use, followed by casual or experimental use, regular use and compulsive use (3,4).

Drug Use by Female Adolescents

Drug use by female adolescents is, in general, slightly less common than by males. The proportion who report use of illicit drugs is roughly the same, however. Prevalence of drug use by females and males is compared in Table 7.1. Slightly more females than males are regular heavy cigarette smokers (half a pack per day or more), a difference which is even greater when occasional smokers are included for comparison. Stimulants are used more by female adolescents, probably for weight loss as opposed to recreational purposes (2,3).

Multiple social and personal factors contribute to drug abuse behavior in an adolescent female. Adolescence is characterized by identification with

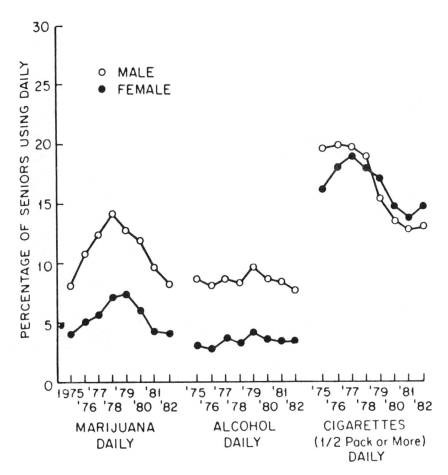

Figure 7.2. Daily use of marijuana, alcohol, and cigarettes by sex. Daily use of alcohol and marijuana is defined as that on 20 or more occasions over a period of 30 days; daily use of cigarettes is defined as smoking a half pack or more a day during a 30-day period. (Reproduced with permission from Johnston JD, Bachman JG, O'Malley PM. *Student Drug Use, Attitudes, and Beliefs: National Trends, 1975–1982.* U.S. Department of Health and Human Services Publication No. (ADM) 83–1260. Washington, DC: U.S. Government Printing Office, 1982.)

peers and rebellion against authority. Indulgence of pleasure-seeking and curiosity may include experimentation with drugs and sex. During these turbulent years, additional developmental crises and disturbances at home or in school strain the adolescent's resources for coping. Some will develop meaningful outlets for this stress; others exhibit destructive coping behaviors, of which pregnancy and drug use are two examples. Female peers may influence drug use; however, women are often introduced to drugs by men, often in groups dominated by males. Disruption of the family is fre-

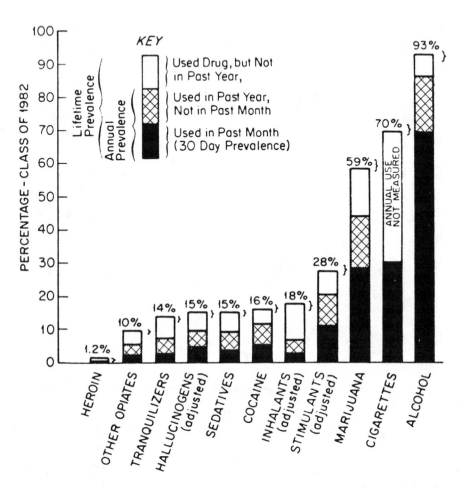

Figure 7.3. Prevalence and recency of drugs used by a high school class of 1982. The bracket near the top of the bar indicates the confidence limits (95%). (Reproduced with permission from Johnston JD, Bachman JG, O'Malley PM. *Student Drug Use, Attitudes, and Beliefs: National Trends, 1975–1982.* U.S. Department of Health and Human Services Publication No. (ADM) 83–1260. Washington, DC: U.S. Government Printing Office, 1982.)

quently cited as a major influence on drug use. Instability in the family because of divorce, death, moving, or because of a troubled parental relationship is likely to affect the behavior of the female adolescent. In addition, parental drug use and abuse, including drinking and cigarette smoking, are significant influences on the drug use behavior of adolescents. Psychological disturbances correlated with drug abuse predate serious drug use, and include anxiety and mood swings; poor interpersonal relationships; distrust of authority; feelings of isolation, loneliness, and alienation; and poorly developed coping mechanisms. These characteristics are manifest as serious maladjustment in the home, at school, or at work. Experimen-

Table 7.1. *Prevalence of Use of 16 Types of Drugs by Sex and Class, 1982*

	Lifetime Prevalence		Annual Prevalence		31-Day Prevalence	
	Male (%)	Female (%)	Male (%)	Female (%)	Male (%)	Female (%)
Marijuana	61.5	55.5	47.2	40.8	31.4	24.9
Inhalants*	15.3	10.4	5.8	3.1	2.0	1.1
Amyl/butyl nitrates	12.4	7.3	5.0	2.3	2.1	0.2
Hallucinogens*	14.4	10.2	9.6	6.1	4.2	2.2
LSD	11.3	7.4	7.4	4.3	2.9	1.6
PCP	7.3	4.7	2.8	1.6	1.3	0.7
Cocaine	18.0	13.7	13.1	9.6	5.9	3.8
Heroin	1.4	0.8	0.8	0.4	0.4	0.1
Other opiates	10.6	8.6	6.0	4.6	2.2	1.5
Stimulants (adjusted)†	26.8	28.2	19.6	20.3	10.2	10.6
Sedatives	16.0	14.1	10.0	8.0	3.5	3.1
Barbiturates	10.7	9.6	5.9	5.0	2.1	1.8
Methaqualone	11.8	9.3	5	5.9	2.5	2.0
Tranquilizers	13.8	14.2	6.9	7.1	2.6	2.2
Alcohol	93.4	92.4	88.5	85.3	74.1	65.4
Cigarettes	67.8	72.0	13.1	14.7	26.8	32.6

*Unadjusted for known underreporting of certain drugs.
†Adjusted for overreporting of the nonprescription stimulants.
Adapted from Johnston LD, Bachman JG, O'Malley PM. *Student Drug Use, Attitudes and Beliefs: National Trends, 1975–1982.* U.S. Department of Health and Human Services Publication No. (ADM) 83–1260. Washington, DC: U.S. Government Printing Office, 1982.

tal or casual use of drugs is influenced by peers; progressively heavier involvement, however, is correlated with personal and family disturbances.

Drug Use by Pregnant Adolescents

Adolescents constitute a population at significant risk for drug use during pregnancy. The extent of serious drug use among adolescent females and the increasing prevalence of drug use at earlier ages in all adolescents adds a serious health care risk to pregnancy. The scope of drug problems among pregnant adolescents is, however, difficult to estimate. Inferences drawn from high school senior survey data are probably underestimations because high school drop-outs (approximately 20% of adolescents by senior year nationwide; higher in urban areas and among blacks) are not surveyed (1,2). Drop-outs have higher than average drug use rates. Among female adolescents, pregnancy is a major reason for leaving high school (5), and thus, while trends in usage may parallel those evident in the surveys, actual prevalence of drug use by pregnant adolescents is uncertain.

Correlation with Sexual Activity

Social circumstances conducive to sexual experimentation and possible conception are similar to those necessary for illicit drug use. Correlates identified by Bachman, Johnston and O'Malley—truancy, recreational evenings out of the house, and, inversely, religious commitment—have in common the degree to which the youth is not under the supervision of adults. The negative correlation between age at first intercourse and the level of cigarette smoking, described by Zabin (7), is strong enough to be statistically significant despite a positive correlation between age at first intercourse and current age. Adolescents who date (two or more dates per month) report use of marijuana and other illicit drugs at significantly greater rates than do nondaters (8). This contrast is evident for those age 12 to 13 years as well as for those age 16 to 17 years. Those who begin sexual involvement early in adolescence are at greater risk for pregnancy in the early months and throughout adolescence (9). Thus, pregnancy in adolescence takes place in a milieu conducive to the use of alcohol, cigarettes, marijuana, and other psychoactive substances.

Consideration of Risks

Concern for exposure of the pregnant woman and fetus to drugs has contributed in part to relatively recent investigations of the extent to which psychotropic drugs are used by women of childbearing age. Studies identifying agents with teratogenic and toxic potential in pregnancy have received widespread publicity and have resulted in recommendations to moderate or avoid drug use during pregnancy. Public awareness of drug-induced risks to the fetus has had a demonstrable effect. In one study (10), responses to interviews regarding drinking and smoking behavior were compared between groups of pregnant women interviewed in 1974–75 (after public announcements about the effects of smoking in pregnancy) and 1980–81 (after widespread publicity about the dangers of drinking in pregnancy). Significantly more women polled in 1980–81 were abstaining from alcohol during pregnancy (58% vs. 19% in the earlier sample) and at the time of conception (35% vs. 20%). Significantly fewer women in 1980–81 reported binges during pregnancy, and a decline was reported in consumption of each type of alcoholic beverage. There was a small but significant increase in the number of nonsmokers (78% vs. 75%) and a decline in the smoking of heavy nicotine cigarettes. The investigators speculate that these results reflect a general increased awareness of the risks of substance abuse in pregnancy, especially among highly educated and older women.

In contrast, the adolescent is often misinformed or unaware of the risks of continuing drug use in pregnancy. Peer pressure may persist, contributing to occasional, casual, or regular use of any one or combination of the psychoactive agents. In a report of an adolescent prenatal program, nonmedical use of drugs was detected by interview and urinalysis at rates comparable to drug use patterns of all youths (11). Cigarettes, alcohol, and marijuana were the substances most commonly detected; use of salicylates was also reported frequently. The effects of continued drug use by pregnant adolescents and young adult women (14 to 23 years) was described in a prospective study (12). There was a statistically significant increase in the frequency of low-birthweight babies (< 2500 g) born to women who continued drug use throughout pregnancy as compared to a control group of non users and to groups of those who quit prior to conception or prior to 20 weeks gestation. Drugs used were not specified, however, and possible differences in lifestyle, nutritional status and health care were not analyzed. Both of these studies, though, indicate that drug use during pregnancy is a problem for adolescents.

Pharmacologic Considerations

The definition of what constitutes substance abuse is dependent on the type of drug, the characteristics of the user, and the circumstances in which the drug is used. For example, nonmedical use of diazepam (Valium) by an adolescent for the same indication that it was legitimately prescribed for an adult family member constitutes abuse. A single dose of heroin is defined by society as abuse, while regular and even heavy use of nicotine, alcohol, or caffeine, though mood altering, is generally accepted or tolerated. Licit drugs can be used illicitly; for example, amphetamines prescribed for weight reduction can be used to inhibit sleep. Over-the-counter drugs as well as prescription drugs, can be abused. Fumes of various household substances such as aerosol propellant, gasoline, cleaning fluid and glue can be inhaled to alter consciousness, constituting abuse. As evidence mounts describing the teratogenic and fetal toxic effects of psychoactive drugs, the nonmedical use of these drugs during pregnancy may be considered abuse by definition (13).

Each drug has expected effects on the user and may have toxic effects (often dose related) or unexpected toxic effects. A licit drug is what it is purported to be, although the user might not be aware of its chemical components, whereas an illicit drug is rarely pure and may be contaminated by substances that have their own toxic effects, depending on dose and route of ingestion. Multiple substance use can precipitate drug interactions that are additive, synergistic, potentiating, or antagonistic and may be complicated by the presence of unknown contaminants in unknown proportions in illicit drug samples (14).

Certain drugs that are abused may induce adaptive reactions in the user. Dependence is defined as a physiologic state whereby a drug is used compulsively to experience its effects or to avoid withdrawal—the physiologic and psychologic disturbances that result when the drug is not taken. Tolerance is a reduced response to a drug, which results from repeated use. When tolerance has developed, the effects experienced at a particular dose may be less, thereby necessitating higher doses to obtain the desired effect. Cross-tolerance to other similar drugs can develop.

Addiction is characterized by an overwhelming need for continuing drug use, resulting in compulsive drug-seeking behavior (15). A fetus chronically exposed to certain drugs in utero can develop physical dependence (not addiction) and will experience a withdrawal syndrome when those drugs are no longer available from the uteroplacental circulation at birth.

Drugs with significant abuse liability are those that affect the central nervous system (CNS). Psychoactive substances have either generalized CNS effects (sedative-hypnotics, stimulants and solvents) or localized CNS effects on emotional, sensory, or perceptual function (tranquilizers, opiates, and hallucinogens) (Table 7.2).

Table 7.2. *Psychoactive Substances*

Generic, Trade Names	Street Name
Depressants	
Ethanol	Alcohol
Barbiturates	"Downers," "Barbs"
phenobarbital	
pentobarbital (Nembutal)	"Yellow jackets"
secobarbital (Seconal)	"Reds"
Sedative-hypnotics	
methaqualone (Quaalude)	"Ludes"
ethchlorvynol (Placidyl)	
hydroxyzine (Atarax, Vistaril)	
meprobamate (Equanil, Miltown)	
Benzodiazepines	
chlordiazepoxide (Librium)	
diazepam (Valium)	
flurazepam (Dalmane)	
Anesthetics	
nitrous oxide	"Laughing gas"
Solvents	
toluene	
naphtha	
benzine	
Cannabinoids	
delta-9-tetrahydrocannabinol	"THC"
marijuana	"Grass"
hashish	"Hash"

Table 7.2 *(continued)*

Generic, Trade Names	Street Name
Stimulants	
Amphetamines	"Uppers," "Speed"
amphetamine (Benzedrine)	"Bennies"
d-amphetamine (Dexedrine)	
methamphetamine (Methedrine)	"Crystal"
Cocaine	"Coke," "Crack"
Caffeine (NoDoz, NoNod, Vivarin)	
Nicotine	
Hallucinogens	
Lysergic acid diethylamide	"LSD"
Dimethyltryptamine	"DMT"
Mescaline	"Cactus buttons"
Psylocibin	"Magic mushrooms"
Phenylcyclidine	"PCP," "Angel dust" (up to 50 street names)
Morphine	
Methylmorphine (codeine)	
Diacetyl morphine (heroin)	
Dihydromorphone (Dilaudid)	
Propoxyphene (Darvon)	
Meperidine (Demerol)	
Methadone	
Pentazocine (Talwin)	
Inhalants	
Amyl/butyl nitrates	"Popper," "Snappers," "Locker room," "Rush"

Adapted from Finnegan LP. *Drug Dependence in Pregnancy: Clinical Management of Mother and Child.* U.S. Department of Health, Education and Welfare Publication No. (ADM) 79–678. Washington, DC: U.S. Government Printing Office, 1979.

Effects of Drugs on Pregnancy

The physiologic changes of pregnancy affect drug absorption, distribution, metabolism and excretion. Absorption is altered by gastrointestinal (GI) disturbances of early pregnancy, decreased gastric secretions, and decreased GI motility. Distribution of drugs from maternal circulation to tissues occurs mainly by simple passive diffusion of lipid-soluble substance. Reduced plasma albumin concentration in pregnancy, however, results in reduced plasma protein binding capacity, thus affecting circulating levels of unbound drugs and the concentration gradient between mother and fetus.

Fluid volume expansion further alters the plasma concentration of drugs. The rate of biotransformation of drugs is reduced due to decreased activity of maternal enzymes, although increased cardiac output and perfusion of the liver counter this effect. Excretion of most drugs is enhanced by increased renal blood flow and an increased glomerular filtration rate. Pulmonary excretion of inhaled gases is greater due to increased respiratory rate and tidal volume. Placental transfer of drugs is influenced by these changes, and is also dependent upon the degree of ionization and lipid solubility of the drug. Nonionized drugs with high lipid solubility are transferred easily, as are drugs of molecular weight less than 600. The rate of transfer is affected by the concentration gradient as well. Characteristics that enhance the psychoactivity of drugs (i.e., ability to permeate the blood-brain barrier), likewise enhance transfer of drugs across the placents (15-17).

The effect of psychoactive substances on the fetus are variable. A drug may have no observable or measurable fetal effects. Alternatively, it may seriously interfere with fetal organ or skeletal development (teratogenicity) or have adverse effects similar to toxic effects observed in an adult (fetal toxicity). Until establishment of placental circulation uniting mother and fetus (approximately 11 days after conception), the embryo is vulnerable to drugs administered vaginally. Later in that first month after conception, any drug ingested by the mother probably has an all-or-none effect on the embryo; that is, the embryo is either unaffected or seriously affected and aborted. Thereafter, the stage of development at the time of exposure to a drug is a major factor in dysmorphogenesis. Organ development occurs at 13 to 60 days, with the development of the CNS at 18 to 38 days, the cardiovascular structures at 20 to 50 days , and limbs at 26 to 48 days. After the first trimester, the development of the genital tract and teeth occurs; CNS development continues to term (18). Adverse drug effects that occur in mid-and late pregnancy are generally toxic reactions, manifested as growth, functional, and behavioral abnormalities. The response of the fetus to passive ingestion of drugs is dependent on the agent, the dose, the duration of exposure, and the genetically determined sensitivity of the fetus. Susceptibility to the harmful effects of a particular substance is also dependent on maternal health status, nutritional factors, and concurrent use of other drugs.

The adolescent is particularly vulnerable to drug-related problems because she may continue to use drugs well into the pregnancy. If her menstrual cycle is irregular, drug use might continue with her unaware of having conceived. Denial of pregnancy and delay in seeking confirmation may postpone contact with a health care provider until after the critical periods of fetal sensitivity to drug-induced effects. Lack of information or misinformation adds to the problem. Personal crises that have contributed to drug use are unlikely to abate and may, in fact, intensify. Despite drug education and counseling in the course of intensive prenatal care, drug use may continue throughout the adolescent's pregnancy.

Effects of Psychoactive Drugs

Determination of risk associated with drugs ingested during pregnancy is based on interpretation of epidemiologic data and experimental animal testing. Proof of teratogenicity can be derived only from evidence of adverse human response. Nevertheless, animal testing provides a means of avoiding unnecessary human exposure to toxic substances.

No one species of animal is predictive of human response. The variance in response may be due to different sensitivity, organogenesis or metabolism of drugs. Types of defects induced in one animal are not always the same as those seen in another animal or in humans. Often, a consistent dose-to-defect relationship cannot be defined. Agents which have not been observed to be teratogenic in humans produce negative results (i.e., no birth defects in only 28% of laboratory animals when all species are tested). Virtually all suspected human teratogens, however, have caused defects in some test species, the mouse being the most likely to show positive results (19). In fact, any drug given in a large enough dose during sensitive periods will affect development (20). Experimentation with large doses, as well as doses within a therapeutic range, is possible in animal testing, providing a basis for estimating human risk from animal teratogenic potency.

Epidemiologic data, on the other hand, can provide proof of increased risk in humans exposed in utero to drugs. Case reports and case studies raise suspicions. Cohort studies are necessary for estimating the relative risk of a particular malformation in an exposed group. The incidence of exposure and the odds of a malformation occurring can be measured in case-control studies. Prospective data rarely are sufficient to identify a significant increase in the occurrance of an adverse effect; for example, the association between chronic maternal alcoholism and fetal alcohol syndrome (FAS) has only rarely been described prospectively. Finally, in interpreting data for counseling purposes, it must be acknowledged that approximately 3 percent of all newborns have congenital defects—many not directly attributable to known human teratogens (20,21).

Effects of Specific Drugs

ALCOHOL

Alcohol is the most widely used drug in the nation. It is the substance most frequently abused by adolescent females. Of high school senior females surveyed, two-thirds reported drinking within the past month and 85 percent during the past year, for a lifetime prevalence of 92 percent (1). Binge drinking within a two-week period was reported by one-third (1). Youths are predominantly binge drinkers, especially on weekends, contributing to dramatic increases in arrests for driving while intoxicated and public drunkenness (22). Young et al. (11) reported detection of alcohol use by one-fourth of pregnant adolescents enrolled in the prenatal program described.

The use of alcohol in association with conception or gestation has been proscribed throughout the ages. The ancient cultures of Carthage and Sparta had laws prohibiting the use of alcohol by newly married couples in order to prevent conception while intoxicated. Biblical prohibition during pregnancy is found in Judges 13:17. In the nineteenth century, abnormalities in pregnancy outcome and characteristics of the offspring of chronic alcoholics were noted, but interest in the phenomenon waned, coincident with prohibition in Great Britain and in the United States (23).

Alcohol has wide-ranging toxic effects on the pregnant user and fetus. It is a CNS depressant readily absorbed in the GI tract and distributed evenly throughout the body, including across the placenta into fetal circulation. It is metabolized primarily in the liver at a rate of approximately 10 to 15 ml of ethanol (±one drink) per hour. Daily consumption of one to two alcohol drinks (or the equivalent in beer or wine) will lead to tolerance (24). In pregnant women, alcohol consumption augments the tendency toward hypoglycemia and ketoacidosis, while also altering lactate, uric acid and lipid metabolism. Dietary deficiencies that result from alcohol consumption in pregnancy include malnutrition due to poor intake, absorption and storage of nutrients, and disturbances in vitamin and mineral metabolism, especially thiamine and folate deficiencies. Chronic alcoholism is associated with disease of the liver, GI tract, cardiovascular system, and hematopoietic and immune systems. Alcohol is frequently abused in combination with other psychoactive substances, especially nicotine, a pattern most common in females and in adolescents (22).

The detrimental effects of alcohol consumption on pregnancy outcome have been clearly established. Drinking 1 ounce of absolute alcohol (AA) or one to two mixed drinks twice a week or more is associated with a risk of spontaneous abortion twice that of nondrinkers (25). An increase in still-births, growth retardation, prematurity, and complications of labor have been reported (26-28). The acute and chronic toxic effects on the fetus have been intensively investigated. Acute toxic effects, hypoglycemia, gastritis, and lethargy, have been observed in neonates of mothers treated with ethanol to inhibit premature labor. Animal studies have demonstrated fetal acidosis associated with binge drinking late in pregnancy. Chronic alcohol consumption by the mother causes alterations in fetal carbohydrate and lipid metabolism, as well as protein synthesis. The fetus is further jeopardized by the indirect effects of poor maternal nutrition, smoking or use of other psychoactive drugs in combination with alcohol, and the psychosocial stress which accompanies alcoholism. In the newborn, blood alcohol levels obtained during an acute episode of maternal alcohol ingestion decreased at a rate only half that of the mothers because of hepatic immaturity (23).

In 1968, the teratogenic effects of alcohol consumption were proposed in a description of congenitally malformed offspring of French alcoholic families (29). These case studies were followed by a definitive description of dysmorphogenesis associated with maternal alcoholism, subsequently termed FAS (30). The incidence of perinatal mortality (17%) , abnormal features suggestive of FAS (32%), and neurologic morbidity (44%) among the surviving 19 to 23 babies born to alcoholic mothers was described the following year (31).

FAS appears in 1 to 2 per 1000 live births, with the incidence of fetal alcohol effects (FAE) or partial expression of the dysmorphic condition in 3 to 5 of 1000 live births (32). Diagnosis is based on finding defects in each of three categories: 1) growth, less than tenth percentile, 2) CNS dysfunction, and 3) facial dysmorphology, at least three signs. The prominent features of FAS are listed in Table 7.3. Other malformations associated with FAS are ocular abnormalities, major cardiac defects, internal and external urogenital defects, hemangiomas, and musculoskeletal malformations. Typically, the syndrome is observed in the newborn, then maternal alcoholism investigated and documented; few cases have been found in prospective studies. In the recent medical literature reviewed by Rosett (23), 245 cases of FAS had been documented worldwide. High concentrations of blood alcohol during critical periods of embryologic and fetal development are probably responsible for FAS or FAE. Facial and skeletal malformations are due to high levels during embryologic development, while growth disturbances probably occur with heavy drinking in the second and third trimester. CNS deficiencies may differ according to the developmental state at which the fetus was exposed to high concentrations of blood alcohol (33).

Table 7.3. *Features of Fetal Alcohol Syndrome*

CNS Dysfunction	Growth Deficiencies	Facial Abnormalities
Mild to moderate retardation	Prenatal <2 SD for length and weight	Eyes: short palpebral tissues
Microcephaly	Postnatal <2 SD for length and weight	Nose: short, upturned, hypoplastic philtrum
Poor coordination, hypotonia	Decreased adipose tissue	Maxillae: hypoplastic
Irritability in the infant		Mouth: thinned upper vermilion, retrognathia in infancy, micrognathia or relative prognathia in adulthood
Hyperactivity in the child		

Adapted from Clarren SK & Smith DW. The fetal alcohol syndrome. *N Engl J Med* 1978; 298:1063–1067.

No safe level of ingestion has been determined. FAS has been associated with chronic heavy consumption of at least 5 ounces AA per day (greater than six mixed drinks), but lower amounts have been associated with other risks to the fetus. Variations seen in the effects of alcohol on pregnancy outcome are probably related to the gestational age at which the fetus was exposed and the pattern of maternal alcohol consumption. Binge drinking during critical developmental periods has been associated with increased risk of FAS or FAE, suggesting that the maximum blood alcohol levels reached may be more significant than daily consumption (23,32). It is possible that a threshold effect, rather than a linear dose-response relationship, is responsible for the variation in outcome.

TOBACCO

Cigarette smoking is a common, socially tolerated habit among people of all ages, and is not generally regarded as substance abuse. Among female adolescents, cigarette smoking is widespread, second only to use of alcohol. After a rapid increase in prevalence in the 1970s, smoking has declined modestly among adolescents. Females, however, now surpass male adolescents in occasional and heavy smoking (1). Cigarette smoking is highly correlated with precocious sexual activity (7). It is often one of a number of substances abused in combination by adolescents. Despite widespread publicity in the mid-1970s about the detrimental effects of cigarette smoking in pregnancy, adolescents continue to smoke. Half of the adolescents enrolled in the prenatal program described by Young et al. (11) smoked at the time of registration for antepartal care. In a three-year prospective study of pregnancy outcome among adolescent primiparae, Hollingsworth et al. (34) reported smoking by 60 percent of white and 37 percent of black adolescents, although only one smoked more than 10 cigarettes per day.

Cigarette smoking produces toxic agents, including nicotine, carbon monoxide and cyanide, and particulate matter. Nicotine, the active alkaloid in tobacco, is a proven carcinogen with direct effects on the central and autonomic nervous systems, and indirect effects on virtually every organ in the body. Nicotine stimulation of the CNS results in tremors, respiratory excitation, antidiuresis, and cardiovascular changes. Stimulation of the adrenal medulla and cortex by nicotine results in the release of catecholamines and corticosteroids, causing an increase in circulating free fatty acids and increases in heart rate and blood pressure. In the pregnant smoker, nicotine may cause constriction in uterine circulation, leading to fetal anoxia. It crosses the placental barrier, and is found in breast milk. Carbon monoxide, a combustion product of tobacco, alters oxygen tension and oxygenation of fetal tissues. Cyanide reduces vitamin B_{12} (35).

Nicotine affects smoking behavior but is not entirely responsible for the dependence that develops. Lighting up and handling the cigarette, oral stimulation, and social feedback enhance the experience. Situational factors influence smoking: while men tend to crave cigarettes when bored or fatigued, a woman's desire to smoke is often associated with stressful situations, suggesting that women may smoke to decrease anger or other negative feelings. There is, however, little consensus concerning the mental health of smokers. The mood-altering effects of smoking are unclear. The compulsion to smoke in order to maintain optimal blood and tissue levels of nicotine is referred to as tobacco use syndrome (35).

During pregnancy, tobacco smoke components are absorbed by the fetus with direct effects on fetal growth, perinatal mortality and the incidence of pregnancy complications. The mechanism by which tobacco by-products are toxic to the fetus is unclear, though probably related to relative anoxia of the fetus and altered maternal physiologic adaptations to pregnancy (36). More than 45 studies of more than 500,000 births have demonstrated the association of cigarette smoking in pregnancy with a reduction in infant birthweight averaging about 200 g. Children exposed in utero to tobacco by-products remain shorter and lighter throughout childhood. There is a dose-related risk of spontaneous abortion, abruptio placentae, placenta previa, premature delivery, premature rupture of the membranes and intrauterine fetal demise.

The risk of perinatal mortality is increased 35 percent for infants of mothers who smoke a pack or more per day; this increase is due primarily to prematurity. Long-term adverse effects on infant growth and development have been demonstrated. Many studies have found a strong association between cigarette smoking and sudden infant death syndrome, suggesting that passive exposure postnatally, as well as prenatally, entails increased risk. No safe level of smoking has been determined, although the risk of adverse effects can be reduced by smoking less or quitting during pregnancy.

MARIJUANA

Marujuana is the most widely used illicit drug in the United States. While primarily associated with youth culture, use is prevalent in all age groups. Among 12- to-17-year-olds, 27 percent have used marijuana, compared to 64 percent of those 18 to 25 years old and 23 percent of those 26 years and older (8).

Use of marijuana by female adolescents is common, though at rates less than males. The use of marijuana during pregnancy was reported by about 10 percent of the adolescents described by Young et al. (11). In any group of pregnant adolescents, however, use might vary considerably from this figure and from nationwide adolescent prevalence because of personal and social circumstances surrounding the pregnancy and opportunities for drug use.

Cannabis is one of the most thoroughly studied of the psychoactive drugs.

It is usually obtained in its street version, marijuana, and smoked to produce tetrahydrocannabinol (THC), the main psychoactive ingredient. Smoking also produces carbon monoxide, hydrocarbons, and particulate matter. THC is obtained from smoking the dried flowering tops of the marijuana plant (1 to 2% concentration of THC) or hashish, the resin of the tops (5 to 8% concentration of THC).

There is no evidence that physical dependence occurs with regular use; however, psychological dependence can develop and may be more difficult to break. Reverse tolerance (increasingly smaller doses creating the desired effect) can develop because of the user's experience and expectations, as well as the long halflife (three days) of this lipid-soluble substance. The usual effects of THC are mild sedation, disruption of recent memory, distortion of time, and increased appetite; hallucinations, lethargy, and diminished motivation may also be experienced (14).

Studies of the effects of THC are, by and large, conflicting and do not provide a basis for definitive counseling of the pregnant woman. Finnegan and Fehr (37) reviewed the scientific and epidemiologic data on the effects of cannabinoids on chromosomes and fetal development. In most studies performed in vitro, cannabis has not been shown to be mutagenic. Laboratory animal response has been inconsistent, as have cytogenetic studies of marijuana smokers. The role of smoke by-products in mutation is questionable. THC crosses the placenta, more in early than late pregnancy, and though fetal levels are low, the fetal CNS has a greater affinity for THC than does maternal tissue. Laboratory animal studies have produced reports of drug-induced abnormalities, growth retardation, and increased perinatal mortality, though replication of results has been generally unsuccessful. Retrospective studies have demonstrated anomalies in offspring of chronic smokers, but use of other drugs by these women confounds interpretation of the results. One such retrospective study, however, demonstrated a significant dose-related negative association between marijuana smoking and infant birthweight; additionally, women who smoked marijuana were five times as likely to have infants with some characteristics of FAS (38). Finnegan and Fehr (37) conclude that it would seem prudent, on the basis of the animal evidence alone, to advocate abstinence from cannabis during pregnancy.

COCAINE

Surveys conducted in the 1970s revealed a dramatic increase in cocaine usage by adolescents. Annual prevalence among high school seniors rose from 5.6 percent (1975) to 12 percent (1979), leveled off between 1979 and 1981, and declined slightly to 11.5 percent in 1982 (1). Regular and daily users, however, were rare. While psychosocial correlates of drug use remained stable during the 1970s, a major shift occurred in the strength of correlation between lifestyle factors and cocaine use as cocaine became a more popular type of deviant behavior among adolescents (6).

Cocaine, a CNS stimulant, is a derivative of the alkaloid found in the leaves of the coca plant grown in South America. In the powder form, called "snow," it is inhaled or "snorted" intranasally and absorbed through the nasal mucosa. When ingested this way, its effect is somewhat limited by the localized vasoconstriction, and use is less likely to lead to addiction. Local ischemia may result in atrophic rhinitis and necrosis of the nasal mucosa.

"Crack" is almost pure cocaine and is sold in chips, chunks, or "rocks." It is smoked in a pipe (free-basing) or is mixed with tobacco and smoked in a cigarette. The effect is similar to intravenous injection or "shooting" of cocaine. The addictive potential of crack is very high. In recent years, there has been a dramatic increase in the use of crack as the drug has become cheaper and more widely available (39).

Because of its high addictive potential, demand for the drug in this form will increase as its use becomes more widespread. An epidemic of cocaine abuse has been documented in a case study in the Bahamas (40), and epidemic use, particularly among adolescents, has been reported in the United States (39,41). Intravenous use is complicated by infection and vasculitis. Hyperpyrexia, seizures, and ventricular arrhythmias, as well as myocardial infarction, have been reported with free-basing and shooting cocaine. Psychic effects include extreme anxiety, hallucinations (tactile), depression and paranoia. Malnutrition and damage to the lungs from smoking are associated with use (39).

Cocaine crosses the placenta, and, while no teratogenic effects have been identified in humans, concern for its toxic effects on the fetus is mounting as use during pregnancy increases. Once recent study (42) demonstrated a significantly higher rate of spontaneous abortion in women who used cocaine during pregnancy. Four of 23 cocaine-using women had onset of labor with abruptio placentae immediately after intravenous injection. While gestational age, birthweight, length, and head circumference were not significantly affected by use, newborns exposed to cocaine during pregnancy demonstrated significant alterations in behavior and response to environmental stimuli.

AMPHETAMINES

While prescription of amphetamines has been curtailed in the past decade, the drug is still available, primarily for use in weight reduction and treatment of narcolepsy. Its abuse potential for an adolescent is particularly great, given its pharmacologic induction of euphoria, anorexia, and insomnia. Tolerance to these effects, however, develops rapidly over several weeks. Amphetamine addiction is a biphasic adaption to prolonged use. During the action phase (several days), multiple daily injections of amphetamines result in euphoria, hyperactvity, and excitability. The reaction phase (24 to 48 hours) that follows is characterized by extreme exhaustion and psychological depression, during which the user may sleep for 48 hours. Each repeated cycle is referred to as a "run." Hallucinations, paranoia, and malnutrition frequently accompany abuse, and multiple drug use is common. Abuse of amphetamines by adolescents is common, surpassed only by alcohol, cigarette, and marijuana use. In addition "look alikes," over-the-counter preparations for weight reduction and staying awake, have become increasingly popular with adolescents.

Studies of amphetamine use in pregnancy indicate a risk of congenital anomalies and alterations in postnatal behavior. Major abnormalities (cardiac defects, microcephaly, biliary atresia, mental retardation and visceral anomalies) as well as oral cleft abnormalities and intrauterine growth retardation (IUGR) have been reported by various researchers (37). The preponderance of amphetamine addicts in Sweden has furnished data on the effects of continued use in pregnancy (43,44). A withdrawal response is sometimes observed in the newborn. Most studies of the response of rats or mice to amphetamine exposure in utero indicate that hyperexcitability is evident in postnatal behavior of the offspring (37). Postpartum adjustment for the mother who continued use during pregnancy is complicated by depression, feelings of inadequacy, inability to cope, and superimposed cycles of euphoria and exhaustion (43).

BARBITURATES

Barbiturate consumption in pregnancy poses a threat to both maternal and fetal health. Tolerance and physical dependence in the mother result from chronic use, while withdrawal can have serious adverse effects on her physical and pyschologic health. Barbiturates cross the placenta, with chronic exposure leading to dependence in the fetus and neonatal withdrawal at birth. Barbiturate withdrawal during pregnancy, unless controlled, can precipitate fetal demise. The teratogenic potential of barbiturates has been reported for mice and isolated cases of human offspring, but concurrent use of other drugs, including anticonvulsants, makes interpretation of the findings difficult (37). Neonatal abstinence syndrome and depressed function in the newborn are evidence of adverse effects on offspring. Use of barbiturates should be avoided in pregnancy.

HALLUCINOGENS

Hallucinogens cause distortion of perception often accompanied by visual hallucinations. The hallucinatory state is distinguishable from a psychotic state in which hallucinations are auditory and awareness of reality is diminished. In addition to cannabis, drugs of this classification include lysergic acid diethylamide (LSD), mescaline, and phenylcyclidine (PCP). Finnegan and Fehr (37) summarized the literature on LSD, noting conflicting chromosomal studies, wide variation in teratogenic susceptibility among laboratory animals, and an association in humans with increased risk of spontaneous abortion and congenital anomalies. The teratogenic potential of other hallucinogens remains to be investigated.

OPIATES

Use of opiates during pregnancy has grave implications for both the mother and fetus. Maternal health is generally poor. Anemia, cardiac disease, hypertension, hepatitis, phlebitis, pneumonia, tuberculosis, urinary tract infections, and venereal disease are all complications of opiate dependence. Malnutrition is common. Abuse of other psychoactive substances is prevalent. Menstrual abnormalities affect a majority of heroin-dependent women. Additionally, the opiate-dependent woman is a poor user of the health care system. During pregnancy, heroin addiction is correlated with spontaneous abortion, abruptio placentae, chorioamnionitis, pre-eclampsia and eclampsia, gestational diabetes, premature labor, premature rupture of the membranes, postpartum hemorrhage, and septic thrombophlebitis. Abrupt opiate withdrawal has been associated with spontaneous abortion, premature labor, and stillbirth. Infants born to heroin-addicted mothers are small for their gestational age. The incidence of congenital defects, however, is not significantly increased. Neonatal complications include prematurity, birth asphyxia, septicemia, and hyperbilirubinemia. The majority of infants born to opiate-dependent mothers experience symptoms of withdrawal in the neonatal period. An association between maternal opiate dependence and SIDS has been suggested. Methadone maintenance and intensive prenatal care have been shown to reduce the incidence of obstetric complications and neonatal morbidity and mortality (37,45).

Care of the Pregnant Adolescent Drug User

The adolescent who continues drug use during pregnancy is in the midst of significant physical, psychological, and social crises. She presents a unique challenge to health care providers. Intensive prenatal care is critical to maintaining her health and assuring an optimal outcome.

Obtaining an accurate report of past or current drug use from the pregnant adolescent is difficult. Fear of detection, resistance to authority, or simply general distrust of the care provider lead to underreporting. Privacy and a nonjudgmental approach are essential to developing the rapport and trust conducive to an honest discussion of drug use. Prefacing questions with a straightforward, simple expression of concern for the adolescent's health and that of the baby may diminish her fears of her drug use being detected, criticized or her being punished. Young et al. (11) suggested the use of urinalysis to complement the interview, stressing that this technique was shown to be more likely to detect the use of alcohol, other CNS depressants and amphetamines. With the consent of the adolescent, this approach might be warranted for initial assessment of drug use problems and monitoring in this high risk group.

Familiarity with patterns of adolescent substance abuse is essential in order to elicit a complete picture of drug use during pregnancy. Alcohol consumption is most common, occurring primarily in binges rather than in chronic daily consumption. Cigarette smoking is prevalent and occurs frequently in conjunction with abuse of other drugs. Marijuana is the most commonly used illicit drug. Familiarity with the street names for marijuana and other illicit drugs is useful to the clinician. Adolescents are generally multiple substance abusers whose involvement, if progressive, is somewhat predictable in its sequence. When the pregnant adolescent admits to use of psychoactive substances, a thorough description of each agent, dose, route of administration, duration of use, and use since conception should be obtained and documented.

When substance abuse has been identified as a problem for the pregnant adolescent, the additional stresses in her environment must be carefully assessed. Adolescents will experiment or use drugs casually for entertainment, relaxation, or curiosity, but progressive involvement is related to personal stress and psychological disturbances predating serious drug use. Instability in the family and serious problems at school may be evident. The relationship with the father of the baby may be tenuous, adding further turmoil to the circumstances of the pregnancy. If possible, drug use by the father of the baby should be assessed when interviewing of the pregnant adolescent. His influence may contribute to her drug behavior. A sense of her life day to day is obtained in order to assess the impact of her lifestyle on rest, nutrition, hygiene, and opportunities for drug use.

Diagnosis of Pregnancy

Diagnosis of pregnancy may be complicated by factors relating to drug use. Marijuana, heroin, methadone, phenothiazines, and antidepressants may cause false positive reactions to be obtained with many of the commonly used urine pregnancy tests (45,46). Early symptoms of pregnancy may be confused with withdrawal by heavy users. Irregular or missed menses are common among adolescents and among women under stress. Amenorrhea is common to narcotic-addicted women. Menstrual abnormalities, unreliable laboratory results, and late registration for care often make assessment of gestational age difficult.

The nutritional needs of the pregnant adolescent are more complex than those of her adult counterpart, for she must support her own physical growth and development as well as that of the fetus. Drug abuse further compromises her nutritional status. Cigarette smoking, for example, may be a means of controlling weight gain. An adolescent's concern for excessive gain in pregnancy may, in fact, intensify her desire to continue smoking, despite advice to the contrary. One study examined the effect of smoking on caloric consumption by pregnant adolescents (47). Nonsmokers consumed more calories per day than light smokers; however, heavy smokers (more than 15 cigarettes per day) consumed more calories than either nonsmokers or light smokers. This finding is suggestive that oral and tactile stimulation needs are important factors in both smoking and eating, and that one activity is not necessarily a substitute for the other. Alcohol consumption alters carbohydrate and lipid metabolism, as well as protein synthesis, augmenting the tendency toward hypoglycemia and hetoacidosis in pregnancy. While maternal diet may be no worse than that of a pregnant nondrinker, absorption and utilization are impaired and result in maternal vitamin and mineral deficiencies, especially folate and thiamine (23). Cannabis is an appetite stimulant, however, its acute effects are not likely to result in balanced, healthful binge eating, and its chronic effects, lethargy and diminished motivation are probably detrimental to maternal intake. Amphetamines are significant appetite suppressants.

The adolescent who uses drugs requires frequent diet assessment and counseling during pregnancy. Multiple vitamin, iron, and folate supplementation as well as enrollment in a food supplementation program are advisable. Weight gain or loss is an important indicator of maternal and fetal nutritional status and should be discussed with the adolescent at each visit, with attention to the interference of drug use in the pattern. Serial complete blood counts will aid in assessing the effectiveness of nutritional intervention.

Risks

Drug users are subject to a variety of infections, some common to pregnancy and adolescence, and others related directly to drug abuse. Regular screening and prompt treatment will avert most adverse effects on maternal and fetal health. Sexually active adolescents are at risk for sexually transmitted diseases, including gonorrhea, syphilis, trichomonas vaginitis, condylomata acuminata, herpes, urethritis and salpingitis. Screening active and former opiate users for syphilis, however, will result in a high incidence of false-positive serologies; therefore specific diagnostic tests (FTA-ABS, TPI) should be used (45). Intravenous drug users are at risk for skin abscesses, cellulitis, phlebitis, tetanus, auto-immune deficiency syndrome (AIDS), and types A, B, non-A, and non-B hepatitis. These users should be screened for the presence of hepatitis-associated antigen (HAA), even in the absence of clinical symptoms of active disease, and may be offered testing for AIDS. Other infectious complications of pregnancy in narcotic-dependent women include bacterial endocarditis and resultant cardiac disease, tuberculosis, pneumonia, bacteremia, septic thrombophlebitis and urinary tract infections.

Fetal growth and development are major concerns for the provider of care for pregnant adolescents. Drug use during pregnancy heightens that concern because of the recognized toxic effects of drugs on the fetus and the detrimental effect of drugs on the fetal environment. Fetal growth is retarded by cigarette smoking, chronic alcohol consumption, use of heroin, marijuana, and amphetamines. Clinical assessment of gestational age and growth, backed by ultrasonographic determinations when indicated, will identify fetuses at risk, in need of additional antepartal surveillance.

Education and Support

Use of scare tactics in hopes of altering the pregnant adolescent's drug behavior "for the baby's sake" will probably be ineffective and may enhance her guilt and fear. In fact, where the effects of drug use in pregnancy can be "disproven" by the experience of a friend or relative, the warning given to a pregnant adolescent who smokes, for instance, must be clear, factual, and nonthreatening or it will be discounted as erroneous. Discovering the extent of and basis for her knowledge may be difficult, but will provide a basis for education and dispel unwarranted fear. The adolescent needs support and encouragement for taking good care of herself and her baby, even if her efforts to reduce or curtail drug use are ineffective.

Assessments of the home and school situations should be made with particular attention to the major sources of stress in each setting. It may be useful to help the adolescent identify ways in which alternatives to drug use can lessen that stress. Helping her to identify the major factors that promote or discourage drug use may help her to avoid those situations. If the father of the baby is involved with the pregnancy, he may be influential in her drug behavior. If he is drug-dependent, referral for substance abuse treatment may benefit both mother and baby. Coordinated, accessible, intensive support from health care providers and social service agencies can have a positive impact on the adolescent and her pregnancy.

Neonatal Care

During pregnancy, the anticipated outcome for the baby is discussed with the mother. To whatever extent possible, the mother needs to be reassured that the baby will be healthy. When drug addiction or chronic heavy use is a problem and neonatal abstinence syndrome a strong possibility, the symptoms and treatment should be discussed, with emphasis on her involvement in the care. Meeting the staff of the nursery or neonatal special care unit and touring the facility during late pregnancy may be useful in preparing her.

Neonatal Abstinence Syndrome

Birth deprives the fetus of drugs to which it may have developed a physical dependence. This abrupt withdrawal results in neonatal abstinence syndrome—generalized symptoms displayed as circulating levels of the psychotropic agent decline. Neonatal abstinence syndrome has been described in association with maternal ingestion of opiates (heroin, methadone, propoxphene hydrochloride, codeine, pentazocine) and CNS depressants (alcohol, barbiturates, chlordiazipoxide, diazepam, and others) (37). Neonatal abstinence syndrome in infants born to amphetamine-dependent mothers has been reported (44). Symptoms most often observed in the neonatal period include tremors, high-pitched cry, sneezing, increased muscle tone, frantic sucking of fists, and regurgitation. In addition, the baby sleeps and eats poorly, is frequently tachypneic and has loose or watery stools (45). The onset of symptoms from heroin withdrawal is 4 to 24 hours after birth, and from methadone withdrawal, within two to three days of birth. Withdrawal from barbiturates or tranquilizers may be delayed. The incidence, onset, and severity of symptoms are difficult to predict. A neonatal abstinence scoring system is used to assess the symptomatology and guide pharmacologic relief of symptoms with paregoric, phenobarbital, or diazepam (45). Treatment is aimed at controlling symptoms in order for the infant to sleep, eat well and gain weight. Drug therapy may take one week to two months, though mild symptomatology may persist longer.

Maternal-Infant Interaction

In the first hours and days after delivery, the mother should be encouraged to hold and care for her infant in order to facilitate maternal-infant attachment. She can be actively involved in the infant's care, learning to recognize and deal with symptoms of withdrawal (45). Ongoing assessment of maternal-infant interaction, the mother's emotional state, and the support she may receive from family is critical in planning for her discharge. Whenever possible, the adolescent mother should be permitted to remain in the hospital during the period required for observation of her baby. If the mother must be discharged during prolonged hospitalization of the infant for management of withdrawal, her active participation in the infant's care should be strongly encouraged, with coordinated efforts made by the nursery staff, the mother's health care provider and social service workers to facilitate her involvement.

Breastfeeding

The adolescent mother who wishes to breastfeed must understand the effect of drug use on lactation. Most drugs taken in therapeutic doses are excreted in breast milk in amounts not harmful to the infant (48). Excessive amounts may affect the nursing infant. For example, alcohol consumption results in milk levels similar to maternal blood levels, although excessive intake can result in vomiting or drowsiness in the infant. Amphetamines may cause tremors or insomnia. Barbiturates may cause sleepiness and decreased sucking. Maternal smoking of 20 to 30 cigarettes per day may significantly decrease breast milk supply and may cause nausea, vomiting, abdominal cramping, and diarrhea in the infant. Heroin and methadone are passed into breast milk in small amounts; therefore, breastfeeding will diminish withdrawal symptoms in the newborn. The effects of stimulants, hallucinogens, cannabis, and other psychoactive substances are virtually unknown. Multiple drug use in varying amounts may aggravate neonatal symptoms. Nevertheless, the advantages of breastfeeding for developing maternal-infant attachment may outweigh the risks when the mother is supported by her primary care provider and well supervised by her drug treatment program. She must be highly motivated to breastfeed in order to overcome the obstacles that poor feeding, hyperirritability and separation due to hospitalization present. The bonding and immunologic benefits derived are significant in the early months. Prolonged breastfeeding is probably inadvisable because of the greater amounts of drugs being ingested in breast milk as the baby's appetite increases. Additionally, the adolescent mother may resume drug activities as her connection with health care providers wanes, thereby exposing the baby to possibly greater amounts and varieties of psychoactive substance.

Postpartum Care

During the postpartum period, a multitude of factors affects the adolescent mother's drug use behavior. Postpartum adjustment includes for her the stress of normal physical changes and fatigue, as well as concern for the baby's health while withdrawing, separation from the baby, and guilt or shame for the baby's condition. Her family's stability may be threatened by the addition of a new, demanding member, requiring realignment of roles within the family structure. Ambivalence may characterize her feelings about returning to school—an area where problems contributing to drug use may persist. Relationships with peers often change profoundly. Involvement with the father of the baby, who may have influenced the use of drugs, may be different. Each of these factors is stressful and may result in the resumption of destructive coping behavior, drug use. In addition, regular contact with supportive health care providers declines, reducing positive reinforcement for drug avoidance. Compliance with drug treatment programs usually declines postpartally.

Contraceptive care of the adolescent is complicated by drug use. Oral contraceptives may be inadvisable for the adolescent with a history of vascular disease secondary to drug use. Heavy smoking compounds this risk. Intrauterine contraceptive devices expose the adolescent user to increased incidence of serious pelvic infections as a result of sexually transmitted diseases, thereby threatening subsequent fertility. Barrier methods are free of risks particular to the drug user, but their appropriateness for the adolescent must be carefully assessed on an individual basis. Counseling on contraceptive methods should include attention to the adolescent's drug use and drug treatment plans, as well as consideration of the affects of drug use on her health and health care.

References

1. Johnston LD, Bachman JG, O'Malley PM. *Student Drug Use, Attitudes and Beliefs: National Trends, 1975-1982*. U.S. Department of Health and Human Services Publication No. (ADM) 83-1260. Washington, DC: U.S. Government Printing Office, 1982.

2. Johnston LD, O'Malley PM, Bachman JG. Statement to the press on forthcoming report. *Drugs and American High School Students, 1975-1983*. Ann Arbor, MI: University of Michigan News Information Services, Feb. 3, 1984.

3. Beschner GM, Treasure KG. Female adolescent drug use. In: *Youth Drug Abuse*. Beschner GM, Friedman AS (eds). Lexington, MA: Lexington Books, 1979:169-212.

4. Green J. Overview of adolescent drug use. In: *Youth Drug Abuse*. Beschner GM, Friedman AS (eds). Lexington, MA: Lexington Books, 1979:17-44.

5. Furstenburg FF. The social consequences of teenage parenthood. *Family Planning Perspectives* 1976;8(4):148-164.

6. Bachman JG, Johnston LD, O'Malley PM. Smoking, drinking, and drug use among American high school students: correlates and trends, 1975-1979. *Am J Public Health* 1981;71(1):59-69.

7. Zabin LS. The association between smoking and social behavior among teens in U.S. contraceptive clinics. *Am J Public Health* 1984;74(3):261-263.

8. Miller JD, Cisin IH. *Highlights from the National Survey on Drug Abuse: 1982*. U.S. Department of Health and Human Services No. (ADM) 83-1277. Washington, DC: U.S. Government Printing Office, 1983.

9. Zabin LS, Kanter JF, Zelnik M. The risk of adolescent pregnancy in the first months of intercourse. *Family Planning Perspectives* 1979;11:215-222.

10. Streissguth AP, Dary BL, Barr HM, Smith JR, Martin DC. Comparison of drinking and smoking patterns during pregnancy over a six-year interval. *Am J Obstet Gynecol* 1983;146(6):716-724.

11. Young DD, Neibyl JR, Blake DA, Shipp DA, Stanley J, King TM. Experience with an adolescent pregnancy program: a preliminary report. *Obstet Gynecol* 1977; 50:212-216.

12. Poland BJ, Wogan L, Calvin J. Teenagers, illicit drugs and pregnancy. *Can Med Assoc J* 1972;107:955-958.

13. Lee RV. Drug abuse. In: *Medical Complications During Pregnancy* (2nd ed). Burrow GN, Ferris TF (eds). Philadelphia: WB Saunders Co., 1982:538-545.

14. Schnoll SH. Pharmacological aspects of youth drug abuse. In: *Youth Drug Abuse*. Beschner GM, Friedman AS (eds). Lexington, MA: Lexington Books, 1979:755-776.

15. Bonica JJ. *Principles and Practice of Obstetric Analgesia and Anesthesia*. Philadelphia: FA Davis Co., 1972.

16. Finnegan LP. Pathophysiological and behavioral effects of the transplacental transfer of narcotic drugs to the foetuses and neonates of narcotic-dependent mothers. *Bulletin Narcotics* 1979;31(3,4):1-58.

17. Juchau MR, Faustman-Watts E. Pharmokinetic considerations in the maternal-placental-fetal unit. *Clin Obstet Gynecol* 1983;26(2):379–390.
18. Moore KL *The Developing Human: Clinically Oriented Embryology.* Philadelphia: WB Saunders Co., 1974;82–84, 116–123.
19. Brown NA, Fabro S. The value of animal teratogenicity testing for predicting human risk. *Clin Obstet Gynecol* 1983;26(2):467–477.
20. Shepard TH. Counseling pregnant women exposed to potentially harmful agents during pregnancy. *Clin Obstet Gynecol* 1983;26(2):478–483.
21. Cordero JF, Oakley GP. Drug exposure during pregnanacy: some epidemiologic considerations. *Clin Obstet Gynecol* 1983;26(2):418–428.
22. Morrissey ER. Alcohol-related problems in adolescents and women. *Postgrad Med* 1978;64(6):111–119.
23. Rosett HL. The effects of alcohol on the fetus and offspring. In: *Research Advances in Alcohol and Drug Problems, Vol. 5. Alcohol and Drug Problems in Women.* Kalant OJ (ed). New York: Plenum Press, 1980;595–652.
24. Cohen S. The pharmacology of alcohol. *Postgrad Med* 1978;64(6):97–102.
25. Kline J, Stein Z, Shrout P, Susser M, Warburton D. Drinking during pregnancy and spontaneous abortion. *Lancet* 1980;2(8187)176–180.
26. Kaminski M, Rumeau C, Schwartz D. Alcohol consumption in pregnant women and the outcome of pregnancy. *Alcoholism* 1978;2:155.
27. Ouellette EM, Rosett HL, Rosman NP, Weiner L. Adverse effects on offspring of maternal alcohol abuse during pregnancy. *New Engl J Med* 1977;297:528.
28. Sokol RJ, Miller SI, Reed G. Alcohol abuse during pregnancy: an epidemiological model. *Alcoholism* 1980;4:135.
29. Lemoine P, Haronsseau H, Borteryu JP, Mennet JC. Les enfants de parents alcoholiques: anomalies observees a propos de 127 cas. *Ouest Medicine* 1968; 25:476–482.
30. Jones KL, Smith DW, Ulleland CN, Streissguth AP. Patterns of malformation in offspring of chronic alcoholic mothers. *Lancet* 1973;1:1267–1271.
31. Jones KL, Smith DW, Streissguth AP, Myrianthopoulos NC. Outcome in offspring of chronic alcoholic mothers. *Lancet* 1974;1:1076–1080.
32. Clarren SK, Smith DW. The fetal alcohol syndrome. *New Engl J Med* 1978; 198:1063–1067.
33. Tennes K, Blanchard C. Maternal alcohol consumption, birth weight, and minor physical anomalies. *Am J Obstet Gynecol* 1980;138(7)(part 1):774–780.
34. Hollingsworth DR, Moser RJ, Carlson JW, Thompson KT. Abnormal adolescent primiparous pregnancy: association of race, human chronic somatomammotropin production, and smoking. *Am J Obstet Gynecol* 1976;126:230–237.
35. Gritz ER. Problems related to the use of tobacco by women. In: *Research Advances in Alcohol and Drug Problems, Vol. 5. Alcohol and Drug Problems in Women.* Kalant OJ (ed). New York: Plenum Press, 1980;487–543.
36. Pirani BBK, MacGillivray I. Smoking during pregnancy: Its effect on maternal metabolism and fetoplacental function. *Obstet Gynecol* 1978;52(3)257–263.
37. Finnegan LP, Fehr KO. The effects of opiates, sedatives, hypnotics, amphetamines, cannabis and other psychoactive drugs on the fetus and newborn. In: *Research Advances in Alcohol and Drug Problems, Vol. 5. Alcohol and Drug Problems in Women.* Kalant OJ (ed). New York: Plenum Press, 1980;653–723.

38. Hingson R, Alpert JJ, Day N, et al. Effects of maternal drinking and marijuana use on fetal growth and development. *Pediatrics* 1982;70(4):539–546.

39. Crack. *Medical Letter on Drugs and Therapeutics* 1986;28(718):69-70.

40. Jekel JF, Podlewski H, Dean-Patterson S, Allen DF, Clarke N, Cartwright P. Epidemic free-base cocaine use. *Lancet* 1986:459-462.

41. Extra-potent cocaine: Use rising sharply among teen-agers. *New York Times;* March 20, 1986:A1, B4.

42. Chasnoff IJ, Burns WJ, Schnoll SH, Burns KA. Cocaine use in pregnancy. *N Engl J Med* 1985;313(11):666-669.

43. Larsson G. The amphetamine addicted mother and her child. *Acta Pediatr Scand* 1980;278 (suppl):1–24.

44. Erickson M, Larsson G, Winbladh B, Zetterstrom R. The influence of amphetamine addiction on pregnancy and the newborn infant. *Acta Pediatr Scand* 1978;67:95-99.

45. Finnegan LP. *Drug Dependence in Pregnancy: Clinical Management of Mother and Child.* U.S. Department of Health, Education, and Welfare Publication No. (ADM) 79-678. Washington, DC: U.S. Government Printing Office, 1979.

46. Hatcher RA, Steward GK, Stewart F, Guest F, Josephs N, Dale J. *Contraceptive Technology: 1972-1982* (llth ed). New York: Irvington Publishers, Inc., 1982, 163.

47. Carruth BR. Smoking and pregnancy outcome of adolescents. *J Adolescent Health Care* 1981;2:115-120.

48. Vorherr H. Drug excretion in breast milk. *Postgrad Med* 1974;56(4):97-104.

8 Preparation for Labor and Delivery

Pregnant adolescents or those who have given birth are an easily identified population. Goals in assisting these adolescents include ensuring them adequate prenatal care, continuing their education, and teaching them good parenting skills. As the adolescent is exposed to the childbirth process, she becomes aware not only of her own bodily changes but also of the realities of contraception and family planning and the care of the normal newborn. A variety of federal and state programs are available to help the adolescent adjust to her pregnancy and childbearing responsibilities. Many federal programs, however, are subjected to cutbacks; the Women's, Infant's and Children's (WIC) feeding program is one of these. State and local governments try to assure financial aid for such programs and also seek clinical assistance from private organizations, consumer groups, childbirth educators, certified nurse-midwives, and physicians.

In some areas of the United States special public high schools for pregnant adolescents are in operation, with day care facilities to encourage continuing education after delivery. Religious organizations also are available to adolescents. Jerry Falwell's Moral Majority program, "Save a Baby," for instance, operates in conjunction with an adoption agency to discourage abortion. Centers such as "The Open Door" in New York City or "The Crittenton Center" in Los Angeles promote contraceptive services to nonpregnant adolescents by exposing them to pregnant adolescents to reinforce the need for birth control. In an effort to promote delayed childbearing and further education, black inner-city adolescents in some areas of the U.S. are being paired with black adult role models who are successful achievers (1).

Childbirth education promotes decision-making skills by preparing and informing the adolescent about the events of childbearing and childrearing. The adolescent is allowed to express freely her thoughts, fears, misconceptions and frustrations in a stable atmosphere. Effective communication in the health care setting may be difficult because of the adolescent's poor verbal and social skills. Role playing, visual aids, discussion (rap) sessions, and visits with other adolescent mothers and their infants all assist the pregnant adolescent in preparing for childbirth.

The pregnant adolescent may be concerned with the present and find it difficult to anticipate the baby's needs. Having the adolescent draw a picture of her baby may sometimes be a revealing exercise. Early adolescents tend to fantasize about pregnancy, and the fetus can appear to them as a power to compete with or to manipulate. During middle or late adolescence, learning becomes more active, and the concepts of child care and development are more easily grasped. Older adolescents may also have the opportunity to practice child care through babysitting at home and in church nurseries or day care centers. In this way the adolescent can rehearse such skills as feeding, diaper-changing, bathing, and playing with a baby. These activities promote the adolescent's confidence and positively reinforce her self-esteem.

While the pregnant adolescent is now receiving more attention and assistance in meeting her needs, the adolescent father remains an "invisible factor," forgotten or excluded by health care systems. Adolescent fathers are assumed to be irresponsible, and therefore they receive little attention or time from the health care system. Many young fathers, however, are not only willing but eager to be a supportive partner and participate in the birth and childcare responsibilities of their offspring. Adolescent fathers are often anxious to attend prenatal and postnatal parenting classes but need support to assume these responsibilities and learn about the role of a father.

New York City's Bank Street College of Education offers vocational services, counseling and prenatal and parenting classes to almost 400 adolescent fathers and prospective fathers in eight cities throughout the United States. At the completion of this two-year program, 82 percent of the adolescent fathers reported daily contact with their children, 74 percent stated they contributed to the child's financial support, and almost 90 percent maintained a relationship with the adolescent mother (2).

In another study, 45 percent to 63 percent of the pregnant adolescents maintained contact with their male partners throughout the pregnancy (3). These growing numbers of adolescent fathers are coping with the conflict between the desire to provide and care for their offspring and doubt or anxiety about their abilities as "providers." These fears can lead the proud adolescent father to lose face or masculinity. Adolescent fathers generally have less education, lower incomes and more children than males who wait until at least 20 years of age to begin having children (2,3). When his girlfriend discovers the pregnancy, the adolescent male often drops out of school and takes a low-paying job. This attempt to be a "good father" by becoming a "provider" traps him in a poor job future without further education. This overwhelming situation is often complicated by the adolescent male's own father being absent. Thus, he lacks an appropriate role model. Without guidelines or social preparation for the fathering role, the adolescent male is filled with feelings of self-doubt, ambivalence, and fluctuations in identity. The responsibilities of fatherhood, particularly financial ones, are difficult to grasp, and feelings of being trapped in a downward spiral are not uncommon. Education is usually the first sacrifice made for financial necessity, although some adolescent fathers manage to juggle both work and school. These demands, however, leave little time for the supportive adolescent father to adjust to his partner's changing body image, sexuality, mood swings and dependency on others. At the same time, the adolescent father may be the target of family anger and blame. He may also genuinely fear for his partner's and baby's well-being as the pregnancy proceeds and childbirth nears. Fears of abnormalities of the baby or difficulties in labor and delivery are common, particularly if there is little knowledge of the normal childbirth process. Concerns about his ability to help his partner may not be addressed and may remain unspoken. These feelings can frighten the adolescent male, forcing him to abandon the situation and let the pregnant adolescent face the responsibilities of childbirth and childrearing alone.

Including the adolescent male in the health care system may alleviate his fears of childbirth and prepare the adolescent couple for parenting. Facilitating communication between the partners and families can promote a more stable relationship and help the adolescents resolve their problems through improved decision-making skills. Exploring fears and misconceptions about parenthood and the reactions of families and friends can help the adolescent identify support areas that can reduce anxiety and helplessness. Health education and anticipatory guidance prepares adolescents for labor and delivery and for their parenting roles. Including the adolescent father in all aspects of childbearing may finally stop the cycle of adolescent pregnancy from repeating itself in future generations.

Childbirth Education

Helping the adolescent deal with the concept of labor is not an easy task. Most pregnant adolescents' idea of labor is "mission impossible." To them its parameters are unknown and their resources are often minimal. The adolescent's peer who has recently gone through labor may offer a less than reliable description of it, and the older generation may either distort their own labor experiences to a level of horror or remain silent about them. Too frequently, a deep-rooted fear develops that could unfavorably affect the labor pattern.

It is well recognized that there is a dark side to labor that frightens all women in some way. This is especially true for the primigravida. Because of the adolescent's psychological age, associated concerns about body image, and the fact that she is generally a primigravida, natural fears are dramatically increased. Consequently, all who attend the adolescent during labor must be sensitive to and tolerant of these factors. This awareness often requires not only the health care provider's patience, but also his or her immense strength and love. Without this, the frightened, unprepared laboring adolescent will be predisposed to a difficult and prolonged labor and may well be the teller of one more tale of woe and horror for the next generation.

Support and proper preparation for labor are obviously the keys to a more favorable psychological experience for most pregnant teenagers.

Two components must be considered in the education process: teaching and preparation. Because tension and anxiety are enhanced by fearful anticipation of the unknown, every attempt is made to strip away unknown factors.

Teaching Adolescents

Teaching adolescents requires flexibility and good humor. Anyone who has taught adolescents about the physiology of labor and delivery is usually acutely aware of their inaccurate knowledge. Maintaining this diversified group's attention, therefore, requires both ingenuity and at times ego strength. Accordingly, it is essential that the teacher be thoroughly familiar with the subject of labor and delivery and be able to present it in a creative, imaginative manner. Unfortunately, the standard approaches used in adult childbirth education classes will not likely appeal the average adolescent. One manifest difference is immediately apparent: Most adolescents are single and may or may not have a committed partner. While every attempt is made by the teacher to include partners or significant others, most adolescents do not have someone who can attend classes with them. Schedules, transportation, motivation, and minority status in the class are all factors. Hence, the instructor accepts that while it is ideal for partners or others to attend childbirth classes, it is not a great loss if they do not. The target for these classes is the pregnant adolescent herself.

Approach

The psychological environment of the class will contribute significantly to a better learning experience. When the environment is comfortable and conducive to relaxed interaction, adolescents are less likely to be bored. If the teenagers consider the teacher a member of the group, the group's comfort and learning levels will increase. The teacher's approach and the students' acceptance of this approach can be a factor in learning.

A friendly and welcoming approach is essential. The teacher begins with an introduction using both her given and surname. Encouraging the adolescent to use first names only facilitates communication, increases trust, and reduces the teacher's impact as an authority figure. This approach also instills an understanding of the professional role of the teacher in the health care system. Without this information, the adolescent may confuse the role with that of other health care providers and subsequently seek out answers from inappropriate sources.

Once the class begins, the teacher may elect to sit with the group or stand in front of them. Sitting with the group in this type of learning situation improves rapport and eliminates the psychological distance between the teacher and the adolescents. When comfortable, the teacher's style, spontaneity and fluency of presentation will improve.

Late arrivals can disrupt or destroy the momentum of the class, so all should be present before class begins. Because adolescents have short attention spans, any interruption is kept to a minimum, and the teaching dialogue moves at a brisk and interesting pace. This requires the teacher to be alert and sensitive to the group's response and interest levels. Inevitably, attention does wander and at times there may be one or two who are obviously bored. However, when a general lack of interest is apparent, it is time to alter the course and change the teaching tactics. An alternative that is often appealing involves role playing.

Role Playing

Role playing is fun and is usually actively enjoyed by the adolescents. Since a partner is needed in the process, it is helpful to choose an adolescent who has good ego strength. To change roles, the teacher becomes a pregnant adolescent and the adolescent becomes the health care provider. Before beginning the role playing set the scene with such descriptive details as where you as the adolescent have been, what you have been eating, what you have been doing, and what you thought when you first felt pain or your "water broke." This scenario is guaranteed to capture interest. Meanwhile, the adolescent, as the health care provider, is working away in the hospital as a busy nurse or nurse-midwife. Describe in detail what she has been doing, but not too extensively that it becomes boring or confusing. Quickly return to your "pregnant" predicament because it is easy for the class to identify with. Have a boyfriend or mother doing or saying funny things. Have everyone arrive with you at the hospital full of questions for your health care provider. If your teaching has been successful, the class will have some answers for your anguished questions. This teaching approach is usually successful. Attention levels are good, receptivity is excellent, and knowledge is retained. In short, acting out the pregnant woman's initial visit to the hospital for labor evaluation or for any other problem is an excellent teaching mechanism to facilitate the adolescent's understanding of early labor and its management.

Phantom Dialogue

If an adolescent is a nonverbal participant in class but does not appear hostile, she might be included as a dialogue partner in a phantom dialogue. In reality, it is a monologue provided by the teacher that simply utilizes the adolescent's name in the exchange. The dialogue can consist of any pertinent topic but it is generally most effective when associated with aspects of the labor and delivery process. An example might be "Mary Brown and I went for pizza the other day and Mary asked me about medicine in labor.

Mary said she had heard that if you have natural childbirth, you can't have medicine." The dialogue continues along the lines of where she had heard this, what her concepts of natural childbirth were, etc. This teaching approach allows the teacher to include the shy and withdrawn adolescent as a participant without the threat of vulnerability or exposure. Additionally, it creates a constant unknown because only the teacher knows what will occur next in the dialogue. This heightens the suspense and attention levels. In short, it is a form of storytelling and has a remarkable propensity for attracting the group interest.

Throwing questions out to the group at large will also generate interest and response and consequently is a good teaching alternative to consider. Every response from the class, whether in the form of a word or a phrase or a question receives positive reinforcement from the teacher. This will encourage further participation and interest and help to maintain a positive learning environment.

Audiovisual Aids

Audiovisuals are another good teaching tool used to help promote additional learning. Many films are available on childbirth and can be selected from film catalogues. Slides may be valuable as well. A tour of the labor and delivery suite is an option many adolescents request. Unfortunately, getting the adolescents collected on a day when the labor and delivery area is quiet is often difficult and sometimes it is impossible. If the area is busy, it may restrict the opportunity to adequately tour the area, answer questions, and explain the purpose of different pieces of equipment. On the other hand, slides made of the labor and delivery area, and its associated equipment, can often fill in the blanks, and if a tour is not possible, can serve as enrichment. Slides shown in class serve the function of answering the many questions that were either left unasked or unanswered on the tour. Slides can be frozen on the screen when desired to allow the teacher to discuss different aspects of the setting shown in each slide. This pictorial approach helps the adolescent to become familiar with the labor and delivery surroundings and familiarizes her with pieces of equipment such as fetal monitors, oxygen masks and birthing mirrors at a time when the adolescent is not feeling threatened or stressed. It also gives the adolescent an opportunity to question the purpose of each object. Slides of birthing rooms, labor rooms and delivery rooms help to acquaint adolescents with the setting, facilitate expression of feelings about the experience of labor and delivery, and reduce their sense of confrontation with an alien environment when labor begins.

Necessary Information

Class discussions about labor include the physiology of labor. Presentations can begin with a definition of the word, which serves as an easy introduction to the topic. The adolescent is also taught the differences between early and active labor, and first and second stage. Since many adolescents have heard about the "mashing" of the adbomen during third stage, they are anxious to have that explained. Clarification of this concern can serve as an effective entry into a discussion of the third and fourth stages of labor. Also the use of medication in labor and the meaning and purpose of an episiotomy are presented. The value of a support person during labor is another area for discussion as is the demonstration of the breathing exercises to be used at different points in labor. A successful finale to classes on the physiology of labor is usually a film showing an actual birth. When showing a film, however, prepare the adolescent for the sight of blood. When not forewarned of the film's content, adolescents have been known to faint while viewing such films. On the other hand, identifying with the laboring women may be too overwhelming for a few pregnant adolescents; hence they are given the choice to attend or not as they desire.

The second component of childbirth education, preparing the adolescent for labor, is provided on an individual basis during the last four to five weeks of pregnancy. Ideally, this individualized instruction is provided by the same health care provider. The continuity of the same teacher for specific adolescents is immensely reinforcing to learning. A one-to-one basis also develops trust, which allows for an easy and free exchange of the adolescent's concerns and anxieties. It is during this period that time is taken to ascertain with each adolescent her level of understanding about the physiology of labor. For example, it is vital that she understand how the contraction pattern develops, its frequency, and the breathing exercises to be used during labor.

The Physiology of Labor

Comprehension of cervical dilation and station is necessary if the adolescent is to cope successfully with the contractions. Explaining this concept is best achieved with a knitted bag and a small doll. It is a graphic way to quickly teach this physiological phenomenon. However, a simple drawing will also suffice. Drawing the uterus as a large bag containing another bag of water in which the baby floats is an adequate analogy. Drawing a placenta on the wall of the uterus and attaching it to the baby via the cord is sufficient to teach about placental circulation. The mouth of the bag can next be identified as the cervix with the vagina extending beyond it as a tube. Most adolescents can rapidly grasp the anatomical landmarks involved with labor when they are described this way. Once cervical dilation is explained, the purpose of the contractions will be better understood, and the fear of contractions reduced accordingly as the adolescent is kept informed throughout labor of the degree of her cervical dilation and progress. This information will be reassuring to her and give her a sense of control over her body. Additionally, the time factors associated with both the first and second stage of labor need to be precisely presented. If the adolescent's comprehension of the length of labor is correct, it will help her to cope more realistically.

The contraction's curve is another area which requires discussion. The adolescent, like her older counterparts, needs information about the intensity of contractions from beginning through peak and deceleration. She is coached on breathing techniques to use throughout the curve. This knowledge is preferably acquired during pregnancy and not once she has commenced labor. If the learning is delayed until labor, the tendency will be to lose control even in the presence of a very strong and supportive coach. In other words, without such learning, she is deprived of an important coping mechanism in labor. Fortunately, with the strong backing of a caring teacher on a one-to-one basis, most adolescents will be motivated to learn the breathing techniques prior to labor and hence have access to an invaluable tool when coping with the contractions and duration of labor.

Describing the concept of station to the adolescent is a difficult task. Most clinic settings do have models of the pelvis. If one is available and the teacher has something round such as an orange or a small ball, the phenomenon of station can be adequately demonstrated. In addition, a grapefruit is ideal for showing pelvic disproportion. However, in the event that a pelvic model is not available, one's hands or a drawing is an alternative.

A balloon filled with water is a good device to explain ruptured membranes. When no balloons are available, a rubber glove filled with water is a reasonable substitute. Pricking the bag with a needle will demonstrate "a leaking bag of water." Puncturing it with a pin or pair of scissors will demonstrate the concept of ruptured membranes. Because management of ruptured membranes varies between individuals and institutions, alert the adolescent to its possible occurrence and significance. Additionally, a common misconception among adolescents is that labor will automatically follow once the membranes have ruptured. This fallacy often results in many adolescents remaining at home anticipating the commencement of labor. When nothing occurs, they reappear in the clinic at their next scheduled appointment and relate suspicions that their bag of water "burst last week." Many also will confuse urinary incontinence and ruptured membranes, resulting in false alarms. Others may not report the incident because they fear "a dry labor," which is a term for an induced labor after the membranes have ruptured. If the membranes are ruptured, these delays may contribute to a difficult and risky situation for both the adolescent mother and her baby; these are avoidable problems, however, when the adolescent is informed and knows to report any leaking or ruptured membranes. Encouraged by her care provider to report any such likelihood and motivated by a commitment developed through this rapport frequently results in a positive response if these problems occur. A quick response will have a direct effect on her pregnancy outcome and will significantly reduce the risk of a possible intrauterine infection for both herself and her baby.

During this interim of preparation in third trimester the adolescent is also informed that vaginal examinations are a necessary part of her labor management. Most adolescents are relieved to learn that these will not include speculum exams unless, of course, there is a question of ruptured membranes. The adolescent also needs to be reassured that in all likelihood her membranes will rupture spontaneously after she has started labor and is in the hospital. Additionally, it will help her if she is already aware that the artificial rupture of membranes is sometimes performed in labor.

The preparation of a pregnant adolescent for labor is an intense period which is best handled on a continuum over the last four to five weeks of pregnancy, and is most successful if it is conducted in a private place on a one-to-one basis.

The "significant other" that an adolescent has identified and might like included in her labor and delivery experience is invited to attend these preparation sessions. This invitation is clearly stated and explained to the adolescent. The inclusion of this individual can greatly enhance the prenatal bonding with the baby for both parties and can increase the opportunity of a favorable labor experience for the adolescent.

Labor and Delivery

Each adolescent is an individual with her own cultural and social background and her own emotional reactions and intellectual abilities, all of which affect her capacity for adaption to hospitalization. The pregnant adolescent who enters the hospital to have her baby experiences a particularly difficult period of transition. It occurs at a time when she is changing from a child into a woman who will care for a new human being. Quite often she has never been in a hospital before, and is unfamiliar with the routines and procedures. On the other hand, she may have had some previous hospital experience through visiting a very ill relative or perhaps undergoing surgery as a child, either of which may not have been a positive experience. The adolescent may have difficulty relating to the hospital staff, especially if she has had little experience with or knowledge of health care facilities. She may be unsure about answering personal questions, filling out forms or signing consents. She may not know how to receive such information or how to express her concerns and fears. There are many opportunities for misunderstanding and misinterpretation.

Even in the postpartum stage, the adolescent may still be trying to adjust to her entry in the hospital and the events that followed—labor and delivery. Also, the pregnant adolescent may enter the hospital for the first time when she is in labor, already a period of distress and uncertainty. The adolescent who has tried to cope with labor and delivery may continue to fear losing control of herself and her bodily functions. She may have attempted to cope with the labor and delivery experiences by acting-out in a rebellious fashion or by panicking. She may not have understood the various routine procedures, an ignorance which may accentuate fears and fantasies carried throughout the pregnancy. Often healthy adolescents feel they are in some way invincible, beyond harm; yet hospitalization may successfully threaten this self-confidence and may lead to feelings of hostility or withdrawal. The adolescent may experience confusing and restrictive procedures such as being confined to bed, or having intravenous fluids, or the presence of a fetal monitor during labor. She may even feel isolated or abandoned, particularly if visiting privileges are restrictive. Her perspective may also be clouded by medications. She may also feel strange and embarrassed about being in hospital clothing, and shy about being examined by hospital staff. Many of these and other unresolved feelings of the delivery experience may persist and color her postpartum course (4).

The adolescent may also be struggling with a range of emotional reactions when entering the hospital. She may have ambivalent feelings about her new role as a mother and provider. She may be facing conflicts at home with her family or perhaps with the father of the baby. Plans to care for the baby may be ill-defined and she may feel ambivalent about further education or work. She may well be concerned about the dramatic bodily changes she is experiencing during parturition, fearing that she is becoming "different," abnormal or even mutilated. She may feel frustrated by these changes in her body image and unsure of its effect on her developing sexuality. She may have difficulty in coping with her own health needs and those of her baby, particularly if the baby is small or unwell. Occasionally, the adolescent may express feelings of denial about the birth experience. She may feel resentment toward the baby who has indirectly brought about these unwelcome changes and who might become a rival object of familial attention.

The adolescent may not have adequate coping mechanisms to adjust to the physical and emotional changes during parturition and hospitalization. The verbal and nonverbal behaviors of the adolescent are often inconsistent. The adolescent may display regressive or dependent behavior, particularly when meeting the needs of her newborn, while at the same time she may demand to be treated as a responsible adult. Noncompliance to health care procedures and advice may also be seen. The adolescent's behavior can also change dramatically during visiting hours when family and peers are present. The attention span may become limited if the adolescent is easily distracted.

While in the hospital, the adolescent will express her need for acceptance and help during this transitional period through a variety of emotional responses from enthusiasm to aggression. Her ability to cope with hospitalization will vary according to her developmental stage, her preparation for childbirth, her support at home, and the flexibility of the hospital staff. She will need assistance in realistically planning for her educational or work goals. She may need practical guidance in solving family and childcare problems. Repetition is often necessary for the adolescent to learn the skills needed in her new role as care-provider for her baby. She may also need to discuss her possible changing relationship with the father of the baby, and she may need help in relating to both old friends from school and other young mothers. During this period of transition she also needs help in order to decrease any fears of isolation, loss of freedom or rejection. Above all, it must be remembered that she is still an adolescent, despite her changing responsibilities, and will need time and acceptable outlets to act as an adolescent.

Prior to admission to the hospital, the adolescent needs a clear idea of what to expect while there. Provision of hospital tours of the labor and delivery unit, postpartum unit and nursery are concrete aids to the adolescent's understanding and adjustment. A clear discussion by health care providers of the choices in childbirth and the adolescent's participation in the decision-making process is an essential preparation. Explanations by the health care staff of all procedures prior to instigating them are imperative as well as such common proprieties as introducing everyone who enters the adolescent's room. The adolescent will need as much time as possible to be able to ask questions and to make decisions regarding her own health care and that of her baby. Particularly with adolescents, the "problem" is often identified and treated, but the adolescent herself may well be forgotton. This may readily occur if a cesarean section has been necessary. Also, the amount of pain medication needed during childbirth may have been increased in the case of adolescence, primarily because of the fear-tension-pain cycle.

The adolescent will probably need assistance with adjusting to her new role as mother and coping with the demands of responsible decision-making for herself and her baby. The hospital staff may or may not be aware of her unspoken fears about caring for her baby which need to be expressed. She requires thoughtful preparation for parenthood to help her understand her own changing requirements as well as those of her baby. New methods of coping must be learned, often by imitation of her health care providers. The adolescent needs time to discuss her hospital experiences with the professional staff to clarify any misconceptions and to ensure positive contact in the future with health facilities and staff. Through staff guidance, the adolescent may evaluate realistically her own expectations and experiences to enable her to accept and adapt these into her normal framework. Before assuming her new responsibilities, the adolescent may become aware of the limits and restrictions necessary for her own health and that of her baby through her discussions with her care givers. She may need assistance in redirecting any feelings of guilt, anger and hostility. Short, informal teaching periods are required to inform the adolescent adequately about the care of herself and her baby, and to reassure her of the normalcy of her experience, a point which needs to be continually stressed. In these teaching periods, the adolescent learns by first observing a new task, next performing the task together with the staff, and finally assuming responsibility for the task on her own. She will look for reassurance and expect the hospital staff to assist her as she accepts more responsibility for the care of herself and her baby.

Knowledge of family influences and support is also extremely helpful and it is advisable in the planned teaching sessions to include family members such as the adolescent's mother or aunt when possible.

The adolescent in the hospital challenges the health care providers to adapt their care to meet the individual needs of these young patients. Despite this creative challange, the hospital staff may find caring for adolescents difficult. Health care providers may or may not be aware of their own opinions and prejudices toward the pregnant adolescent or young mother. The adolescent responds positively when approached with sensitivity toward her different needs, influences, coping mechanisms and abilities. The health care provider's primary task is to be able to listen to the adolescent and respond appropriately. The adolescent will be looking closely to see that the staff is not hiding behind barriers of uniforms, desks or hospital policies. They want health care providers who are giving of themselves on a personal level and assurance as to the confidentiality of their medical experiences. They expect and deserve a nonjudgmental approach in order to develop a mutual respect and understanding. Communication through verbal and nonverbal cues grows over time in an atmosphere of trust. Such health education often involves the evolution of self-respect, which clearly reinforces the adolescent's attitude toward her new responsibilities.

Meeting the Demands of Labor

In the final analysis, the adolescent goes into labor. Her labor is physiologically the same as it is for any woman. Consequently, clincial management will not be discussed here, but some suggestions will be made regarding support approaches geared especially to the adolescent.

Ideally, the most obvious positive support approach is the presence of a "significant other" and the care provider, with whom she has had consistent contact throughout her pregnancy and with whom she has developed a meaningful rapport. In the event that a happy mix occurs, she is well on her way to a positive labor experience. Once their special relationship is established it will dictate its own individual support system. In most cases, adolescents are not fortunate and the staff is uninvolved with their care. The adolescent is a stranger to the hospital staff and in this painful situation, frequently a stranger to herself. Accordingly, trying to cope with labor may become a problem for all. There are some approaches, however, which are simple and basic and often helpful.

The adolescent requires a health care provider who is understanding and likes adolescents. This individual needs to be familiar with the prenatal teaching content offered in the clinic, and able to encourage and help the adolescent to utilize this learning as a coping mechanism through each contraction. Every effort is made to praise and encourage the adolescent. Frequent comments about her progress will help her to realize that she is making progress. A calm, gently supportive and nonpunitive health care provider will help the adolescent to regain composure and refocus on the coping mechanisms (such as her breathing techniques) during contractions. When a "significant other" is present and attempts to relate to the adolescent in a caring but uninformed way, the staff can redirect his behavior to be supportive and oriented to approaches that are calming and comforting. Frequently the significant other may require as much reassurance and support as the laboring adolescent. These others are often ignorant of the physiology of labor, but once they are informed and reassured, they can become a vital link in the management of the adolescent's anxiety level and help her to maintain control.

Some adolescents will inevitably lose control. When this occurs, a firm hand may be required, but in a nonpunitive and nurturing fashion. On occasion, an exasperated care provider can be heard challenging the adolescent with such comments as "you should have thought of the labor pain before you got pregnant." Obviously this approach lacks any rationality. Nothing whatsoever is achieved in such an exchange except the ventilation of the clinician's frustration. The adolescent's response, if any, is most likely to be negative as the only rational alternative to such a challenge. As a result, the distance will widen between the adolescent and the clinician. The adolescent may feel that she has been rejected by the health provider and consequently is a failure as a laboring woman. This potential is a real threat and may ultimately interfere with a successful bonding between the adolescent and her child.

Once the baby is born, the beauty of the baby must be ackowledged but never to the exclusion of praise for the adolescent's wonderful efforts in labor. In short, she needs to know what she has achieved as a woman, how well she managed through the laboring process, and what a successful young woman she is. This will help her to express her feelings about her labor experience and resolve any negative emotions when they are present. The step of praising the adolescent after delivery cannot be stressed enough. If her thoughts subsequently reflect a positive attitude about her capability to cope with labor, her ability to mother may be directly affected as well as her enjoyment of future pregnancies.

The labor and delivery experience for the adolescent is often a time of fear and uncertainty. The pregnant adolescent and her offspring are vulnerable to a variety of risks and complications during the perinatal period. The most common problems are anemia, pre-eclampsia, prematurity, and low birthweight. Abnormalities in labor are seen in failure to progress, amnionitis, abruptio placentae and uterine dysfunction. Uterine dysfunction may take the form of hypertonia, prolonged labor, prodromal labor, or precipitous labor. The incidence of cesarean section delivery may be increased because of a small or contracted pelvis, the angle of inclination, lack of engagement, breech presentation or other factors of cephalopelvic disproportion (CPD). Genital lacerations are also common in the adolescent population. These complications dramatically affect infant outcomes. Increases in infant morbidity and mortality rates are signaled by an increase in low Apgar scores, growth retarded newborns, stillborns, physical and mental handicaps, low IQ, decrease rate of growth during childhood, suboptimal school achievement, disordered behavior and interactional difficulties between mother and child (5, 6, 7).

Two major factors in neonatal mortality rates are low birthweight and prematurity. The neonatal mortality rates in white mothers less than 15 years of age are 48 per 1,000 as compared to 28 per 1,000 in white mothers ages 15–19 and 22 per 1,000 for white mothers ages 20–24. The infant mortality rate for nonwhite infants is greater than white infants at each maternal age. Also, the higher the socioeconomic status at any maternal age, the lower the perinatal mortality rate. These effects of low birthweight and prematurity are not solely related to maternal immaturity but are also influenced by maternal race, pre-pregnancy weight, weight gain in pregnancy, marijuana use, gestational age of the infant, infant gender, low socioeconomic status, inadequate prenatal care, and use of cigarettes, alcohol and illicit drugs (5). Other adolescent activities associated with poor neonatal outcomes are poor diet, third trimester coitus, poor compliance with health care regimens, and continuation of exertive physical activities or sports during pregnancy which result in injuries. However, pregnant adolescents tend to smoke fewer cigarettes, use fewer psychoactive drugs, and drink less alcohol than older women, but they develop poor health habits by entering prenatal care later, suffering more gonorrheal infections and having lower pre-pregnancy weights (5).

Although there is no adverse perinatal outcome for pregnant adolescents greater than 16 years of age if adequate prenatal care is accessible, outcomes for those less than 15 years of age continue to be poorer despite prenatal care (5). Maternal nutrition, as seen in pre-pregnancy weight and pregnancy weight gain, is a critical factor in the incidence of low birthweight. A lower birthweight is associated with a low pre-pregnancy weight and a young maternal age because there is competition for nutrients between the growing fetus and normal adolescent growth. Gynecological age, the difference between chronological age and age at menarche, is also a factor in low birthweight. A gynecological age of less than two years is associated with an increase incidence of low birthweight infants (5). The young pregnant adolescent, because of her own growth needs, is required to gain more weight than the older adolescent or adult of similar body size to produce an infant of appropriate weight.

Factors Affecting Perinatal Outcomes

Perinatal outcomes for young adolescents are primarily affected by socioeconomic factors, inadequate nutrition and unsound health habits as opposed to the presence of any intrinsic biologic behaviors. Many complications of adolescent pregnancy are related to an indifference to health care services and delayed or little prenatal care. Adolescent childbearing also results in long-term limitations on the quality of life for the adolescent parents and child (children). Stunted education and few skills result in a lack of job opportunities and welfare dependence. Early childbearing can result in large families, a likelihood of single parenthood, and a life of poverty.

The single adolescent faces a variety of stresses during her pregnancy, both physical and psychological. It may be difficult for her to consider the needs of her unborn child while it is unseen. Her perspective of time may be present rather than future oriented, making the end of pregnancy and the eventual labor and delivery appear unreal. Her changing body image prior to and during labor may arouse fears of mutilation or unrealistic fantasies raising her anxiety level. She may or may not have the support of her family or the father of the baby. If she has been rejected by her parents and her boyfriend, she may be unable to cope alone with the unknown of labor, requiring constant attention and possibly further medication. She may have had to choose between her parents and the father of the baby and now wants the support and comfort of the missing loved one.

Cultural influences can be seen in the adolescent's response to the labor and the health care setting. These cultural and socioeconomic variations affect her expectations and reactions to the childbirth experience. She may fear injury to herself or her baby, pain and even death. She may also be anxious when left alone in a small, dark room or when she hears other women giving birth. Her ability to verbalize her fears may help her maintain control in the stressful situation. If the adolescent can have a positive birth experience, her self-esteem will increase and her response to her baby will be more positive.

Arriving at the hospital for the birth of her child may be the first time the adolescent is away from home and separated from her parents. Everywhere she looks there are strange people, clothing, equipment, rooms, lights and noises. Medical procedures such as examinations, intravenous fluids and fetal monitors are foreign to her. She may fear threats to her body or violation as well as the discomfort of the birth. Cooperation and compliance with hospital regimens will be more readily apparent when the care givers include the adolescent in their management plans, working with her. Giving the adolescent knowledge of her progress and the well-being of her baby will also elicit a positive response while diffusing anxiety.

During early adolescence, the onset of labor can reactivate the denial mechanism in the young adolescent who is unprepared for participation in labor and whose body is less physiologically mature. Conceptualization and problem solving are at beginning levels, making decisions regarding the labor and delivery process difficult for the young adolescent. In middle and late adolescence, cognitive development increases as well as problem-solving skills. The older adolescent is more receptive to childbirth preparation and is better prepared for the labor and delivery experience. When the older adolescent receives adequate prenatal care and preparation for birth, she has a more realistic grasp of the situation and can cope better with the demands of the labor and delivery experience (8).

The Adolescent's Reactions

Some of the adverse results of adolescent pregnancy may be related to missing or inadequate emotional, economic and social supports during a time of developmental changes in which the physical and psychological demands of childbirth and parenting have been superimposed. The pregnant adolescent feels confused and embarrassed about the fluctuating feelings and conflicts between dependent needs and independence. Inconsistent and unpredictable reactions are common. Some of the adolescent behaviors seen during the labor and delivery experience are anger, withdrawal, regression or childlike behaviors, hostility, inappropriate language, silence, depression, panic, threats, critical remarks, helplessness, hyperactivity, talkativeness, sensational stories, flippancy, indifference, playfulness and stoicism. The behaviors are related to the adolescent feelings of loss of control and alienation causing her to react in a "fight or flight" pattern. The adolescent may also feel abandoned and become manipulative and demanding to ensure a physical presence, not to be left alone—even to the point of grabbing the health care provider.

The Adolescent's Concerns

The adolescent needs a supportive, flexible and facilitative environment. She and her partner need to feel accepted, not threatened or punished for being pregnant. During labor, she needs to have as much control over herself and her health care decisions as possible. Even being allowed to wear her own nightgown can be reassuring and comforting. Adolescents require praise and encouragement for their efforts and constant reassurance of normalcy for themselves and their baby. They will need concrete and clear descriptions of procedures and explanations and introductions to all health care providers and equipment. Dependent needs will likely occur and can be met efficiently in a warm, supportive, nonjudgmental way. Although the adolescent is a minor, her informed consent is required for all treatments and procedures. She also retains the option to refuse treatment.

In early labor, adolescents often respond well to ambulation, liquids or even a hot bath or shower. If there is an early labor lounge available with a television, the adolescent and her partner may feel more relaxed in this less stressful setting. Often, the adolescent will arrive in the delivery suite with a special request, such as playing her own music or having several family members and friends attend her during labor. Whenever possible, within reasonable limits of the facility, these options are explored and granted.

The adolescent may be concerned about her privacy and the confidentiality of her experience. Reassurance can be given as well as consideration of the number of staff participating in her care. Careful attention to draping the adolescent during examinations and procedures and knocking before entering her room will reinforce this respect.

The childbirth experience is a time to foster self-esteem and personal development. Health care providers can assist the adolescent during childbirth by being compassionate and responsive to her needs, direct with information, and able to set limits when necessary. Letting the adolescent and her partner know about appropriate behaviors in the health care setting can be accomplished in a firm but supportive manner. Acceptable social interactions are promoted instead of negative reinforcement of acting-out behaviors.

Adolescents and their behaviors are frequently stereotyped, particularly pregnant adolescents. This is a mistaken assumption as each adolescent is a unique individual and will respond to childbirth in her own way. Flexibility and tolerance are necessary as the adolescent struggles with the physical demands of labor. Many adolescents, though indecisive, have strong belief systems. Given some time and understanding, these values can be communicated to the health care providers. All communications with the adolescent and her partner are attuned to the level of their understanding, particularly in the use of medical or technical terminology. A team approach, utilizing nursing, nurse-practitioners, nurse-midwives, social workers, nutritionists and physicians will enable these varied needs of the adolescent to be met. The adolescent's concerns include not only the childbirth experience but also her future plans for school, finances, childcare, peers and relationships with her family and partner.

As previously mentioned, the pregnant adolescent is more at risk for complications during childbirth. Often these factors result in the indication for a cesarean delivery. Major abdominal surgery is normally a cause for anxiety and apprehension, especially when the adolescent is unprepared or caught in an emergency situation. A cesarean delivery evokes the adolescent's fears of disfigurement and concerns regarding appearance and body image. Fear of pain and anesthesia are legitimate concerns that require discussion and time for the adolescent to express her feelings. She may become more childlike and dependent in her behaviors. Her immediate reaction may be one of panic followed by a hostile reaction, particularly if there is fetal distress and the decision is made rapidly. Opportunity to go over the events leading up to the cesarean, the surgery and recovery period is necessary for the adolescent to resolve her situation. Also the immediate post-cesarean adolescent mother needs time and support with her newborn to allow bonding to take place and to breastfeed the baby if desired and possible.

When an adolescent's newborn needs to stay in the special care unit, the adolescent will require information regarding the baby's status and reassurance of normal progress. Transportation to the special care unit is provided frequently to encourage the adolescent to get to know her baby and begin to meet normal child care needs. Discussions of why the baby is unwell and treatment procedures are important factors of the post-delivery follow-up. Assistance at home with child care is an important factor to discuss and arrange with the adolescent prior to discharge from the hospital.

In the case of a spontaneous vaginal delivery, the adolescent will also have adjustments to make to her changing body image and in response to her baby. Many adolescents are afraid to hold their newborns until they have been cleaned of any blood or vernix. They may be afraid to touch the baby unless the baby is first secured in a blanket. Adolescents are often happier watching the baby rather than interacting with the baby through touch and voice. They may need practice and encouragement in stimulating their newborns and in interacting appropriately with them. Adolescent mothers require immediate guidance in learning to approach their newborns with gentle stroking, cuddling, kissing and patting versus an aggresive touch seen in pricking, poking, pinching or jostling (9).

During the immediate post-delivery period the adolescent may also be coping with family conflicts, acceptance of her childbirth experience, her responsibilities to the baby and her own normal self-absorption. Yet, the new adolescent mother will also benefit from the same services as older mothers, such as rooming-in, child care classes and feeding instructions. The adolescent mother may need more encouragement and reassurance to accept these options but they will help her to focus on her new tasks ahead as a care provider to her baby.

Postpartum

The postpartum period for the young adolescent mother is a time of rapid change and adjustments. The Parenting Enhancement Program (PEP) has been developed to promote the abilities of parents to care for themselves and their offspring. It is a program of health preservation and promotion (10). Adolescents particularly need such programs to assist them in becoming safe parents and preventing a cycle of child neglect and abuse. Adolescents may not have had an adequate parenting role model or experienced good parenting themselves. Adolescents have limited parenting skills and abilities, and time and effort is spent learning these new behaviors while in the hospital or at home. Initially, adolescent parents may not have the skills or resources for coping successfully with the demands and frustrations of childcare responsibilities. During the perinatal period, there is the opportunity to enhance and encourage positive relationships and allow confidence to develop naturally. Beneficial attitudes and behaviors of the family unit can be fully developed, and preventable negative influences can be averted. Efforts are made to discuss and improve the home situation and to provide alternative ways of coping with parenthood. Stimulation of the adolescent/ newborn bond is vital because adolescents generally are less likely to remain with their children as primary care givers or to be interested in the child's progress. Also, when childbearing begins at an early age, more children are produced, forcing the adolescent parent(s) into a further distractable and dependent position (5).

The adolescent is encouraged in her self-care efforts and self-esteem is promoted when the PEP model is used. Personal decision-making skills are strengthened as well as an awareness of personal responsibilities within society. A plan of care is developed that adapts to the individual family situation. Family relationships are evaluated, strengths are emphasized, and coping mechanisms are introduced with PEP. The adolescent's family are allowed time to express their feelings and concerns, enabling them to make their own decisions and to assist their daughter in her decision-making.

The postpartum adolescent may experience a wide variety of emotions including loneliness, sexual desires and a wish to be loved. Peer associations may change as the demands of childcare curtail social activities. Such social isolation can lead to stress and rejection of the baby. The physical health of both the adolescent mother and her baby will affect their abilities to interact and respond to each other. During this period of adjustment and possible isolation, there is a greater risk of sudden infant death syndrome in children of adolescents as well as a risk of the baby being either underfed or overfed. There is also an increase risk of mortality in children of adolescents during the first year of life from external events such as accidents, violence or infections (5).

The postpartum adolescent is herself at greater risk of developing such complications as fever, anemia pre-eclampsia, urinary tract infections, endometritis and other infections. Episiotomies are more routinely performed and cause pain and discomfort in the early postpartum period. Feeding techniques, hygiene, nutrition, sexuality, contraception and parenting skills are also part of the postpartum education plan.

While in the hospital, the postpartum adolescent is encouraged to participate in educational services for the care of herself and her newborn. However, whenever possible, the adolescent is allowed to follow her own timetable when caring for her baby. Flexible hours are also given to meet her needs of sleep, nutrition and visiting, allowing for freedom and choice within the hospital boundaries.

A thorough description of expected body changes is also discussed with the adolescent about changes in her breasts, abdomen, vagina, bleeding, and weight. Comfort measures for normal postpartum complaints are given and danger signs are outlined. Whenever possible, a 24-hour "hot line" for concerns and questions that the adolescent may have about herself or her baby is available. The necessity of family planning services and a six-week examination is also emphasized. Often the adolescents are seen for a two-week "social" postpartum visit to observe their adaptations and adjustments to parenthood.

Meeting the adolescent's needs and those of her family during the perinatal period is a challenging and rewarding task. Adolescents today seek honest and informed interactions with society as they try to meet the demands of daily life in an ever changing world. The adolescent parents we are seeing now are making choices about the quality and direction of their lives. It is essential that health care providers are open to the needs of adolescents, listen to what they are saying, and help them meet their goals to begin their life as responsible parents.

References

1. Wallis C. Children having children: Teen pregnancies are corroding America's social fabric. *Time* Dec. 9, 1985;78–90.
2. Stengel R. The missing-father myth. *Time* Dec. 9,1985;90.
3. Panzarine S, Elster AB. Prospective adolescent fathers: stresses during pregnancy and implications for nursing interventions. *J Psychosoc Nurs Ment Health Service* 1982;20(7):21–24.
4. Daniel WA. An approach to the adolescent patient. *Med Clin North Am* 1975;59 (6):1281–1287.
5. Zuckerman BS, Walker DK, Frank DA, Chase C, Hamburg B. Adolescent pregnancy: biobehavioral determinants of outcome. *J Pediatr* 1984;105(6):857–863.
6. Tyrer LB. Oral contraception for the adolescent. *J Repro Med* 1984;29(suppl) (7):551–556.
7. Tyrer LB, Josimovich J. Contraception in teenagers. *Clin Obstetr Gynecol* 1977; 20(3):651–663.
8. Mercer RT. The adolescent experience in labor, delivery and early postpartum period. In: *Perspectives in Adolescent Health Care.* Mercer RT (ed). Philadelphia: JB Lippincott Co., 1979;302–347.
9. McAnarney ER, Lawrence RA, Aten MJ, Iker HP. Adolescent mothers and their infants. *Pediatrics* 1984;73(3):358–362.
10. Porter LS. Parenting enhancement among high risk adolescents. *Nursing Clin N Am* 1984;19(1):89–102.

Bibliography

Adams BN. Adolescent health care: Needs, priorities and services. *Nurs Clin N Am* 1983;18(2):237–247.

Bennett DL. Worldwide problems in the delivery of adolescent health care. *Public Health* (London) 1982;96:334–340.

Daniels MB, Manning DA. Clinic for pregnant teens. *AJN* 1983;83(1)68–71.

Elster AB, McAnarney ER, Lamb ME. Parental behavior of adolescent mothers. *Pediatrics* 1983;71:494–503.

Elster AB, Roberts D. The financial impact of a comprehensive adolescent pregnancy program in a university hospital. *Adolescent Health Care* 1985;6(1):17–20.

Foote JA. Special needs of teenage cesarean patients. *Association of Operating Room Nurses Journal* 1981;34(5):855–858.

Howe CL. Physiologic and psychological assessment in labor. *Nurs Clin N Am* 1982;17(1):49–56.

Mercer RT. Assessing and counseling teenage mothers during the perinatal period. *Nurs Clin N Am* 1983;18(2):293–301.

Petrella JM. The unwed pregnant adolescent. *JOGN Nursing* 1978;Jul/Aug:22-26.

Roosa M, Fitzgerald H, Carlson N. A comparison of teenage and older mothers: a systems analysis. *J Marriage Fam* 1982;44:367-379.

Russell JK. School Pregnancies—medical, social and educational considerations. *Br J Hosp Med* 1983;Feb:159-166.

Santangeli B. Adolescent pregnancy. *Nursing Mirror* 1984;158(11)32-34.

Savedra M. The adolescent in the hospital. In: *Perspectives in Adolescent Health Care.* Mercer RT (ed). Philadelphia: JB Lippincott Co., 1979;172-185.

Smith DL. Meeting the psychosocial needs of teenage mothers and fathers. *Nurs Clin N Am* 1984;19(2):369-379.

Wallace HM, Weeks J, Medina A. Services for pregnant teenagers in large cities of the United States, 1970-1980. *JAMA* 1982;248(18):2270-2273.

9 Adolescent Parents

LOIS SIEBERT SADLER

Introduction

A discussion of adolescent parenthood begins with the acknowledgment that adolescent mothers and fathers are inherently different from older parents. This difference is largely due to their age, which weaves ever-present threads of conflict through their struggle to accept and assume parenting roles. This difference is the basis for understanding, assessing, and managing the care of these young families.

This chapter is concerned primarily with mothers from low socio-economic urban populations, although the phenomenon of adolescent parenthood is not limited to this group. Adolescents in many different cultures have been giving birth to children for centuries, which raises the question of why do we now see adolescent parenthood as a "problem" (1). This chapter focuses on the particular stresses and needs that adolescent parents in the northeastern United States who live in urban poverty face in the 1980s.

Nationwide Trends

Before examining specific dynamics and clinical situations involving adolescent parents, it is useful to take a broader look at the nationwide trends and characteristics of these special mothers and fathers and their children. In the 1980s, much publicity has been given to the epidemic nature of adolescent pregnancy and parenthood. However, when one examines the data more closely, one sees that certain subgroups of adolescent parents do demand our increased attention and help (1, 2). When one looks at the origins of adolescent parenthood in the 1980s, it is necessary to acknowledge that adolescents are becoming increasingly sexually active at younger ages. The phenomenon of adolescent parenthood is seen across all socioeconomic and ethnic groups; it is not limited to the poor, inner-city minority groups, but this group of adolescent mothers seems to have received the most publicity and has been studied most thoroughly. Adolescents under 15 years of age are at the highest risk for physical, emotional and social problems affecting mother, child, and extended family. The overall decline in adolescent birth rates owes to the increased availability and use of contraception and abortion services by adolescents. One can only speculate on the tragic and far-reaching effects of any social or political attempt to make these services less available or, at worst, nonexistent for this group of young women.

Researchers (3) do not agree as to how adolescent pregnancy affects social emotional, and cognitive development of offspring. While researchers and clinicians have noted that adolescent mothers tend to have fewer verbal interactions with their infants, it is not clear that this type of interaction has any significant long-term effect on the child's social and emotional development. Furstenberg, Sandler, Dryfoos, and others (4) have begun to study aspects of cognitive development in the children of primarily poor black adolescent mothers. The tentative results seem to indicate that children exposed to caretakers other than their adolescent mothers score better on a variety of cognitive tests. This theme was amplified in a report by Field et al. (5) in which a subgroup of adolescent mothers received on-the-job childcare training in the day care setting in which their children were enrolled. In a two-year follow-up analysis, the children of these mothers had higher Bayley motor and mental scores than did children from a control group or children from home visiting intervention programs (5).

Studies that attempt to answer the question of whether children of adolescent parents actually are at higher risk for abuse and neglect show some disturbing trends, but few, if any, conclusive findings (6). In Leventhal's (7) indepth critique of 22 case-controlled child abuse studies, he found that while this body of research is fraught with methodological flaws, young maternal age at birth does seem to be a risk factor for child abuse. Researchers and clinicians have noted that adolescent parents seem to have young children who experience more accidents and are perhaps at higher risk for injuries resulting from inadequate supervision (8–11). Adolescent parents seem to have less knowledge about infant and toddler motor and cognitive capabilities. In addition, many adolescent parents seem to believe that young children, even infants, are responsible for their own actions, and therefore that it is their own fault if they get hurt (12). Social isolation, depression, and disorganized living situations add to the potential for adolescent parents to mistreat their offspring. The well-documented pattern of parents who were abused as children growing up to repeat such abusive behavior with their own children completes the grim picture. The tendency for male adolescents to express more abusive parenting attitudes than do female adolescents is an interesting but discouraging finding (12).

Family Patterns

Adolescent parenthood seems to recur with each new generation; patterns of adolescent childbearing, single parenthood, and prolonged dependence on the maternal extended family seem cyclic (13). Reported trends (13) indicate that adolescent mothers and fathers are likely to have had adolescent parents themselves.

Many pregnant adolescents tend to appear chronically depressed, and this may be linked to the cyclic tendency of adolescent pregnancy. A review of the family history of the pregnant adolescent may reveal that her mother gave birth in her teens. This child was probably cared for by the maternal grandmother until the mother finished her own adolescence. When the mother either decided or was told that she needed to assume the role of primary caretaker, the child may have already become quite attached to the maternal grandmother. The child may have considered the sudden transition from grandmother to mother a deep loss, potentially resulting in childhood depression.

This depression may become the foundation for a more chronic feeling of poor self-worth, possibly leading the individual to early sexual experimentation in an attempt to find attention and affection. Thus the script is written for the next generation of adolescent parents. Adolescent girls bear the children, grandmothers raise the children until a certain age, and the children are confused as to whom they really belong. These dynamics may contribute to the cyclical nature of adolescent parenthood and may provide clues toward comprehensive understanding of the problem.

The younger the adolescent has a baby, the more time and chance she has to have additional children before completing her teens. For a variety of reasons, adolescents have significantly more children than do women who postpone childbearing until after adolescence (13). Clearly, these repeat pregnancies only amplify the financial, emotional, and family stresses for the adolescent parent.

The trend over the past decade has been for adolescent mothers who have not elected abortion, to keep and raise their babies. Adoption has declined in popularity to a point where it is a choice that few adolescents of any cultural background would select (13). National trends also indicate that fewer white and black adolescents are choosing to marry to legitimize the birth of a child. If marriage does occur, it is three times more likely to end than for couples who marry past adolescence (13). Lorenzi's (14) study of adolescent parents indicated that, for that sample of inner-city youth, 26 months after the birth, 23 percent of the mothers had married the fathers, 23 percent were seeing each other regularly, 18 percent only saw each other occasionally, and 35 percent of the mothers either never saw the fathers or had married someone else.

Adolescent Fathers

Much descriptive and statistical information has been accumulated concerning the adolescent mother, but relatively little is known about the adolescent father. Perhaps some of the same factors which make him such a difficult person to study also have importance for how he perceives and fulfills the paternal role. Much of the available literature consists of studies in which the adolescent mother reports on various characteristics of her partner (15). There are a much smaller group of studies in which limited numbers of paid volunteer adolescent fathers are directly interviewed (16–19).

Factors which may contribute to the adolescent father's elusiveness as a parent and a research subject probably are related to the strength of the adolescent couple's relationship as well as his desire to protect his anonymity for economic reasons. Many young fathers are reluctant to show themselves to members of the health care system, which in their minds, may be linked to the welfare system. In most cases, the welfare system will provide financial support to a child if the father is out of the picture. Unlike the adolescent mother, the father really has no physical need to be tied into the prenatal, intrapartal, and pediatric health care setting. It therefore becomes much more of a challenge to enlist the trust and participation of young fathers in these health care arenas. Even though clinicians may not see or hear much from the adolescent father, he is not nearly as invisible to the young mother. His existence has important effects on nuclear and extended family members.

Characteristics of Adolescent Fathers

Some attempt can be made to outline the demographic characteristics of the adolescent father from the available data. Early studies indicated that adolescent fathers who were willing to be interviewed were mostly in their late teens and early 20s (14, 20). More recent data suggest that, indeed, much younger males are becoming fathers as well (18, 19, 21). Clincial experience indicates that the adolescent father is usually the same age or several years older than his female partner. If there is a trend for younger girls giving birth then we will also see younger and younger fathers.

The available data on average age of first intercourse for adolescent males tell us that growing numbers of black and Hispanic males in urban settings begin their sexual experiences around the age of 12 years (19, 22, 23). For white youths in urban settings the average age of first intercourse is between 14 and 15 years of age (22). These data combined with the findings which describe the sporatic use of male contraceptives by these populations lead one to realize that very young adolescent fatherhood is probably not as rare as we once thought.

Longitudinal data collected on a random sample of U.S. high school students from 1960 through 1971 indicate that adolescent fathers do have significantly less education and lower status jobs than males who postponed their families until after adolescence (24). In a more recent study of black adolescent fathers two groups from Tulsa, Oklahoma and Chicago were described (17). In the Tulsa group (N=20) the fathers were likely to be employed, have completed twelve or more years of school, and to have come from families with a median income of less than $10,000. The Chicago group (N=27) reflected less education, more unemployment (74%), but families with medium incomes of $10,000 or more. In both groups the mean age at conception was between 17 and 18 years of age (17).

Rivara and others (19) studied 100 black inner-city adolescent fathers and compared them with 100 age-matched urban black nonfathers. Subjects had a mean age of 17.5 years. Significant findings included that more nonfathers perceived pregnancy as disruptive to their own future plans and that more adolescent fathers had mothers who had been adolescent mothers themselves (19).

No conclusive studies are known to either support or refute the presence of depression and or poor self-image in adolescents who become fathers. Attempts have been made to link low self-esteem with early sexual activity in males, but not specifically with the subgroup of adolescent fathers (16, 25).

There are no studies which clearly implicate father-absence as a factor in adolescent paternity; however this pattern does emerge from many clinicians' experiences. Many young fathers have lacked consistently present fathers in their lives. This may have relevance for these boys' own development as well as their lacking a positive role model on which to pattern their own fathering behavior. At this point it is only possible to speculate about this phenomenon and its potential for becoming a pattern which repeats itself from generation to generation.

The issue of multiple paternity, while not greatly documented in the literature, is one that surfaces in clinical work. Within certain proximal neighborhoods or high school communities, the same father may have more than one child with several partners. Among some male peer groups it is highly valued to have fathered children from multiple sexual partners. Such situations provide the male with concrete proof of fertility in addition to the perceived increase in peer group status gained from simultaneous sexual relationships. While these cases do not seem to be the norm, they occur frequently enough to account for a significant amount of rivalry among the involved girls, resulting in verbal and physical fights. Statements such as "She had her baby by him" give some clues as to the nature of these relationships and roles, but much is left to be learned about this issue.

The Adolescent Couple

A far more common situation is the picture of the adolescent couple struggling to define and understand their own relationship while in the midst of the tempest created by a new baby and the extended families. Since many adolescent couples do not marry when they conceive a child, usually the adolescent mother continues to live with her own family. The amount of financial and emotional support offered by the adolescent father varies greatly among individuals. Often times, conflicts arise between the adolescent father and the mother's parents. In some cases the parents may restrict or try to stop the father from seeing the baby and the baby's mother. Sometimes these conflicts are able to be completely or partially resolved through a family meeting with an objective clinician, where visitation contracts and schedules are arranged. In some cases the maternal family is successful in enforcing de facto exclusion of the father even though this violates his legal rights for visitation. In these cases, the father's feeling of attachment and commitment to the mother and baby tend to fade with time. An alternative outcome of the father being excluded is that the young mother may attempt to move out of her family's home with the baby and go to live with the baby's father. This forces the couple to then face the stormy course of financial problems, child care and school demands, as well as household responsibilities.

Many adolescent fathers, especially if they are young, are likely to be living with their own family of origin. In many cases, if both adolescent parents are still living with their own families, then both families become involved in caring for the baby. This arrangement can either be helpful or likened to a competitive playing field on which the baby is thrown back and forth between teams.

The strength of the relationship between the young parents is probably one of the best predictors of how involved the adolescent father will be with his child. Tentative, ambivalent, and narcissistic relationships are seen most often between very young adolescent parents. This experimental kind of young adolescent romance most always has difficulty withstanding the stressful crises of early parenthood. At the birth of the baby many adolescent fathers will describe a romantic picture of their new family and their own sense of ongoing responsibility to the child and mother. Over time, however, as the relationship with the baby's mother fades, the commitment to the child also weakens.

Adolescent fathers have to wrestle with the inherent mismatch of their position (26). Society expects fathers to provide resources for their partners and offspring, both in terms of economic and moral support. In many cases the adolescent father is doomed to failure on both accounts. If he is a student, unemployed, or only partially employed, he is severely limited in the economic support he can offer. If he is still at a point in his cognitive development where he is thinking in concrete terms, then his inability to provide his baby with tangible things means that he is a failure as a father. The more abstract contributions he may be capable of giving, such as emotional support or time spent with mother and baby, may not measure up in his own mind to the things he is unable to give them. This feeling of failure as a provider may certainly contribute to his waning involvement and may even be linked to feelings and behavioral manifestations of depression in the young father.

The question of involvement and commitment raises the question of whether or not to recruit and actively involve adolescent fathers in educational and health care programs for young parents. Anecdotal reports and preliminary findings indicate that when adolescent fathers feel comfortable enough to present themselves to various members of the health care system, they want to talk, want to be included, and do have important questions about their roles as fathers (16, 17, 18, 20). It is also clear from clinical experience that many adolescent fathers either do not wish to surface or are not involved enough with the new family to become actively engaged in health and educational programs for young parents.

Some researchers caution that the adolescent couple who marries has a greater chance for a second pregnancy while they are still in their teens (14, 24). This raises a further issue of how counselors and health professionals sanction the development of the relationships of these young couples. While the solution to this dilemma is not an easy one, it does seem reasonable to invite fathers to participate in the health care of the young mother and child. Fathers who respond and come with their girlfriends to prenatal visits, classes, and pediatric visits should be warmly acknowledged and encouraged to participate in these and other educational programs for adolescent parents. Clinicians and researchers are beginning to design alternative outreach projects in neighborhoods and schools to try to reach the adolescent father who is otherwise invisible to the health care system.

Prenatal classes and hospital labor and delivery orientation sessions should be offered to adolescent fathers, as they are offered to older fathers. If the young father remains in contact with the mother throughout the pregnancy, the issue of his presence at the birth should be discussed with the couple during the prenatal visits. In many cases, the girl may prefer to have her mother or other important woman present with her for the birth, and this may cause the father to feel angry or slighted. Every attempt should be made to change hospital policies or have exceptions made so that the father of the baby *and* the maternal grandmother or other support person can both participate in labor support and share in the birth experience. If these issues can be brought up, discussed, and planned for before the labor begins, the scenario of adolescent father and maternal grandmother battling over labor room visitation on the labor and delivery unit may be avoided. As with older fathers who choose to be present for the delivery, the adolescent father needs preparation and support during the birthing process.

In the case where the clinician is meeting the adolescent mother for the first time during the immediate postpartum period, one of the important questions to be asked is "Are you still seeing your baby's father?". This question is phrased in such a way as to be nonthreatening to the mother no matter what her situation is. Depending on her answer, follow-up questions can then be asked concerning the extent of the father's involvement prenatally, during labor and delivery, and since the birth. If the father is involved with the mother and baby, every effort should be made to include him in the postpartum teaching discussions and the baby's pediatric visits. His questions, concerns and fears about the newborn are not so different from those of the father who is beyond his adolescent years.

Grandmothers

Mothers of adolescent mothers play an important and often little-recognized role in the phenomenon of adolescent parenthood. They have the formidable task of coping with their own reactions to their daughter's situation while, at the same time, coping with the hectic daily routines of a teenager taking care of a small child. The grandmother may feel confused about her responsibilities toward her daughter and grandchild. In the case of most adolescent parents, the role of grandmother calls for limitless patience and the negotiating skills of a seasoned diplomat.

Although little has been written about the grandmothers of babies born to adolescent parents, clinical experience indicates that there is a wide range of reactions, emotions, and patterns of behavior that these women experience. The spectrum of reactions encompasses joy, disappointment, guilt, anger, and sadness, perhaps linked to memories of the grandmother's own pregnancy experiences, possibly during adolescence as well.

Poole (27) described a group of 44 grandmothers surveyed through a series of interviews. She found that most had negative feelings towards the babies' fathers. All of these grandmothers loved their grandchildren, yet their primary concerns about the new role of grandmother divided them into three different groups. The first group felt trapped into caring for their grandchildren because they felt their daughters did not care enough or spend enough time with their babies. The second group put rigid demands on the daughters as the primary caretakers, thereby restricting their other interests and activities. The third group felt their daughters were accepting an appropriate amount of responsibility for the babies and also felt able to negotiate with their daughters. All of the grandmothers surveyed would have welcomed some counseling regarding their new role.

The process of grandmotherhood begins when the adolescent's mother discovers that her daughter is pregnant. This discovery may come through a direct conversation with her daughter where the pregnancy announcement is made, or through vastly more circuitous routes. Bryan-Logan (28) describes a series of adjustments which the mother and adolescent go through while the possibility of pregnancy is being confirmed. The "silent phase" includes the time when the mother thinks the daughter is pregnant but does not verbalize this concern. This is followed by the "question-denial" phase where mother questions and daughter denies that anything is wrong. After the disclosure of pregnancy occurs, many mothers then go on to accept the pregnancies through processes of rationalization and negotiation. The negotiations concern issues of the daughter's relationship with the baby's father, the paternal family's involvement, and arrangements for prenatal care and continuing education.

The ways in which adolescents and their mothers work out the daily division of labor needed for infant care may be related to the quality of the underlying mother-daughter relationship as well as the extent to which the daughter is involved in adolescent rebellion. Both of these conditions may cause the adolescent to turn away from her own mother and look towards another woman in her life for help and support. Alternative role models such as aunts, godmothers, or grandmothers may fulfill this role for the adolescent. What is most important is, how the adolescent mother and the older woman get along together after the baby's birth. A strong caring relationship is necessary to withstand the many negotiations involved in raising a young child.

How Are Adolescent Parents Different?

When working with the adolescent mothers, it is crucial to remember that the adolescent was still a teenager when she became a mother. She finds herself in the midst of two difficult developmental crises, adolescence and parenthood. In addition, she also is experiencing at least one situational crisis, that of integrating a new baby into the family. If the clinician keeps these three crises in mind, it becomes easier to see why adolescent mothers experience such stress and manifest certain characteristic behaviors.

Adolescence is usually divided into three overlapping subphases: early adolescence, middle adolescence, and late adolescence. Early adolescence, ages 12–15, is considered to be the stormiest phase as issues of sexuality, rebellion, cognitive changes, and peer involvement are explored and tested by the individual. Similarly, the process of parenthood may be divided into early, middle and late subphases. The phase of early parenthood extends from pregnancy until the child is of school age (29). It is also thought to be one of the most challenging phases of parenthood, with all the behaviors, skills and emotions which must be incorporated into the new role of parent. When early parenthood occurs simultaneously with early adolescence the potential for problems with both processes is amplified (30).

A developmental framework has been derived from clinical experience and is presented in Table 9.1 (30). The developmental processes of adolescence and parenthood are conceptualized as occurring simultaneously. For each adolescent developmental task, there seems to be a parental task which may cause direct conflict for the individual caught between them. The ultimate goal is for the teenager to continue to develop along both axes, as a parent and as an individual. In most cases, the actual outcomes seem to resemble clashes between the two areas but in some cases, there may be accelerated development along both axes. A closer examination of each task

Table 9.1. *Conceptual Framework of Parallel Developmental Continua*

Adolescence	Parenthood
Narcissim	Empathy with child
Egocentrism	Mutuality between mother and child
Identity formation	Maternal identification
Moratorium; role experimentation	Maternal role definition
Sexual identity formation	Body image changes of pregnancy, labor and delivery, and the postpartum period
Emancipation from family	Family role reassignments
Cognitive development; i.e., transition from concrete to formal operations	Problem-solving and future-planning skills necessary for childrearing

will provide a framework for the understanding and the clinical management of the adolescent mother-infant dyad.

Narcissism and egocentrism are normal characteristics of early to middle adolescent development, yet they may severely interfere with the adolescent mother's ability to form an empathic understanding of her baby. The normal self-centeredness of early adolescence brings about two issues of clinical importance for the adolescent mother. The first is that it may be quite difficult for the mother to put her own feelings and needs second to those of the baby. This is seen clinically as the mother feeling that she is in competition with the baby for the attention of family and friends. She may notice that after the birth she is no longer pampered as she may have been during pregnancy. In fact she may openly admit "My baby gets all the attention now."

This situation dictates that the clinician use an approach which lets the adolescent know that she is still important. The message that she is important and has needs besides those related to her new role as mother, will serve to establish the beginning trust and cooperation that is otherwise often difficult to develop between clinicians and adolescents. The clinical strategy which accomplishes this purpose is a simple one. The clinician can begin the interview with the adolescent mother in a fashion similar to the way in which one could begin talking to any adolescent. Nonthreatening topics which are important to the adolescent and easy for her to discuss are discussed first. Thus, when meeting the adolescent mother for the first time, the clinician takes a few minutes to talk about her school, friends, family and outside activities before asking more specific questions about medical or nursing issues. On the postpartum unit, most newly delivered adolescents need to talk about their own reactions and feelings about the recent labor and delivery process, before they can begin to discuss the newborn or other aspects of postpartum care. In addition to discussing her reactions to the birth, it is helpful to find out who was with her for the birth, who she plans to have help her with the baby, and what plans she has for returning to school or work, and staying in contact with peers. This kind of information is also useful in assessing the young mothers social support system. The few minutes it takes to cover these areas is time well spent. The clinician who is sensitive to the adolescent's needs will continue to use the approach of beginning the interview by focusing on the mother as an individual throughout the well child care series of pediatric visits.

The second clinical issue related to the mother's egocentrism is the possibility that the mother cannot separate her own thoughts, feelings, and needs from those of the baby. Again, the early adolescent is most likely to have the cognitive problem of understanding that she and her baby have very different characteristics and needs. Many teenagers have a great deal of difficulty understanding that babies think very differently from mothers. Adolescents may attribute all kinds of sophisticated problem-solving and memory abilities to infants. Young mothers may talk about their young infants being spoiled, or crying deliberately to get back at the mother, or the need to discipline infants so they will learn right from wrong.

This phenomenon is also seen when discussing infant nutrition. "My baby doesn't like the taste of that formula" may be an indication that the baby needs something to eat which tastes better to the mother. Some adolescent mothers try to feed their infants foods, in their first year of life, which are derived from their own preferences, e.g., soda, hot dogs, potato chips, beer. In many cases these foods may not only be inappropriate sources of nutrition but also unsafe foods because of the risk of choking.

It is very difficult to try to translate the abstract reasons why babies think differently and have different needs into concrete terms for the adolescent mother. It requires patience on the clinician's part to explain simply and concretely that babies have different nutritional needs, digest foods differently and cannot chew foods as the mother can. Specific foods can be listed which are unsafe for any young child because of the risk of choking, including the fact that babies can not swallow pills.

The issue of cognitive differences between babies and adults can be illustrated with the example of hiding a toy the baby is playing with under a blanket. Once the toy is out of sight, the baby forgets about it. This demonstration may help the clinician to teach the mother about the baby's limited memory regarding issues of spoiling, discipline, and safety.

In the areas of identity formation and role experimentation, most adolescent mothers are still struggling to define who they are and where they are going in life. Before the issue of identity formation reaches some stage of closure, most adolescents feel the need to spend a great deal of time with their peers and to try out a wide variety of roles, styles, and behaviors. The freedom to be with one's friends and experiment with various roles is curtailed severely if one has to assume the 24-hour duties demanded by the maternal role.

This obvious conflict of interests occurs in most adolescent mothers. The ways in which the conflict is resolved seems to vary according to how much help the adolescent has from her family or others. At one end of the spectrum is the adolescent mother who is forced to assume the entire responsibility for child care. This individual, whether still living at home, alone with the baby, or with the baby's father is at high risk for the fatigue and overwhelming feelings any new mother has, coupled with feelings of depression and isolation from the loss of her friends, school, and social life. Aside from the obvious risks associated with depression, these mothers are also more prone to repeat pregnancies and the babies are at higher risk for failure to thrive, neglect, and abuse.

The other end of the spectrum of outcomes is represented by the adolescent mother who abdicates her maternal role and returns entirely to her prepregnant lifestyle. Her abdication may be by choice or because she surrenders to the pressure from her mother or other family member who wishes to take over the care of the new baby. If the latter is the case, the adolescent may give up and perhaps become pregnant again to replace her "lost" baby.

In the former case, if there is another dedicated family member, usually the baby's grandmother, who is willing to assume responsibility for the baby's care, then many times the mother and baby will assume more of a sibling relationship. If there is no other family member who can assume the baby's care, then again the child falls into an extremely high risk category for abuse and neglect. These may be instances when the state must assume protective custody and place the child in foster care until the mother is ready to care for her child.

In the middle of the spectrum is the situation where the mother and grandmother share the baby's care in a way which allows the adolescent mother to strike a balance between the activities which are important to her adolescence and the responsibilities and rewards of motherhood. Such a delicate balance involves a grandmother who will supervise and help out with the babysitting without monopolizing the baby. In even the most congenial relationships, the adolescent usually expresses concern at some point about who the baby will call "mommy." This concern usually goes deeper into issues of competition with the grandmother and feelings of guilt from having to be away from the baby because of school or work. These mothers need much reassurance in this area, as well as concrete suggestions as to how they can spend available time with the baby in positive ways, and which names they want the child to use when addressing them and the grandmother.

It becomes clear just how crucial the relationship is between the adolescent mother and her helper (aunt, godmother, baby's grandmother). The assessment of this relationship must take into account the flexibility of the adolescent's helper regarding child care schedules, childrearing practices and making decisions about the baby. It is also helpful to know if the adolescent mother sees her helper as a good parental role model. Many times adolescent mothers will be quite verbal about the shortcomings they see in their own parents as mothers and fathers. Some of this complaining may certainly be related to adolescence, but some of it may indeed be justified. These girls may not want to pattern their own parenting on what they consider to be the mistakes of their parents, yet they may not have access to alternative positive parental role models. This is where special educational and supportive community and school programs become vitally important. Virtually all adolescent mothers need support and understanding from interested professionals. The girls who lack positive parental and adult role models in their own immediate environments especially need the services of parent aid-homemaker programs, special classes in school, and a supervised time, such as a playgroup, where teachers spend time with the mothers interacting with their children. These are the kinds of positive approaches which help mothers to see the options they have as parents and as young adults.

Sexuality

The adolescent mother, in most cases, is still in the process of forming her sexual identity. Depending on her age, she may be still struggling with issues of accepting her pubertal body changes. At the same time, she may be deciding how she sees herself as a sexual being and how she wishes to participate in sexual relationships. The fact that she has given birth to a baby does not mean that she has resolved any or all of these issues. She may even lack a very basic understanding of how her body functions with regard to reproduction.

The clinician must avoid making any assumptions about how knowledgeable or comfortable the adolescent mother may be about her sexuality. It is imperative to find out from each individual mother what her understanding is of the body changes associated with pregnancy, lactation, and postpartal involution. Adolescents may have disappointingly inappropriate expectations about postpartum weight loss and how soon they can return to their designer jeans. It is also necessary to assess each mother's understanding of postpartum fertility and plan for the resumption of sexual activity and contraception.

The issue of breastfeeding may serve to illustrate the adolescent's own degree of comfort or discomfort with her changing body. Egocentrism again seems to play an important role in this issue. The adolescent, who is normally more focused on her body than the adult woman, may be more concerned with the bodily changes associated with childbearing. This concern with her distorted body may lead her to avoid prolonging the breast enlargement and leaking associated with breastfeeding. She simply may not be comfortable enough with her own body to consider the possibility of breastfeeding. Clinicians, although recognizing the advantages of breastfeeding, need to be aware of this developmental factor as they are counseling the adolescent mother about her plans for feeding the baby. Additional factors which need to be considered are the mother's own state of nutrition or malnutrition and her postpartum dietary patterns as well as the logistics of breastfeeding schedules, manual expression of breast milk and school schedules. Many adolescent mothers find this combination of factors too discouraging. Common reasons that adolescents give for not breastfeeding are either the initial discomfort or the fear of the baby needing a feeding when they are in a public place. However, in clinical experience, about 10 percent of adolescent mothers elect to breastfeed and continue to nurse their infants through the first several months of life. These mothers who are able to succeed seem to be more mature and accepting of themselves in general. They all have a good understanding of how breastfeeding works and why it is beneficial. Perhaps most important to their success is that each of these young women has identified a close supportive family member who has helped and encouraged her with her nursing efforts. With breastfeeding as with other parenting behaviors, the issue of positive role models seems to be a critical factor.

Independence vs. Dependence

The concept of adolescent emancipation is a particularly troubling one for the adolescent parent. The adolescent years are traditionally the time when the individual seeks to become independent from the family and particular family members. The adolescent mother certainly feels this need for independence, but at the same time her dependence on her family is increased because of the need for help with child care and support. These struggles of independence and dependence are always present even though they may be well hidden or camouflaged. Many times, the simple question, "What is it like to be a mother and a daughter at the same time," will bring forth a torrent of complaints and descriptions of arguments over who cares for, takes responsibility for, and decides about important issues for the baby. Many adolescent mothers realize they need help with caring for a baby or toddler, but their own independence struggle makes it difficult or impossible to ask their mothers for help, or take the help if it is offered. This dilemma is equally frustrating when experienced from the perspective of the baby's grandmother.

In cases where the emancipation struggle leads to open warfare, the clinician may need to assume the role of mediator. Family meetings can be helpful, where all sides of the conflict may be heard. Often times, compromise can be arrived at through the use of concrete schedules and agreements whereby the infant's care is planned for and divided among mother and other family members in the most fair and consistent way possible. This process is never an easy one, but it proceeds more smoothly if both the adolescent mother and the grandmother feel they have a chance to express their views openly.

Cognitive Development

Finally, the issue of cognitive development must be considered in the adolescent mother. Most adolescents proceed from a stage of concrete thinking in early adolescence to a stage of more conceptual or abstract thinking in late adolescence and early adulthood. In simple terms, the concrete thinker relates to what she can see, hear, and feel in her present environment, while the abstract thinker is more capable of considering concepts, hypothetical alternatives, and future implications of actions.

It is possible for the clinician to determine the stage of cognitive development of the adolescent mother through the data collected in the social and developmental history. Chronological age, school progress and achievement, peer activities, and future goals are all areas which supply the clinician with important clues as to how the adolescent thinks. The clinician will utilize this assessment to determine the well child care teaching content and strategies to be used with each individual adolescent parent.

In the immediate postpartum period, the adolescent mother who is still in a concrete stage of thinking will require very clear information and actual demonstrations regarding infant feeding techniques, schedules and formula preparation, skin and diaper care, use of a rectal thermometer, and the care of the umbillical cord and genital area. A bedside newborn exam performed with the mother is extremely useful to illustrate some of these tasks.

The same series of postpartum teaching sessions might look somewhat different with an adolescent mother who is a more abstract thinker. Here, the clinician could add more conceptual information about the baby's reflexes, different cries and cues, and temperament during the newborn bedside exam.

These individualized teaching strategies carry over into the anticipatory guidance which is given during the baby's well child care visits. The mother who is a concrete thinker needs to be seen with her baby more often, perhaps monthly, for the baby's well child care. This allows the clinician to teach her about her baby on a here-and-now basis regarding issues of feeding, stimulation, play, and most importantly safety. Aside from actually demonstrating the skills and techniques being discussed, it is also helpful to use the approach of role playing with the mother. This is particularly useful, as the child approaches toddlerhood and engages the mother in independence struggles.

Mothers who have more abstract thinking abilities may profit from discussions of present as well as future behaviors in their children in relation to development, play and safety. These mothers usually are capable of thinking about issues of spoiling, discipline, and their child's emotional development in more future-oriented terms.

The success of matching the teaching approach to the mother's level of thinking is easily seen in individual patient teaching as well as parent education in groups or formal high school classes. With all adolescent parent classes it is essential to allow the learning to occur through active rather than passive methods (31). Presentation of material about child rearing or child development through lectures and reading assignments is not likely to be successful with this population of young parents. However, presenting this same content by using charts and photo journals, debates, case discussions, and role plays greatly increases the interest and participation of the class members.

Conclusion

The process of adolescent parenthood is never an easy one. Adolescent developmental characteristics such as egocentrism, identity formation, sexual identity formation, emancipation struggles, and cognitive developmental stages all complicate the already difficult process of early parenthood. Clinicians need to appreciate the developmental reasons why adolescent parents think and behave differently from older parents and use their knowledge to plan specific strategies for helping adolescents to care for their children. This approach implies a challenge for clinicians and a potentially growth-promoting process for the adolescent parent.

References

1. Vinovskis M. An "epidemic" of adolescent pregnancy: some historical considerations. *J Family History* 1981:58–101.
2. Scott K. Epidemiological aspects of teenage pregnancy. In: *Teenage Parents and Their Offspring.* Scott K, Field T, Robertson E (eds). New York: Grune & Stratton, 1981:43–63.
3. Roosa M, Fitzgerald H, Carlson N. Teenage parenting and child development: a literature review. *Infant Mental Health J* 1982;3:4–18.
4. Baldwin W, Cain V. The children of teenage parents. *Family Planning Perspectives* 1980;12:34–43.
5. Field T, Widmayer S, Greenberg R, Stoller S. Effects of parent training on teenage mothers and their infants. *Pediatrics* 1982;69:703–707.
6. Leventhal J, Egerter S, Murphy J. Reassessment of the relationship of perinatal risk factors and child abuse. *Pediatrics* 1983;71:672–675.
7. Leventhal J. Risk factors for child abuse: methodologic standards in case control studies. *Pediatrics* 1981;68:684–690.

8. Taylor B, Wadsworth J, Butler N. Teenage mothering, admission to hospital and accidents during the first five years. *Arch Dis Child* 1983;58:6–11.

9. Rothenberg P, Varga P. The relationship between age of mother and child health and development. *Am J Public Health* 1981;71:810–817.

10. Phipps-Yonas S. Teenage pregnancy and motherhood: a review of the literature. *Am J Orthopsychiatry* 1980;50:403–431.

11. Fontana V. Child abuse: prevention in the teenage parent. *NY State J Med* 1980;80:53–56.

12. Bavolek S, Kline D, McLaughlin J, Publicover P. Primary prevention of child abuse and neglect: identification of high risk adolescents. *Child Abuse and Neglect* 1979;3:1071–1080.

13. *Teenage Pregnancy: The Problem That Hasn't Gone Away*. New York: The Alan Guttmacher Institute, 1981; 30–36.

14. Lorenzi M, Klerman L, Jekel J. School-age parents: how permanent a relationship? *Adolescence* 1977;12:13–22.

15. Robinson B, Barret R. Issues and problems related to the research on teenage fathers: A critical analysis. *J School Health* 1982;52:596–599.

16. Earls F, Siegel B. Precocious Fathers. *Am J Orthopsychiatry* 1980;50:469–480.

17. Caparulo F, London K. Adolescent fathers: adolescents first, fathers second. *Issues in Health Care for Women* 1981;3:23–33.

18. Hendricks L, Montgomery T. A limited population of unmarried adolescent fathers: a preliminary report of their views on fatherhood and the relationship with the mothers of their children. *Adolescence* 1983;18:201–208.

19. Rivara F, Sweeney P, Henderson B. A study of low socioeconomic status, black teenage fathers and their nonfather peers. *Pediatrics* 1985;75:648–656.

20. Pannor R, Evans B. The unmarried father revisited. *J School Health* 1975;45:271–273.

21. Elster A, Panzarine S. Unwed teenage fathers. *J. Adolescent Health Care* 1980; 1:116–120.

22. Finkel M, Finkel D. Sexual contraceptive knowledge, attitudes, and behavior of male adolescent. *Family Planning Perspectives* 1975;7:256–260.

23. McQuade S. *Sexual and Contraceptive Knowledge, Attitudes and Practices of Adolescent Males*. Unpublished thesis New Haven, CT: Yale University, 1981;156–160.

24. Card J, Wise L. Teenage mothers and teenage fathers: the impact of early childbearing on the parents' personal and professional lives. *Family Planning Perspectives* 1978;10:199–205.

25. Offer D, Offer J. Normal adolescent males: the high school and college years. *J Am College Health Assoc* 1974;22:209–215.

26. Elster A, Lamb M. Adolescent fathers: A group potentially at risk for parenting failure. *Infant Mental Health J* 1982;3:148–155.

27. Poole C, Hoffman M. Mothers of adolescent mothers: how do they cope? *Pediatr Nurs* 1981;7:28–31.

28. Bryan-Logan, Dancy B. Unwed pregnant adolescents: their mothers' dilemma. *Nurs Clin North Am* 1974;9:57–68.

29. Benedek T. Parenthood in the life cycle. In: *Parenthood: Its Psychology and Psychopathology*. Anthony E, Benedek T (eds). Boston: Little, Brown & Co., 1970:185–208.

30. Sadler L, Catrone C. The adolescent parent: a dual developmental crisis. *J Adolescent Health Care* 1983;4:100–105.

31. Catrone C, Sadler L. A developmental model for teen-age parent education. *J School Health* 1984;54:63–67.

Bibliography

Hayes C. (ed). *Risking the Future.* Washington, DC: National Academy Press, 1987.

McAnarney E (ed). *Premature Adolescent Pregnancy and Parenthood.* New York: Grune & Stratton, 1983.

10 Setting Up an Adolescent Health Care Program

LOIS SIEBERT SADLER, *coauthor*

Introduction

The concept of a comprehensive health care program for the adolescent is not one that receives priority in the health care community. The issue of poor health simply is not one that is commonly associated with the adolescent population. The stereotype of the adolescent is one of bouncing good health, relentless vitality, and an outlook on life which is mildly askew but benignly tolerable.

While the vast majority of adolescents do not have the conventional health problems which afflict the older population, they do have health needs which are uniquely associated with their age group. Problems such as venereal disease, misuse and abuse of drugs, and adolescent pregnancy are health needs which require health care as well as health education. They are a group of patients who especially need education and help with issues of adequate nutrition and exercise, most acutely during pregnancy. A less recognized but equally serious health need is that of depression. Adolescents may not manifest the classical signs of depression. The use of drugs or the appearance of a pregnancy often are overt clues of a depressed adolescent.

Other health needs as reiterated in the chapter on complications of pregnancy, include the adolescent's propensity to develop anemia and its frequent association with infections. This may be seen in innumerable encounters with chronic vaginal infections and low grade kidney and bladder infections. In addition, diet patterns which are low in vital components such as iron, folic acid, and plasma zinc require correction at an early age, as does the excessive use of salt and foods high in cholesterol.

The ultimate goal of adolescent health care is a healthy population. A population that learns good health care habits early in life is more likely to have good health maintenance throughout life. An investment in developing health care programs which are uniquely designed to introduce the adolescent to health care issues may be costly initially, but a healthier population will emerge over time, and the ultimate result will be a significant reduction in health care costs and health maintenance for the individual and the community.

The focus of this book is adolescent pregnancy, so the concept of total comprehensive health care for the adolescent will not be discussed. Instead, the concept of comprehensive health care for the pregnant adolescent will be discussed. Before constructing an ideal composite program, it is useful to look back on previously developed health programs for pregnant and child-rearing adolescents.

Programs Developed for Pregnant Adolescents

The first programs for pregnant teenagers were based in the residential homes for unwed pregnant girls which were common in the decades of the 1950s and 60s. Some of these homes were in operation prior to the 1950s, and several of the homes are still operational today. In fact, a survey of services available to pregnant teenagers in the 1970s documented at least 20 of these residential centers in large cities in the United States (1). Traditionally, pregnant teenagers would live in these homes until they delivered, at which time many of the babies were placed for adoption. During the decades of the 1950s and 1960s, the educational system responded to the pregnant teenager either by excluding her from classes or by providing home-bound tutoring programs. These policies, by and large, added the problem of being a high school drop-out to the already dismal plight of the isolated, lonely teenage parent.

Beginning in the 1960s, it appeared that the numbers of teenagers who became pregnant were on the rise, and that these young mothers and their infants were subject to some unique health and social problems (2,3). In response to these concerns, hospitals and eventually schools began developing specialized programs for pregnant adolescents.

Hospital-based programs for pregnant teenagers were developed because of the need to consolidate and improve the health services required by the adolescent parent. These programs have been set up most often in urban hospitals or medical centers serving an inner city population. Although each program varies individually, the services provided generally include special clinics for prenatal and postpartum care, social services, nutrional services, pediatric care for mother and child, and family planning services. A current survey of health care services available to pregnant teenagers indicates that most large cities in the United States do have some of these specialized services in place (1). Selected programs will be briefly reviewed to provide a general overview of the different types of services that have been developed for this population of teenagers.

The Cincinnati General Hospital Infant Stimulation/Mother Training Project serves an adolescent population from the inner city as well as from the Appalacians (3). The program collaboration among pediatric, social work, and psychology departments focuses on a series of weekly parenting classes which are held for teenage mothers and their babies until the infants are six months old. The classes are run by nurses and early education specialists and focus on health, well-baby care, nutrition, and infant stimulation. Both mother and infant have access to health care in the same setting in which classes are held.

The San Francisco General Hospital's adolescent maternity program has been in existence since the late 1960s (3). This comprehensive program features vocational education, general guidance, and a high school diploma equivalency program in addition to the prenatal, contraceptive, and parenting components of the program.

Columbia Presbyterian Hospital in New York offers the Young Parents Program which is run by a specialized staff of nurse-midwives, pediatric nurse practitioners, nurses, and social workers who serve both adolescent mothers and fathers. In addition to health education services, this program features a staff training component which seeks to educate staff members about the unique needs and characteristics of the sexually active and childbearing adolescent (3).

The Young Mothers Program at Yale New Haven Hospital has been in existence since 1966 (4). Its core is a prenatal and postpartal clinic run by nurse-midwives for girls 18 years of age and younger. Social service access is one of the keys to its success. Also important are its liaisons with pediatric and adolescent health services, and the local public health school for pregnant teenagers, the Polly T. McCabe Center.

The McCabe Center in New Haven, Connecticut, was established in 1966 by the public school system as a pilot project and prototype for similar specialized schools (4). The center serves middle and high school students who become pregnant. The school's offerings include academic courses in addition to prenatal and postpartum classes, social services, vocational counseling, and liaisons with necessary health care agencies. After delivering, teenagers usually attend classes at McCabe for one to three months, before returning to the public high schools. Once the student mother returns to her high school, she has the educational and supportive services of the New Haven High School Parenting Project (5).

This specialized project provides parent education classes as well as individual counseling for student parents who have returned to their normal academic schedules. The specialized teacher-counselors who run this project are sensitive to the stresses and problems common to young mothers who are trying to adjust to the high school setting. Both the McCabe Center and the Parenting Project have recognized the importance of retaining the adolescent in the educational system for the prevention of future repeat adolescent pregnancies (4,5).

Another well-known and successful specialized school for pregnant teenagers is the New Futures School, which is part of the Alberquerque, New Mexico Public School System (6). This comprehensive program for childbearing adolescents began in the early 1970s. It offers an academic curriculum in addition to a parent education curriculum. After students deliver their babies, much emphasis is placed on follow-up counseling and support groups for the new mothers, fathers, and grandparents.

The St. Paul Maternal and Infant Care Project has offered multidisciplinary general and prenatal health services to junior and senior high school students within school clinics located in St. Paul, Minnesota (7). These innovative and well-utilized clinics provide direct health services in addition to health education and day care for student parents. This project has been able to document many successes, two of which are decreased pregnancy rates and improved obstetrical outcomes for students who do become pregnant (8,9).

A growing number of programs for adolescents who are pregnant or who are parents have been developed beyond the scope of the hospital and school-based programs. Outreach teen-advocate programs using a big sister/little sister model have been developed and tried in both urban and rural settings. Multi-service teen drop-in centers such as The Door in New York City, feature contraceptive, prenatal, and general health education in addition to their academic, legal, and recreational programs (3).

Field and colleagues (10) have developed home-based and day care center-based infant stimulation programs for adolescent mothers. The home-based model includes home visits to the adolescent mother and infant where a series of infant stimulation exercises are taught to the mother twice a week for the first six months of the infant's life. The day care center program employs adolescent mothers as part-time teacher's aide trainees caring for their own infants as well as other infants under the close supervision of an experienced day care teacher. Both programs seem to have positive and important effects for the teenage mother and on the infant's growth and development.

While there are a variety of models which have been used to meet the special needs of the pregnant and child rearing adolescent, some central themes emerge from them all. Adolescents do not negotiate complex systems very well. They require well-prepared, sensitive people to help them obtain the services they need during pregnancy and parenthood. Successful program design and staff training involve a solid understanding of adolescent development and behavior in the context of pregnancy and early parenthood.

Program Policies

The design of an ideal comprehensive health program for pregnant teenagers and teenage parents involves the concept of consolidation. Adolescents who are either pregnant or who are parents generally need support and understanding from trained professionals. Realistically, they require more health, educational, and supportive services than most older parents.

And finally because they are teenagers, they are less able to negotiate multiple complex systems and health care providers than more mature individuals. They will be more consistent in seeking the care they need if they can obtain that care in a single setting from a familiar small group of people. These observations of teenage behavior would argue for the consolidation of educational, health care, counseling, and day care services for adolescent parents under one roof.

With such an ideal school-clinic-day care arrangement, access would be much easier both from the perspective of the adolescent and the clinician or educator. The teenager could easily arrange the health care appointments she needed for herself or her child within the setting she daily attended for her academic classes. The clinicians, teachers, and counselors would have a readily available population as they sought to provide the necessary health, educational, and supportive services needed by these young families. It would seem that fewer individuals would be lost to follow-up care. Many educators in school settings report high rates of absenteeism for student parents on hospital prenatal or well-child clinic days. Such absenteeism would be significantly reduced if clinics were located within schools. In the same manner, it would also circumvent absenteeism in clinic attendance. Absenteeism is a chronic problem in many prenatal clinics today and has a substantial effect on pregnancy outcome. Thus, opening clinics in the school setting might create an acceptable alternative for most adolescents and subsequently contribute to improved compliance with their prenatal management.

A common educational/health services setting would also facilitate the clinicians' ability to assume active and visible roles as health educators. Childbirth preparation and parenting classes could be taught under the same roof by the same people who were actually managing the adolescent's health care. This model would ultimately include an on-site infant day care-learning lab setting for the infants of student mothers. This day care proposal addresses the monumental double-edged problem of adequate day care for infants of teenage mothers, and the issue of young mothers observing, learning, practicing and reinforcing positive infant care skills.

While such an educational health care/day care complex appears quite attractive from a theoretical standpoint, there are several important drawbacks to such an undertaking. Some of these involve administrative difficulties which arise between board of education values in certain communities, and a reluctance to offer any or all of the needed health services in connection with an academic setting. School administrators and community sentiments vary regarding the role of the public school system in relation to providing student services other than a strictly academic curriculm. In some communities, there is the unfounded fear that the provision of services for teen parents encourages future pregnancies.

Another drawback of such a complex are the limited diagnostic and back-up medical services available in a hospital setting. Many of these clinics simply refer the student to contraceptive clinics if she wishes to use a prescription contraceptive such as the pill or IUD. Furthermore, the health services available in school-based clinics are generally not available at night, on weekends, or during school vacations (11). Hence the school-based clinic is apt to function more as an adjunct clinic to the community-based clinic and in many cases replicates its services. This, of course, raises the issue of cost effectiveness. However, because the school-based clinic improves attendance for prenatal care and educates the young about contraceptive techniques, a major savings to the community is bound to occur.

The use of certain medications or antibiotic intramuscular injections are, of necessity, restricted to hospital or medical settings because of the risk of anaphylaxis. Obtaining blood specimens and transporting the cultures, Pap smears, and blood work to the laboratory must also be arranged. If a cooperative spirit exists, however, and the medical and educational communities are committed to the school health care concept, such complexities are not insurmountable.

An additional drawback is often a perceived lack of privacy experienced by adolescents involved in a multi-service setting. The adolescent who is worried about pregnancy or a sexually transmitted disease, for example, may not wish to visit a health care clinic connected to the school fearing that everyone in the setting would learn her problem. This adolescent fear is usually associated more with the individual's stage of egocentricism or belief in the imaginary audience than with an actual breech in confidentiality (12).

Neighborhood clinics are another alternative deserving consideration. These clinic settings often lack the stigma associated with hospitals. The personnel are usually selected from the community; hence, many members of the staff are known to the patients. While it has been theorized that this familiarity may act as a detriment—i.e., no one wants his neighbors to know his personal business—no substantial data have been collected to support that theory. If this hypothesis were true, it would be of particular concern in adolescent health care as the adolescent's sense of vulnerability and concerns about her self-image might limit her utilization of such health care sites. However, the opposite appears to be the case in prenatal care. For this particular type of care, many adolescents select these sites because of their personal flavor.

Another alternative is, of course, the traditional hospital setting. There are many practical factors which favor this choice. Obviously, the location facilitates the procedural aspects of health care, such as consultation and laboratory testing, and creates an easy access to the hospital's technology and emergency facilities, including immediate hospital admission when indicated. Certainly, the proponents of the hospital setting may argue that the medical advantages far outweigh the disadvantages. The major disadvantage lies in the fact that it may be considered an alien and threatening environment and thought of as impersonalized and institutionalized in its approach to people. For some adolescents, this fear may culminate in a decision not to enter the health care system at all until forced to by circumstances such as an emergency illness or an advanced pregnancy. If an adolescent is already in a hospital clinic setting, she may resent being removed from the familiar clinic and referred to a new prenatal clinic. She may feel lost and alone in a new situation without the support of her familiar clinic and health professionals. In short, she may feel she has been thrown out by that system when she needed it most. Her reaction may be to become a medical drop-out. The reassurance that the unknown setting has "nice people" is hardly adequate in helping her to cope. Why should she exert the mental and emotional energy necessary to establish a rapport with yet another group of health care providers who, nine months down the line, will discharge her to another clinical service?

The final results of such a dilemma contribute to a poor pregnancy outcome. Many hospital-based health care providers may have difficulty recognizing that the structure of their health care facilities may contribute indirectly to such an outcome, at least from the adolescent's perspective.

Program Proposal

One compromise in the organization for a multi-service program would involve a separation of clinical services from formal educational and day care settings. The clinical services would be located in a hospital or medical center in close proximity (within a few blocks) to the specialized educational setting. This arrangement would assume a close liaison between the staffs and administrations, possibly including some clinicians or educators being jointly employed by the two programs.

Goals of such a program would be the provision of general health care, prenatal care, postpartum care, mental health services, and pediatric care for children of adolescents in one setting with one specialized core of nurse-midwives, pediatric nurse practitioners, nutritionists, doctors, and social workers experienced in working with adolescents. In addition to the specialized service such a staff would provide, there would be the opportunity for training future adolescent health care practitioners and a site and population for clinical research.

Such a comprehensive program would curtail the necessity to refer the adolescent to different settings for general versus prenatal care, for example, and would therefore increase the likelihood of patient compliance. Services which would be available to all adolescents attending the center would range from general or primary care, including gynecological and contraceptive care, pregnancy diagnosis, prenatal, intrapartal and postpartal care, and pediatric care of the children of adolescent clients. While the adolescent health care clinic would not offer academic curricula, there could be health education classes in nutrition, childbirth preparation, and parenting. Specialized support groups would also be possible, such as for young fathers, adolescents' family members, and others. Because the academic setting would not be included in such a center, it would be necessary for the staffs of the health center and the school for pregnant teenagers to communicate closely with one another.

The proposed comprehensive health center would require a staff who first and foremost enjoyed adolescents and had a solid theoretical appreciation of the adolescent process. Individuals would need to be specialists in the sense of adolescent health care, but generalists in the sense of being able to manage the myriad physical, emotional, developmental, and family concerns which emerge with teenage patients.

Clinic Staff Members

Pediatric nurse practitioners, certified nurse-midwives, and a social worker would comprise the front line staff of a clinic for adolescents. Pediatric nurse practitioners are well suited and prepared to establish and maintain the relationship necessary for engaging adolescent patients in the health care setting. With phone consultation and occasional on-site consultation from a pediatrician specializing in adolescent medicine, most medical problems occurring in adolescent patients could be easily managed.

Certified nurse-midwives would manage the prenatal, intrapartal and postpartal courses of teenagers who became pregnant. Nurse-midwives are particularly well-matched to the needs of the pregnant adolescent because of their emphasis on patient education and preparation, and their philosophy of care. Even though all adolescent pregnancies technically fall into the high-risk category, experience has shown that certified nurse-midwives manage the vast majority of these young pregnant women extremely well. Phone consultation and occasional on-site consultation from an attending obstetrician would be necessary when indicated in the prenatal, labor and delivery, and postpartal management of teenage pregnancies.

The role of social worker is an essential one for such an adolescent program. Families and support networks of teenagers who become pregnant or who have children are often stressed to their limits. There are often family issues which need attention as the adolescent seeks the health care he or she requires. These families and teenagers may require assistance as they negotiate the various economic, bureaucratic and social welfare systems they must use. The social worker with a background in pediatrics and adolescent health care is an integral member of the health care team.

The nursing staff of the proposed adolescent clinic would have an enormous opportunity to design and implement creative patient education programs. This effort could take the form of various special interest groups for general clinic patients in areas such as weight control, sports health care, CPR, or contraception. It would be feasible for the clinic nursing staff to organize and conduct childbirth preparation classes, and postpartum mothers and fathers groups for pregnant patients. These programs could occupy waiting room time and space or be conducted at separate times.

Another important front-line member of the clinic staff is the secretary or receptionist who answers the phone. This team member is usually the first person to meet the adolescents as they enter the clinic. It is essential that this staff member have a solid understanding of adolescent behavior and sincerely likes teenagers.

Additional clinic staff members would include a nutritionist, a community outreach worker for difficult patient follow-up situations, and a peer counselor. The nutritionist would play an important role as liaison with state and federally funded nutritional programs for pregnant teenagers and their children. She would also be a valuable consultant for prenatal nutritional management plans and teenage parent education programs for infant and toddler nutrition.

The role of peer counselor or peer advocate has great potential in such an adolescent setting. Various school and clinic health programs have trained and utilized the services of peers for reaching out to teens in such areas as contraception, substance abuse prevention, and pregnancy. Some programs have had successes, others have had problems, and to date peer counselors are not used extensively (13). However, it appears that the concept has merit and with careful selection and training, such an individual could act as a valuable liaison between the adolescents and clinic staff members. The role of the counselor could take many forms, including functioning as a sounding board, or as an older "sister" or "brother" or as a health teacher.

In such a proposed clinic setting, a female adolescent might enter the system at age 12 or 13 for a school physical examination and be seen and followed by a pediatric nurse practitioner or nurse-midwife for whatever episodic, contraceptive, or routine gynecological care she needed until she reached her early 20s. If a patient entered the system concerned about pregnancy, she would be seen by a pediatric nurse practitioner or nurse-midwife who could diagnose and counsel her about pregnancy. In the event she elected to have the baby, she would be referred to the nurse-midwife in the clinic for prenatal, intrapartal, and postpartal care. During the pregnancy, she would be able to maintain contact with her primary pediatric nurse practitioner whom she could elect to provide the pediatric care for her baby. After the baby's birth, she would be able to see the pediatric nurse practitioner for the baby's care as well as her own general care. The pediatric nurse practitioner would subsequently follow through on the contraceptive care plan initiated by the nurse-midwife during the postpartum period.

Because the clinic would be a general one, males would also be seen for general care visits or episodic health problems. It would, therefore, be important to have male clinic staff members available as many teenage boys prefer to see male clinicians just as many girls prefer to see female clinicians. The fact that the clinic would be open and available to teenage males for general health care might make it a more appealing site for the boyfriends of pregnant teenagers. These boyfriends might also become more visible in such a clinic as they assume their roles as new fathers.

A clearly stated goal of such a program is to limit the total number of practitioners the adolescent encounters to as few as possible. Adolescents, because of their developmental stage, often have difficulty establishing trusting clinical relationships with adults who are strangers to them. In addition, many adolescents are either unfamiliar with or intimidated by the health care system, and, therefore, require clinicians who will orient and educate them about the process as they go along. These two adolescent characteristics—difficulty in negotiating relationships with new clinicians and naivete about health care systems—can be important factors which influence not only what the adolescent has to say during a clinic visit, but the quality and appropriateness of the care she or he receives. Therefore, once the adolescent does establish a working relationship with a clinician, efforts need to be made to make as few referrals to additional clinicians as possible. When a specialized problem comes up, a reasonable alternative to referring the patient is for the clinician to obtain consultation from the appropriate specialist for guidance or perhaps joint management of the patient's problem.

In this particular field of health care, there is another important variable to consider. Adolescents, especially adolescents who are pregnant or who have children, are an extremely demanding patient population. The developmental tasks of adolescence coupled with complicated social and family situations can lead to many large and small crises. The "here and now" orientation of many teenagers underscores these crises. Consequently, it can be exhausting for clinicians to be continually available to such a population. Because of issues related to staff burn-out, it is recommended that staff members are provided with significant free time away from the clinic setting or hot line. This implies the necessity of a cross-coverage or team system whereby a small group of practitioners relieve one another in the clinic setting. Because of the aforementioned difficulties that adolescents have with multiple care givers, the size of such a team is limited and team members must maintain similar philosophies of care and approaches with patients. Adolescent patients are able to successfully receive care from several members of a small group of clinicians who share the goals and approaches common to competent adolescent health care. Maintaining sincere interest in the adolescent as a person, keeping adolescent developmental characteristics in mind, and involving and educating the adolescent concerning health care procedures and decisions are all components of the adolescent-oriented philosophy of care which members of the health care team have in common.

Obstacles

Adolescents generally use the health care system most when they have a crisis. Consequently, a medical emergency, sexually transmitted disease, recognition of pregnancy, or an abscessed tooth will find them making every attempt to seek available help. But for routine comprehensive health care, the effort is not nearly as impressive and there are many obstacles.

One obstacle includes the fact of their adolescence. The adolescent's developmental tasks and chronological age may be a deterrent to seeking comprehensive health care. If the adolescent comes from a lower socio-economic status family, there may be another problem. Studies done among the lower socioeconomic status adult population show that health care rates low in value (14). Studies also show that most health values and behaviors are learned and reinforced by role models such as parents (15). Thus, learned behaviors• may become another obstacle for the lower socio-economic status adolescent in seeking comprehensive health care.

When discussing obstacles to health care, one must also consider finances. The recent publicity about adolescents demonstrates that they are the last to be hired and first to be fired. In a capitalistic society the resulting im-plications are obvious. For example, the pregnant adolescent registering for prenatal care in many clinics is requested to make a down payment toward her total hospital bill. This is usually obtained in small amounts at each pre-natal visit. As she enters her last trimester, the number of prenatal visits in-creases until they are on a weekly basis. With this increase there is a corres-ponding increase in requests for money. Since many of the adolescents cannot produce the required funds, they suffer a significant degree of em-barrassment, and feel trapped in situations over which they have little con-trol. Unfortunately, the repercussions are often reflected in poor clinic attendance.

Another obstacle for adolescents seeking health care in family planning and abortion services is that of conern and fear that their parents will be con-tacted. Indeed, to quote Goldstein and Wallace on the availability of family planning for teenagers:

> In one fifth of the clinics . . .it was indicated that there was an age restriction; in one fifth parental consent was required; and in one in nine there were legal restric-tions (16).

Abortion is another story. The associated constraints are illustrated in the following incident:

A young woman, 17 years old, had one child aged 3 months. She and the baby's father were sharing parenting responsibilities. He was in a local college; she was still in high school so they alternated days for babysitting and parenting. In this way they were able to pursue their respective goals and maintain their parenting roles. Then a calamity occurred when the mother feared she was pregnant. Her contraceptive method, an intrauterine device, had apparently failed. The dilemma she faced was the requirement that she needed parental consent to obtain an abortion at her local health institution. The need for parental consent was as unacceptable to her as was the thought of a repeat pregnancy within a year. Through the help of social workers, it was finally arranged for her to go to another city where she could obtain an abortion without her parents' consent. Her boyfriend was to borrow a friend's car so they could go together. At the last minute the car was unavailable and frantic attempts to obtain transportation were made. Eventually she had the abortion. This illustration emphasizes the impact that such clinic policies can have on the adolescent's decision to seek appropriate health care. Clinics that mandate parental consent before granting an abortion or contraceptive services to an adolescent may be an obstacle to the adolescent who desires an alternative to pregnancy. This is also true for the private sector. A recent study reported that half of all physicians offering abortion services would not perform one for a minor without parental consent, nor would 18 percent of private-practice obstetricians/gynecologists prescribe contraceptives for minors without parental consent (17).

How then does one introduce the adolescent to the health care system? The clinic must be structured so that the adolescent does not encounter hostile personnel and endless red tape. Adolescents have difficulty tolerating the frequent financial interviews, waiting, and hostile treatment from some clinic personnel. Unless these areas are improved, adolescents will continue to use clinics only for crises rather than for preventive health care.

Adolescents can be taught that health care is a value. To achieve this goal, clinics must be truly "theirs," as well as be interesting and informative. Too often clinic settings have dull waiting rooms with blank walls, rows of chairs, outdated magazines, and a few pamphlets seemingly designed to guarantee the reader's boredom. Music, if offered, is frequently piped in from the local FM station and is unappealing to the adolescent age group. Attention to these aspects will create a more inviting environment in clinic settings for adolescent patients.

The school is critical in the introduction of health care to the adolescent. It is only through the educational system that there is any realistic hope to reach large numbers of adolescents. Unhappily, the current quality of much health education is reported to correlate directly with the teacher's commitment to the topic. Since many schools rotate responsibility for health courses on a semester basis from teacher to teacher, the commitment level and content will vary. Additionally, teachers frequently emphasize too little the topic of pregnancy, the physiological changes associated with it, and the physiology of labor and delivery. In short, adolescent pregnancy and its complications are not generally considered a priority in such classes. The obvious irony is that the very group that needs to hear the most on the subject hears the least. Furthermore, if and when the subject is presented, it is frequently presented in medical language which is less than comprehensible to the adolescent. Such a presentation is one of covertness, in that this language acts as a barrier to learning and hides the substance of the content. When this occurs, the normal reaction is not to listen, which is exactly what most adolescents will do. The need to create a dialogue in these classes which will be informative and stimulate the adolescent interest is obvious. The lecture-type approach utilized to teach health care must end, but until then, the threat of an incomprehensible and boring introduction to health care will remain a reality for most adolescents.

Innovative approaches to health care introductions can be developed. Outstanding ideas include concepts such as those developed by a group called "Looking In," located in Hartford, Connecticut. It consists of a group of teenagers who perform improvisational skits about significant health issues confronting today's adolescents. This same approach could be used when introducing adolescents in the school system to health care issues, and would make the learning experience effective, meaningful and more interesting.

Introducing health care to adolescents at community meetings at neighborhood clinics and local "Ys" is also effective. Such meetings often attract good attendance and advertising slogans such as "Adolescents for Health" or "Begin a long life when you are young" attract interest and promote the concept of adolescent health care. Movies are always popular and can stimulate discussion when shown at a community meeting. Pantomimes developed to simulate common health care crises can activate the audience's participation by identifying the medical problems involved, and indicating what might have been done to prevent the problem from developing. The same results can also be achieved in school groups. Innovative approaches are as varied as the individuals involved; every situation can create its own particular set of needs and thus sets forth its own unique circumstances and responses.

Clinical Strategies

Familiarizing the adolescent with the clinic setting, its equipment and its procedures is a vital feature in the overall introduction to health care for the adolescent. An opportunity to visit the clinic setting may be offered through the health course taught in the school system and be conducted by one of the health care providers in the clinic during a time set aside by the clinic schedule. The tour group should be kept small and the tour conducted at a time when no clinic is actually in session. This will give each adolescent the chance to view and touch the equipment and to discuss its use.

Some adolescents may fear needles to the extent that they refuse to allow anyone to take blood samples. This creates a problem in clinical management. Giving these adolescents an opportunity to discuss their fears beforehand, and to see the needles and equipment may help reduce some of their anxiety. On the other hand, if the fear remains, it may help them to know that "needles" are not a routine part of most clinic visits. It is also appropriate in this introduction to inform them that friends or family may accompany them to any clinic visit. Knowing there is an ally present frequently helps them to cope with their fears and may reduce their anxiety.

For many adolescents, seeking health care is a new and threatening experience. There are, however, simple but important measures that the clinician in an adolescent clinic can use to reduce the perceived threat. To help the adolescent establish a sense of security it is helpful to ask first about such topics as friends, school, or family members, and then to inquire about the physical complaint or the reason for the visit. This prelude provides the clinician with important social and developmental data and gives the adolescent a chance to talk about nonthreatening topics before discussing health concerns. This also emphasizes to the adolescent that the clinician is interested in the whole person and not just an isolated health problem.

As the visit progresses, the clinician can orient the teenager to the various aspects of the health history, explaining why specific questions are asked or discussed, and in this way help the adolescent to become an effective and informed health care consumer.

The process of orientation to the clinical visit is continued during the physical examination. Most adolescents are inherently focused on their changing bodies, and thus can benefit from simple explanations and reassurances as the clinician performs the examination. This participative approach not only educates the adolescent about her body, but also reduces the stress associated with a physical examination. A major fear the female adolescent experiences is the pelvic examination. An attempt to allay this fear is begun at the clinic introduction session where the examination can be discussed and reviewed with the adolescent. Allowing teenagers to see on a model how the speculum is inserted will help them understand both their anatomy and the purpose of the examination. During an actual pelvic examination, especially if it is the first, the clinician can provide a mirror so that the adolescent may see her own anatomy.

The fact that many adolescents refer to the pelvic speculum as "clamps" reveals connotations suggestive of pain, stretching and pinching. For this reason the adolescent should be allowed first to handle the instrument to determine how it operates before the examination is begun. For some the fear of the pelvic exam may actually prevent the clinician from performing it. It cannot be emphasized enough that if this occurs the pelvic exam should not be forced on a frightened or unwilling teenager. Adolescents, as well as older patients, require a patient and supportive approach in this situation. One method is to help the teenager through a desensitization process. In this process, the clinician works closely with the adolescent patient to build up trust and the reassurance that she will not be hurt during the procedure. The clinician may begin this process by having the patient insert first "a Q-tip," then one, then two fingers, or even a tampon into her own vagina at home. This approach helps the patient to develop control and gives her an opportunity to acquaint herself with the physical sensations associated with a pelvic examination.

Unfortunately, much of what adolescents have heard about pelvic examinations is inaccurate information passed along from mother to daughter or from adolescent to adolescent. An introduction to the pelvic examination gives the adolescent an opportunity to discuss these misconceptions and subsequently correct erroneous ideas. This new, integrated information will help to reduce the potential for a traumatic experience at her first pelvic examination. Moreover, the adolescent who is comfortable at her first pelvic examination is not apt to be frightened by the prospect of future exams and hence will return for annual Pap smears and gynecology visits throughout her life.

An adolescent's introductory visit to a health clinic can deal with many other of her fears as well, or at least give her the opportunity to express them. Conducted at a time when a clinic appointment has not yet been made, there is no immediate sense of vulnerability and no preoccupation with anticipated pain. Hence, the adolescent is able to concentrate on what she is being told. Indeed, if successful, the ramifications are significant in promoting the adolescent's commitment as a consumer of preventive health care.

Any clinic designed to care for adolescents must address the need for a pregnancy diagnosis service. This service is required on an emergency as well as on a routine basis. A weekend is a long time to wait if you are an adolescent and fear the possibility of pregnancy. Therefore, the clinic's services ideally need to offer pregnancy testing seven days a week.

In addition, the clinic's service needs to include extensive and intensive postpartal follow-up for pregnant adolescents. Although it remains the one least frequently offered, this service is probably the most frequent recommendation made by health professionals in the field of adolescent health care. The importance of this service is highly relevant to the health status of both the adolescent and her baby. Many adolescents and their babies fall through the cracks of the health care system during the postpartal year; and too frequently when they return to the clinic, it is because of a repeat pregnancy. Poorly nourished, anemic, and totally unprepared to begin parenting a second child, they present a tragic picture. This sad state is generally compounded by a depressed state of mind and a low socioeconomic status.

Extensive postpartal contact with those who cared for the adolescent throughout her pregnancy may help avert this tragedy. As stated earlier in this book, an adolescent who begins childbearing in her teens is at risk to have a second child as a teenager, but extended postpartal follow-up utilized in a few prenatal clinics for adolescents has reduced this recidivism.

In such clinics the adolescents are scheduled for routine appointments throughout the first postpartal year for both their own care and the baby's well child care. These visits give the health care providers an opportunity to monitor the new mother's physical and emotional health status and give positive reinforcement of her parenting skills, success with contraception, and maintenance of life goals. Contact throughout this period also provides opportunity to identify early signs of depression, poor maternal/infant adjustment and acting-out behaviors. Successful intervention at an early point in these situations can make a crucial difference in these outcomes. Extended follow-up care also includes individual group counseling sessions for career counseling, discussion of childcare, boyfriend/girlfriend issues, conflict problems with parents, and other concerns the adolescent identifies.

The concept of a hot line is another item to be considered when discussing total comprehensive health for pregnant and all adolescents. Although hard to administer, this is a vital service. The adolescent population is crisis-oriented, therefore, the existence of a hot line is undisputedly a major need and advantage. Systems utilizing nurse-midwives can solve the administrative problems of a hot line if the nurse-midwife on call is willing to accept all incoming calls regardless of whether or not they concern labor. Hot lines also contribute to the adolescent's sense of trust and security which is essential for establishing credibility.

The final strategy to develop is that of team conferences. To the reader, this may appear to be an obvious need. However, too many clinics try to function without taking time for this necessary review. The quality of care will automatically improve when the entire group of health care providers meets to share concerns, information and the management proposed for each adolescent in the system. Conferences also reduce the tendency to treat the clinical problem and ignore the individual adolescent's total needs. Of course, clinic conferences need to occur on a regular basis, and sufficient time must be scheduled to allow a comprehensive review of the entire caseload at each conference.

A comprehensive adolescent prenatal and general care clinic will provide both physical assessment and psychosocial services to the adolescent over an extended period of time. It also includes extensive follow-up in the first postpartal year and longer when possible. The ultimate goal of such a clinic is to promote a healthy society and to help the young learn to appreciate the value of good health care.

References

1. Wallace H, Weeks J, Medina A. Services for pregnant teenagers in the large cities of the United States, 1970-1980. *JAMA* 1982;248(18):2270-2273.
2. Klerman L. Programs for pregnant adolescents and young parents: Their development and assessment. In: *Teenage Parents and Their Offspring.* Scott T, Field T, Robertson E (eds). New York: Grune & Stratton, 1981;227-248.

3. Garrett C. Programs designed to respond to adolescent pregnancies. In: *The Adolescent Parent.* Anastasion N (ed). Baltimore: Brookes Publishing Co., 1982; 67–82.

4. Klerman L, Jekel J. *School-Age Mothers: Problems, Programs and Policy.* Hamden, CT: The Shoe String Press, Inc., 1973.

5. London K. Mainstreaming the adolescent mother. *Issues in Health Care for Women* 1981;3:7–22.

6. Gaston C. Parenting education at the new future school. *Health Education* 1978;11(4):13–15.

7. Edwards L, Steinman M, Arnold K, Hakanson E. Adolescent pregnancy prevention services in high school clinics. *Family Planning Perspectives* 1980;12(1):6–14.

8. Edwards L, Steinman M, Arnold K, Hakanson E. An experimental comprehensive high school clinic. *Am J Public Health* 1977;6(8):765–766.

9. Berg M, Taylor B, Edwards L, Hakanson E. Prenatal care for pregnant adolescents in a public high school. *J School Health* 1979;49(1):32–35.

10. Field T, Widmayer S, Greenberg R, Stoller S. Effect of parent training on teenage mothers and their infants. *Pediatrics* 1982;69(6):703–708.

11. Dryfoos J. School-based health clinics: A new approach to preventing adolescent pregnancy. *Family Planning Perspectives* 1985;17(2):70–75.

12. Elkind D. Egocentrism in adolescence. *Child Development* 1967;38:1025–1033.

13. Jay M, DuRant R, Schoffitt T, Linder C, Litt I. Effect of peer counselors on adolescent compliance in use of oral contraceptives. *Pediatrics* 1984;73(2):126–131.

14. McKinlay J. The help-seeking behavior of the poor. In: *Poverty and Health.* Kosa J, Zola I (eds). Cambridge, MA: Harvard University Press, 1976;224–273.

15. Kane R, Kasteler J, Gray R. Poverty, illness and medical utilization: An overview. In: *The Health Gap.* Kane R, Kasteler J, Gray R (eds). New York: Springer Publishing Co., 1976;3–24.

16. Goldstein H, Wallace HM. Services for and needs of pregnant teenagers in large cities of the United States, 1976. *Public Health Rep* 1978;93:46.

17. Orr M, Forrest J. The availability of reproductive health services from U.S. private physicians. *Family Planning Perspectives* 1985;17(2):63–69.

11 The Pregnant Adolescent Speaks

Pregnant adolescents in the Young Mothers Program (YMP) at Yale-New Haven Hospital consented to discuss their feelings about pregnancy and associated matters if they could do so anonymously. The staff agreed and designed a portfolio of questions to which the adolescents responded. Since the participants were attending a prenatal clinic, they were either pregnant or 6 weeks postdelivery. Convenience sampling was used.

The natural inclination in the adult world is to wish that sexually active adolescents had values more like adults, primarily because these values generally include the use of contraceptives. Such a value does exist among adolescents, but so do factors such as peer pressure, minimal information about contraceptives, sporadic sexual activity, pressure to maintain a relationship, and age-related social values. Unfortunately, these factors also play a role in the frequency with which adolescent pregnancy occurs, and collectively they are less easily dealt with than is a conscious decision not to use any contraceptive method.

A frank observation the staff made was the adolescents' inability to discuss contraception while they were pregnant. Here and there, they acknowledged contraception but seemed reluctant to discuss it in any depth during pregnancy. Once they had delivered, their responses were more relaxed and informative. Negative feelings were expressed frequently about oral contraceptive pills (OCP), with "Can it cause cancer?" being the most commonly expressed fear. The intrauterine contraceptive device was even less favored than were OCP. The adolescents believed that the device "falls out," causes infertility, "it hurts" (which it should not), and that "he feels it" (which can occur if not properly inserted or the strings are left too long or cut too short). The idea of foam was "OK" but "a mess," and the adolescents really did not have much patience for the time required for proper use. Condoms were an acceptable alternative if "he remembers," but chances of that seemed remote. The diaphragm, to most adolescents, seemed an enigma. Consequently, their attitudes about contraception appear to be ambivalence and a fluctuating level of commitment to its use.

The staff asked the girls what advice they would give to a younger sister or a teenage daughter about boys, sex, and getting pregnant. The answers were filled with a painful wisdom. About a third said that as parents of a teenage daughter, they would talk with their daughters, encourage them to get "protection," and help them to find it. In short, they would accompany them to clinics and respond to their contraceptive needs in a nonthreatening manner. All agreed they would not want their daughters to be pregnant at a young age. Their admonitions to their hypothetical daughters included getting "protection," and a strong dictum not to go to bed "without it." The pain in this, of course, is reflected in their own situations. Most of these adolescents did not talk with their parents or older female siblings about sex. They had little or no reliable information about birth control, and they were either intimidated by the health care system and subsequently did not utilize its resources or lacked the insight to evaluate their own contraceptive needs.

Many adolescents expounded on the level of advice they would give their daughters to include the need to assess what one "really wants out of life" and the "need to take your time." A few even suggested "waiting for marriage." While most did not accept that philosophy, there was general agreement that it is best to be careful "who you mess around with" and a strong inference, reflecting significant psychological growth, was recognition of the fact that this must be something "you [yourself] want to do." In addition, many cautioned about the need to stay with "one boy." They believed more than one partner reduced the level of commitment both to contraception and the relationship, and significantly reduced support aspects in the event of pregnancy. One pregnant adolescent was pathetically straightforward in her advice: "Don't make all the wrong moves like I did."

When asked what they would do if they had this to do all over again, responses varied. Some said they would have "stayed on the pill," while others were less succinct, but allowed that they would have "been more careful because it is not easy being a parent." A few stated they definitely would not have become pregnant, while others expressed ambivalence about that possibility. One adolescent reacted with a truly negative response and said she would "cry, scream, or go crazy." At the other extreme, one who was enjoying pregnancy said "she would be proud to do it again." None of these adolescents, if confronted with the same situation again, discussed the possibility of abortion.

About a third of the group acknowledged that they had considered an abortion because of fears about 1) their capabilities to raise a child by themselves, 2) being "too young to have a child," or 3) their capabilities to cope with family/peer reaction to their pregnancy ("I was so frightened I didn't know what to do"). The rest of the group actively voiced opposition to abortion. While most said they did not believe in abortion, much of their discussion reflected their mothers' opinion on the subject; "My mother doesn't believe in it and neither do I." Some even referred to it as "killing." But the majority seemed to feel that the conception was "not the baby's fault." "It came out of pleasure," hence abortion was not a fair alternative for the baby.

When they initially found out they were pregnant, the first person most frequently informed was "the father of the baby." It was interesting that that was a consistent phrase and only one referred to him as "my boyfriend." Mothers were rarely told first, and fathers were never selected. However, when asked who helped most during the pregnancy, the response overwhelmingly favored mothers or a mother figure such as an aunt. The family member most adolescents did not want informed about the pregnancy was their father or father figure such as a grandfather. This may reflect a genuine absence of trust in the role men play in the family life of many of these pregnant adolescents.

The boyfriend's reaction to the pregnancy was described as "happy" by about half of the group. One even recalled her boyfriend's response: "He was so thrilled . . . jumping up and down. He always wanted to be a daddy and me a mommy." Others described reactions which were "strange" and "different" and "panicked." The behaviors and attitudes of adolescent fathers are not well documented in the literature. Little practical information is available, but for all of the adolescents who participated in this group the boyfriend or "the baby's father" played an important role in the total experience of her pregnancy. The fathers may not have been a positive role, but there was a definite articulation that he was expected to be involved. When this did not occur, the adolescent either expressed feelings of loss or identified an inability to discuss her feelings in a meaningful way with significant others, including her health care provider.

When they discussed love-making during pregnancy they were thoughtful. About half of the group stated they had no comments. Others varied in their opinions. A frequent concern revolved around the baby's well-being and the fear that sex might hurt the baby. This is, of course, a common anxiety shared by pregnant women of all ages and, therefore, not an unusual response. Others felt "funny" about it during pregnancy, and at least one third stated they were "not interested." They also identified concerns about sex after the baby's birth, feeling it might be a strange experience "like starting all over again."

When the adolescents were asked what helped most upon learning they were pregnant, they identified love and acceptance. By far the most important source of love was their mothers. Boyfriends were the second most significant group. About 80 percent of the goup did not properly predict their mothers' reaction. Of this group, 50 percent stated their mothers reacted positively when they expected a negative response. The reverse was also true for 40 percent of the group. Only 10 percent accurately predicted their mothers' reaction. For that group, the negative response they anticipated occurred but later resolved itself in acceptance. Those who were surprised by their mothers' negative response described her reaction as one of "disappointment," "shock," and "disbelief." The fact that these adolescents were later able to talk about their mothers' initial feelings was an important step in helping them to resolve their own feelings. Family situations that allow for honest and nonpunitive expression of feelings are generally capable of resolving their own conflicts; such seems to have been the case for most of these adolescents.

When asked what the best things were about being pregnant the responses varied. Approximately one third of the group addressed the issue of parenting. They were excited and spoke enthusiastically about the role. The remaining two thirds, however, were definitely self-focused in their responses. They spoke about the attention they received and rated it in "the best" category. One declared "it was best" "because you are treated like a baby." Such an answer raises two concerns: 1) Was this adolescent so deprived of parental love that pregnancy was percieved as a means to recover this loss? and 2) Was she apt to develop a feeling of sibling rivalry with her own child when the focus of attention shifts to her newborn after delivery?

Difficulties related to teenage pregnancy were identified as loneliness, finding transportation, and the physiological discomforts associated with pregnancy. About a third also felt a loss because they could not participate in sports or social activities. A few said they were forlorn about their lifestyle: "All I ever do is watch TV, sleep, and eat"; "All I do now is stay in the house." What they said they missed most was the company of friends. Some elaborated and said all the criticism was trying, as was the recognition that the baby's father was not reliable. Others in the group said nothing had changed and did not feel pregnancy imposed any particular problems for their age group.

Almost half of the group did not think having a baby would change any plans they had for school, careers, or marriage. Some simply stated, "It won't change anything." Others were more realistic. A small portion said pregnancy would change school but that was OK because they wanted "to stay home anyway." A few honestly admitted they "didn't know" how a baby would change their future. Three said they knew it would change school, but they didn't know how, and the remainder believed that having a baby would "encourage them."

Finally, they were asked what advice they would give health care providers caring for them. They were uniform in their responses. Ideally, they suggested health care providers put themselves in their position and *talk* with them. They wanted encouragement and reassurance that *"it* will be OK, and at all costs to "be friendly" to them.

Other researchers have obtained similar responses in adolescent populations they have surveyed. In 1976, Zelnik and Kanter (1) did a nationwide overview on the subject of adolescents' failure to use contraceptives. Half of their population stated no use occurred because they did not think they could become pregnant at the time of intercourse. Other reasons given included unexpected intercourse, nonfamiliarity with resources for birth control, a nonreceptive partner, and perceptions that contraception is dangerous to health, is uncomfortable, and hard to use.

Kisker (2) reported on the focus-group discussions developed in 1983 by The Alan Guttmacher Institute. There were 10 of these focus-groups nationwide; in most cases the participants were sexually active, predominantly white, middle- and lower-middle-class teenagers. Of the 10 groups, two were made up of male teenagers. The purpose of these groups was to identify and explore reasons why adolescents in the United States failed to use contraception. The reasons given by these groups for such a failure included no anticipation of first intercourse, inability to discuss birth control with a new partner, fear that expressed concern about pregnancy risk is interpreted as immature, fear a partner will go elsewhere if she doesn't comply, and fear that contraception in some way will destroy the sexual experience (2). A few others said they were willing to risk pregnancy, while others trusted their partners to be careful.

The male teenagers in the focus groups believed that introducing the topic of birth control to a new partner might be a "turnoff," and one New York City teenager, who was older, believed that there was no need to discuss it with a new partner because it was "her problem" (2). Moreover, most of the young women agreed that birth control is the female's responsibility especially if it's a "one-night stand" (2).

These participants did not feel they could discuss sex and contraception with their parents. They described themselves as too embarrassed and scared to do so. This was true even when an adolescent's mother offered to help her daughter obtain proper contraception (2). The need for this guidance was pathetically obvious when they discussed the different methods of contraception in such an uninformed manner. It is obvious, therefore, that adolescents have developed a myriad of barriers to the use of contraceptives.

Adolescent fathers have been a difficult population to reach. As a result, they are frequently stereotyped as irresponsible with little or no commitment to their children, and in the words of one researcher (3) "hit-and-run victimizers of women." This researcher goes on to report that this stereotype does not apply to all young fathers. Two years ago, eight pilot projects funded by the Ford Foundation and coordinated by the New York-based Bank Street College program were set up nationwide to help the teenage father develop a relationship with his child through childbirth classes, counseling about schools and jobs, child development clinics, and family planning help. These programs are known as Teen Parent Programs and, to date, claim 395 teenage fathers as participants. When interviewed, these fathers spoke of the need to stay in touch with their children throughout their lives. One commented he had never known his father and did not want his child to have that experience (3).

The obvious conclusion is that pregnant adolescents are really no different from the rest of us. The pregnant adolescent is human, needs love and reassurance, is frightened but not overwhelmed, and is sometimes confused. Like all mothers she wants something better or at least different from what she had for her child. Just as with adults, some adolescents are better prepared to be parents than others. Some will be highly successful parents, others will not. Some can be helped to become better parents, and in these cases the health care provider and programs such as Teen Parents can make a difference. Recognizing and reaching these adolescents is a major aspect of the health care provider's role. This professional can influence outcomes physically and psychologically for pregnant adolescents, adolescent parents, and the children they bear.

References

1. Zelnik M, Kanter J. Sexual activity, contraception use and pregnancy among metropolitan area teenagers, 1971-1979. *Family Planning Perspectives* 1980;12: 230.
2. Kisker E. Teenagers talk about sex, pregnancy, and contraception. *Family Planning Perspectives* 1985;17(2):84.
3. Reaching out to unwed teenage fathers. *The New York Times* Oct. 7, 1985;B12.

Index